A Practical Approach to Prenatal and Postpartum Care

Editor: Josephine Buren

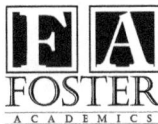

FA FOSTER
ACADEMICS

www.fosteracademics.com

www.fosteracademics.com

FA FOSTER
ACADEMICS

Cataloging-in-Publication Data

A practical approach to prenatal and postpartum care / edited by Josephine Buren.
    p. cm.
Includes bibliographical references and index.
ISBN 978-1-63242-664-2
1. Prenatal care. 2. Postnatal care. 3. Maternal health services. 4. Obstetrics.
I. Buren, Josephine.
RG940 .P73 2019
618.24--dc23

Foster Academics,
118-35 Queens Blvd., Suite 400,
Forest Hills, NY 11375, USA

ISBN 978-1-63242-664-2 (Hardback)

Contents

Preface

Prenatal care is a form of preventive healthcare concerned with the facilitation of appropriate care to mothers during the course of the pregnancy to prevent potential health issues. It strives to promote healthy lifestyles that benefit mother and child. Pregnant women are informed regarding physiological and biological changes during pregnancy, and the need for prenatal nutrition. Routine prenatal screening and diagnosis can significantly reduce the chances of miscarriages, low birth weight, maternal death, birth defects and neonatal infections. The postpartum period refers to the first six weeks after childbirth when the mother's body gradually returns to its non-pregnant state. This period can be divided into three stages, namely the initial or acute phase, subacute postpartum period and the delayed postpartum period. This book contains some path-breaking studies in the field of prenatal and postpartum care. It outlines the principles and practices of prenatal and postpartum care in detail. Those in search of information to further their knowledge will be greatly assisted by this book.

The researches compiled throughout the book are authentic and of high quality, combining several disciplines and from very diverse regions from around the world. Drawing on the contributions of many researchers from diverse countries, the book's objective is to provide the readers with the latest achievements in the area of research. This book will surely be a source of knowledge to all interested and researching the field.

In the end, I would like to express my deep sense of gratitude to all the authors for meeting the set deadlines in completing and submitting their research chapters. I would also like to thank the publisher for the support offered to us throughout the course of the book. Finally, I extend my sincere thanks to my family for being a constant source of inspiration and encouragement.

Editor

Prevalence of Abortion and Contraceptive Practice among Women Seeking Repeat Induced Abortion in Western Nigeria

Mustafa Adelaja Lamina

Maternal and Fetal Health Research Unit, Department of Obstetrics and Gynaecology, Olabisi Onabanjo University Teaching Hospital, PMB 2001, Sagamu, Nigeria

Correspondence should be addressed to Mustafa Adelaja Lamina; ademustapha_2003@yahoo.co.uk

Academic Editor: Justin C. Konje

Background. Induced abortion contributes significantly to maternal mortality in developing countries yet women still seek repeat induced abortion in spite of availability of contraceptive services. The aim of this study is to determine the rate of abortion and contraceptive use among women seeking repeat induced abortion in Western Nigeria. *Method.* A prospective cross-sectional study utilizing self-administered questionnaires was administered to women seeking abortion in private hospitals/clinics in four geopolitical areas of Ogun State, Western Nigeria, from January 1 to December 31 2012. Data were analyzed using SPSS 17.0. *Results.* The age range for those seeking repeat induced abortion was 15 to 51 years while the median age was 25 years. Of 2934 women seeking an abortion, 23% reported having had one or more previous abortions. Of those who had had more than one abortion, the level of awareness of contraceptives was 91.7% while only 21.5% used a contraceptive at their first intercourse after the procedure; 78.5% of the pregnancies were associated with non-contraceptive use while 17.5% were associated with contraceptive failure. The major reason for non-contraceptive use was fear of side effects. *Conclusion.* The rate of women seeking repeat abortions is high in Nigeria. The rate of contraceptive use is low while contraceptive failure rate is high.

1. Introduction

Unintended or unplanned pregnancy poses a major economical, psychological, social, and/or religious challenge in women of reproductive age, especially in developing countries. It has been estimated that, of the 210 million pregnancies that occur annually worldwide, about 80 million (38%) are unplanned and 46 million (22%) end in abortion [1]. More than 200 million women in developing countries would like to delay their next pregnancy or even stop bearing children altogether [2], but many of them still rely on traditional and less effective methods of contraception or use no method at all.

In Nigeria, unintended intercourse is the primary cause of unwanted pregnancies, and many women with unwanted pregnancies decide to end them by abortion [3]. Since abortion is illegal in Nigeria (unless medically recommended to save a mother's life), many abortions are carried out clandestinely, and often in an unsafe environment [4].

Induced abortion is not only widespread in Nigeria but is also provided and practiced in a number of different settings, from traditional medical practitioners, herbalists, and private practicing clinicians to modern pharmacists [5]. The consequences of these clandestine abortions are grave and can be life-threatening, often leading to maternal death. Abortions account for 20%–40% of maternal deaths in Nigeria [4–6].

The leading contributory factor to unwanted pregnancy in Nigeria is low contraceptive usage [7–9]. The current prevalence rate for contraceptive use in Nigeria is approximately 11%–13% [10]. This rate is very low in spite of the high rate of sexual activity (the average age of sexual debut ranged between 12 and 20 years, with a mean age of 16 ± 1.2 years) and widespread awareness of the various contraceptive methods (ranging between 29% and 69% depending on the method) among Nigerian adolescents and youths [10, 11]. Several studies in Nigeria have shown that more than 60% of women with unplanned pregnancies were not using contraception. The consequence of low contraceptive use among Nigerian women leads to an estimated 1.5 million unplanned pregnancies every year, with half of these resulting in elective abortions [4, 12–14].

It has also been noted that some women use abortion as a means of child-spacing instead of using modern contraception [3]. Fear of future infertility was the overriding factor in adolescents' decision to rely on abortion rather than contraception [3]. Many perceived the adverse effect of modern contraceptives on fertility to be continuous and prolonged, while abortion was seen as an immediate solution to an unplanned pregnancy [3].

Hence, the aim of this study was to determine the rate of repeat induced abortions and the related contraceptive practices among women in private health care facilities in Western Nigeria.

2. Subjects and Methods

2.1. Study Setting. Nigeria has a population of about 170 million people, 70% of whom live in rural areas [9]. Ogun State as one of the 36 states in Nigeria is located in the western region of the country. Ogun State has a land area of 16,762 square kilometers and a population of a little over 1 million. It has 20 local government areas, six urban and 14 rural. The Institutional Ethics Review Committee of Olabisi Onabanjo University Teaching Hospital, Sagamu, Ogun State, Nigeria, gave the approval to conduct this study.

2.2. Study Design and Participants. The current study was a prospective hospital-based study. The sample was drawn from the list of private hospitals/clinics in Nigerian Medical Directory [15]. Thirty-two private health institutions were selected, 18 in urban and 14 in rural local government areas. These institutions were located in the most and least urbanized areas of local government in Ogun State. Every fourth hospital was selected in the urban local government areas while all the hospitals in the rural local government areas were chosen (because there were fewer hospitals in the rural areas than urban areas). The medical officers in these institutions who provided the abortion care were then approached and their cooperation solicited in view of the sensitive and legal nature of the procedure. They were assured of confidentiality and anonymity and the fact that the information obtained would be used for research purposes only.

A semistructured questionnaire was developed for the purpose of this study and was pretested among 25 abortion care seekers a month preceding the commencement of the study in 2011. After pretesting, the questionnaire was modified according to local traditions and cultural sensitivity. The questionnaire sought information on sociodemographic and educational characteristics of abortion care seekers; number of previous abortions; contraceptive practice; and reasons for not using contraception.

The medical officers administered a questionnaire to every abortion care seeker in the institutions from January to December 2012. Trained medical officer interviewers, who visited the hospitals regularly, assured that the forms were

TABLE 1: The age distribution of women seeking first and repeat induced abortion.

Age group (years)	First abortion seekers		Repeated abortion seekers	
	Frequency	Percentage	Frequency	Percentage
15–19	142	6.3	78	11.6
20–24	703	31.1	213	31.5
25–29	626	27.7	185	27.4
30–34	391	17.3	101	15.0
35–39	296	13.1	61	9.0
40–49	99	4.4	35	5.2
50 and above	2	0.1	2	0.3
Total	**2259**	**100.0**	**675**	**100.0**

properly filled out. After this assurance, the forms were collected and double-checked by a senior doctor. The senior doctor took the filled forms to the principal investigator for storage. Each trained medical officer covered eight hospitals and there were two supervisors for all the twenty local government areas.

The participants were assured that information provided by them will be kept confidential and will not be used against them. They were also assured that their names will not appear on the questionnaires and their responses will not cause them any harm neither will it prevent them from receiving the best of care from the hospital.

2.3. Data Analysis. Data analysis was by both descriptive and inferential statistics at 95% confidence level using *SPSS software for Windows version 17.0.* Frequency tables were generated for relevant variables. Proportions were compared with the Pearson chi-square test. Relationships were expressed using odds ratio and confidence intervals.

3. Results

Of 2934 women seeking abortion within the one-year study period, 675 presented for repeat induced abortion, giving a rate of 23%.

The age range for those seeking repeated induced abortion was 15 to 51 years while the median age was 25 years. Majority of women (70.5%) seeking repeated induced abortion were aged less than 30 years while 43.1% were within 15 to 24 years of age (Table 1).

Of the 675 women seeking repeat induced abortion, 47.9% were single and 51.6% were married. Table 2 shows a cross-tabulation of number of repeat abortions and marital status of women seeking repeat induced abortion. A woman presenting for second- or higher-order repeat induced abortion is statistically significantly more likely to be single than married (43% versus 22%, odds ratio = 2.67 {1.38 < OR < 5.20}, 95% confidence limits, p-value = 0.0015225).

All the women had some form of formal education, with 97.6% having a minimum of secondary education. The bulk of the women were students (33.2%) and traders (32%).

The number of previous abortions ranged from 1 to 6, with a mean of 1.44 and median and mode of 2 each,

TABLE 2: Number of repeat abortions versus marital status of women seeking repeat induced abortion.

Number of previous abortion(s)	Marital status				Total
	Single	Married	Separated	Widowed	
1	183	270	1	3	457
2	103	60	0	0	163
3	27	13	0	0	40
4	6	4	0	0	10
5	4	0	0	0	4
6	0	1	0	0	1
Total	**323**	**348**	**1**	**3**	**675**

TABLE 3: Number of previous induced abortions.

Number of abortions	Frequency	Percentage	Cumulative percentage
1	457	67.7	67.7
2	163	24.2	91.9
3	40	5.9	97.8
4	10	1.5	99.3
5	4	0.6	99.9
6	1	0.1	100.0
Total	**675**	**100.0**	

TABLE 4: Contraceptive use among women seeking repeat induced abortion.

Method	Frequency	Percentage	Cumulative percentage
Emergency contraceptives	43	6.4	6.4
Condom	33	4.9	11.3
Oral contraceptive pills	31	4.6	15.9
Injectable contraceptives	18	2.6	18.5
Intrauterine contraceptive device	2	0.3	18.8
Rhythm method	5	0.7	19.5
Withdrawal method	2	0.3	19.8
Lactational amenorrhoea	1	0.2	20.0
Periodic abstinence	1	0.2	20.2
Traditional methods	9	1.3	21.5
No contraceptive method	530	78.5	100.0
Total	**675**	**100.0**	

TABLE 5: Reasons for non-contraceptive use among women presenting for repeat induced abortion.

Reason	Frequency	Percentage
Fear of side effects	291	54.9
Lack of adequate information/misinformation	79	14.9
Not thinking about using contraceptive	53	10.0
Objection from partner	31	5.9
Objection from family members	21	4.0
Conflicts with religious beliefs	5	0.9
Not having sexual intercourse to have a baby	36	6.8
Unplanned sexual intercourse	14	2.6
Total	**530**	**100.0**

respectively. About one-third of the women (32.3%) seeking repeat induced abortion have had 2 or more previous induced abortions (Table 3).

Of those who had had one or more abortions, the level of awareness of contraceptives was 91.7% while only 21.5% used a contraceptive at their first intercourse after the procedure, and of the 145 who chose contraception, 87.6% used modern methods of contraception: emergency contraceptive, condom, oral contraceptive, and injectable contraceptive (Table 4). Out of 11.3% of the women that used emergency contraceptive (6.4%) and condom (4.9%), only 10.5% used them consistently and correctly; 78.5% of the pregnancies were associated with non-contraceptive use while 17.5% were associated with contraceptive failure (mainly due to incorrect/inconsistent use of condoms and emergency contraceptives).

The reasons for not using contraceptive among women seeking repeat induced abortion are as shown in Table 5. About 70% of the women did not use any contraception because of fear of side effects and lack of adequate information/misinformation about contraception. About 10% of the women did not use contraception as a result of objection from partner and family members.

Figures 1 and 2 show the relationship between education, number of abortions, and contraceptive usage of women presenting for repeat induced abortion. Figure 1 shows the relationship between educational level and number of abortions in women presenting for repeat induced abortion. The number of repeat abortion increased with educational level. Figure 2 shows the relationship between educational level and contraceptive usage of women presenting for repeat

induced abortion. The contraceptive usage rate increased with increased educational level.

There is a direct relationship between the educational level of the women and the number of abortions and their contraceptive use. The number of abortions and contraceptive use increased with increase in educational level.

4. Discussion

Many Nigerian women of reproductive age experience an unwanted pregnancy and resort to abortion [3]. Unwanted pregnancy is the leading cause of unsafe abortion in Nigeria. Abortion law is restrictive in Nigeria. Therefore, induced abortions are carried out clandestinely, and sometimes under unsterile conditions and by unskilled personnel [10]. Abortions contribute to 20%–40% of all maternal deaths, constitute an economic drain on the Nigerian health system, and are expensive for women [16], especially for those who develop complications leading to pelvic inflammatory disease (PID), infertility, and/or ectopic gestation [16].

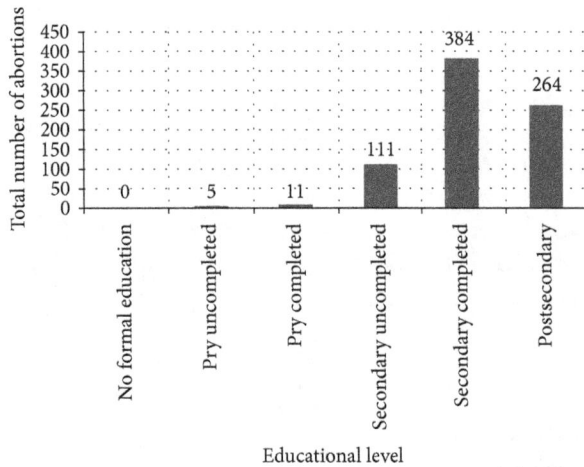

FIGURE 1: Educational level and total number of abortions of women with repeated induced abortion. Footnotes: pry uncompleted: primary school uncompleted; pry completed: primary school completed; secondary uncompleted: secondary school uncompleted; secondary completed: secondary school completed; postsecondary: postsecondary school.

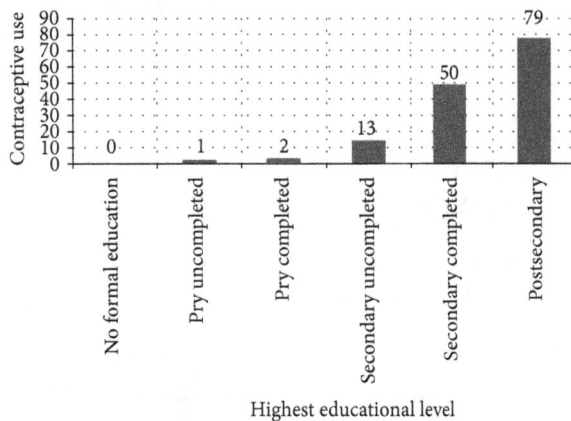

FIGURE 2: Educational level and contraceptive use of women with repeated induced abortion. Footnotes: pry uncompleted: primary school uncompleted; pry completed: primary school completed; secondary uncompleted: secondary school uncompleted; secondary completed: secondary school completed; postsecondary: postsecondary school.

The rate of repeat induced abortion of 23% from this study is slightly lower than rates of 33% and 35% reported in China [17, 18]. However, having close to a quarter of women who had had one or more previous abortions presenting for repeat induced abortion is worrisome. This is a reflection of nonincorporation of postabortion contraceptive counseling in abortion care (as part of comprehensive abortion care), poor postabortion contraceptive counseling, or poor contraceptive uptake by the women presenting for repeat induced abortion [18].

More than two-fifths of the women presenting for repeat induced abortion were young women (age group within the 15–24 years) while adolescent constituted 11.6%. This rate in the adolescents is similar to 13.1% reported from a study in

India [18] and lower than 23.7% in an earlier study from Nigeria [12]. This is attributable to nonconsensual sex, early initiation of sexual activity, high sexual activity, and low contraceptive use among the adolescents [12, 19, 20].

The observation that a significant proportion of women presenting for repeat induced abortion were youths (15–24 years) and the fact that a woman presenting for second- or higher-order repeat induced abortion is more likely to be single than married are worrisome. This is born out of the fact that the level of knowledge and awareness of contraception is high among the youths. But paradoxically, contraceptive utilization rate is low among the youths as reflected in this study and others [12, 17–20]. Ambivalence and discomfort among health providers in communicating with unmarried youths and providing contraceptives to them and their right to privacy and confidentiality are some of the factors militating against contraceptive uptake among the youths [10, 21].

However, this procedure is not exclusively an activity of unmarried/young women, as a significant number of older/married women in the reproductive age group also sought abortion. This is consistent with the findings of studies from South-Western Nigeria [5, 12]. This is a reflection of low contraceptive use among the older/married women who desired child-spacing and limited family size in view of present economic hardship in Nigeria [10, 12].

It has also been noted that some women use abortion as a means of child-spacing instead of using modern contraception [3]. Fear of future infertility was the overriding factor in adolescents' decision to rely on abortion rather than contraception [3]. Many perceived the adverse effect of modern contraceptives on fertility to be continuous and prolonged, while abortion was seen as an immediate solution to an unplanned pregnancy [3].

Majority of the respondents (97.7%) were aware of some methods of contraception. This compares well with 91.3% reported from South-Western Nigeria [5]. Despite this high level of awareness, only 21.5% of the women had tried contraception after the last abortion, showing a great gap between awareness and usage; the overall conclusion would be that knowledge does not necessarily translate into attitudinal change where contraception usage is concerned [22].

The reasons given by women presenting for repeat induced abortion for not using contraceptives in this study are similar to those reported in other studies [3, 7–9, 23]. These included fear of side effects, lack of adequate information/misinformation, objections from their partners, conflicts with their religious beliefs, objections from family members, not thinking about using contraceptives, not having sexual intercourse to have baby, and unplanned sexual intercourse. All the reasons depicted a basic problem, which is lack of proper information on contraception. Public enlightenment on contraception can start from antenatal and gynaecological clinics. This can be extended to other outpatient clinics which men are part of, so that the information on contraception will spread to as many people as possible. This will reduce the magnitude of misconception/misinformation on contraception to a minimum level and increase contraceptive use.

Despite the high association between education and usage rate of contraception, this same group also had a high association with abortion. This compares with similar findings from Lagos and other parts of the world, indicating that women who had used contraception are more likely to have had abortion than women who had not used contraception [5, 13, 24].

Limitations. The number of previous induced abortions could have been underestimated due to the fact that women are usually reluctant to own up to having had induced abortion. The effect of this factor has been minimized considerably by assuring and ensuring high degree of confidentiality and anonymity; and the fact that women easily volunteer previous history of induced abortion at antenatal clinics.

Recommendations. Lack or ineffective postabortion contraceptive counseling could contribute to high rate of repeat induced abortions. Therefore, there is a need to incorporate postabortion contraceptive counseling as part of comprehensive abortion care. In a study carried out in USA, it was reported that women having a second- or higher-order abortion were over twice as likely as women having a first abortion to indicate interest in long-acting reversible contraception [25]. Training of health care providers in abortion care is also a prerequisite to providing abortion care services of good quality. However, an advocacy for change in abortion policy in Nigeria (from being restrictive to liberal) is mandatory in order to provide a supportive environment for both health care providers and clients.

The low contraceptive utilization among the youths can be improved upon by providing adolescent-friendly sexual education and reproductive and contraceptive services to the unmarried youths. Moreover, evidence had shown that many unmarried young women presenting for repeat induced abortion were ready to receive postabortion contraception at abortion clinic [25].

There is also a need to translate high contraceptive awareness to an increased use in order to bridge the large gap of unmet need. There is a need to dismystify misinformation about contraception. A significant component of any family planning program for Nigeria would have to be concentrated on community health education to reduce misconceptions about the side effects of modern contraceptives, which is the most common reason for nonuse of modern contraceptives in Nigeria. Another component would be the involvement of men in family planning and use of the radio for information dissemination.

5. Conclusion

There is abundant information that contraceptive knowledge and awareness are high among the Nigerian population. This awareness has not been translated into contraceptive use, with the end-result being very low contraceptive prevalence in Nigeria. This low contraceptive prevalence correlates with high levels of unplanned pregnancies and abortions, leading to increases in the maternal mortality ratios, especially in the rural areas in Nigeria.

The medical technology is known, and the sociocultural, religious, family, misinformation, and male-dominant factors impeding contraceptive use in Nigeria societies have been identified. What is lacking is the generation of political priority for family planning and safe motherhood as well as the political will and commitment to make this change on a large scale. With the commitment of financial and human resources as well as assistance from international organizations, public-private sector collaboration, community-oriented knowledge, acceptability, and availability of a wide range of modern contraceptive choices, the contraceptive prevalence rate will increase and should contribute to the reduction of the prevalence of unwanted pregnancy and induced abortion and the worst maternal health crisis in Nigeria and sub-Saharan Africa. This will ultimately lead to substantial reduction in population growth and poverty reduction. At the existing rate of population increase, Nigeria will become a failed state because institutions cannot be built/maintained if the population keeps increasing with nearly 3% a year, which means a population doubling rate of a little more than 20 years [26].

Appendix

Prevalence of Abortion and Contraceptive Practice among Women Seeking Repeat Induced Abortion

Semisructured Questionaire

(1) Age ...

(2) Marital status:

   (i) single
   (ii) married
   (iii) separated
   (iv) divorced
   (v) widowed

(3) Level of education:

   (i) none
   (ii) primary
   (iii) secondary
   (iv) tertiary

(4) Occupation ...

(5) Religion ...

(6) Parity ...

(7) Gestational age ...

(8) Age ...

(9) Marital status:

   (i) single
   (ii) married
   (iii) separated

(iv) divorced

(v) widowed

(10) Level of education:

(i) none

(ii) primary

(iii) secondary

(iv) tertiary

(11) Occupation . . .

(12) Religion . . .

(13) Parity . . .

(14) Number of previous termination of pregnancy(ies) . . .

(15) Gestational age (weeks) at previous termination of pregnancy . . .

(16) Type of contraceptive used to prevent previous pregnancy:

(i) male condom

(ii) oral pills

(iii) emergency contraception

(iv) rhythm method

(v) withdrawal method

(vi) periodic abstinence

(vii) lactational amenorrhoea

(viii) intrauterine contraceptive device

(ix) injectable

(x) traditional method

(xi) non

(17) Type of contraceptive used after previous termination of pregnancy:

(i) male condom

(ii) oral pills

(iii) emergency contraception

(iv) rhythm method

(v) withdrawal method

(vi) periodic abstinence

(vii) lactational amenorrhoea

(viii) intrauterine contraceptive device

(ix) injectable

(x) traditional method

(xi) non

(18) Type of contraceptive ever used:

(i) male condom

(ii) oral pills

(iii) emergency contraception

(iv) rhythm method

(v) withdrawal method

(vi) periodic abstinence

(vii) lactational amenorrhoea

(viii) intrauterine contraceptive device

(ix) injectable

(x) traditional method

(xi) non

(19) If no contraceptive was used, kindly state the reason . . .

Consent

The study has been well explained to the patient who fully understands the content of the research.

Conflict of Interests

The author declares that there is no conflict of interests.

Acknowledgment

The author wishes to thank the medical officers who assisted in the interviewing of respondents.

References

[1] WHO, *Safe Abortion: Technical and Policy Guidance forHealth Systems*, World Health Organization, Geneva, Switzerland, 2nd edition, 2012, http://apps.who.int/iris/bitstream/10665/70914/1/9789241548434_eng.pdf.

[2] H. B. Peterson, G. L. Darmstadt, and J. Bongaarts, "Meeting the unmet need for family planning: now is the time," *The Lancet*, vol. 381, no. 9879, pp. 1696–1699, 2013.

[3] V. O. Otoide, F. Oronsaye, and F. E. Okonofua, "Why Nigerian adolescents seek abortion rather than contraception: evidence from focus-group discussions," *International Family Planning Perspectives*, vol. 27, no. 2, pp. 77–81, 2001.

[4] O. M. Abiodun and O. R. Balogun, "Sexual activity and contraceptive use among young female students of tertiary educational institutions in Ilorin, Nigeria," *Contraception*, vol. 79, no. 2, pp. 146–149, 2009.

[5] B. A. Oye-Adeniran, I. F. Adewole, A. V. Umoh, E. E. Ekanem, A. Gbadegesin, and N. Iwere, "Community-based survey of unwanted pregnancy in Southwestern Nigeria," *African Journal of Reproductive Health*, vol. 8, no. 3, pp. 103–115, 2004.

[6] V. K. Oriji, I. Jeremiah, and T. Kasso, "Induced abortion amongst undergradute students of University of Port Harcourt," *Nigerian Journal of Medicine*, vol. 18, no. 2, pp. 199–202, 2009.

[7] B. A. Oye-Adeniran, I. F. Adewole, K. A. Odeyemi, E. E. Ekanem, and A. V. Umoh, "Contraceptive prevalence among young women in Nigeria," *Journal of Obstetrics and Gynaecology*, vol. 25, no. 2, pp. 182–185, 2005.

[8] U. Amazigo, N. Silva, J. Kaufman, and D. S. Obikeze, "Sexual activity and contraceptive knowledge and use among in-school adolescents in Nigeria," *International Family Planning Perspectives*, vol. 23, no. 1, pp. 28–33, 1997.

[9] "Nigeria 2008: results from the demographic and health survey. National population Commission; ICF Macro," *Studies in Family Planning*, vol. 42, no. 1, pp. 51–56, 2011.

[10] E. Monjok, "Contraceptive practices in Nigeria: literature review and recommendation for future policy decisions," *Open Access Journal of Contraception*, vol. 2010, no. 1, pp. 9–22, 2010.

[11] United Nations and Department of Economic and Social Affairs-Population Division, *World Contraceptive Use*, 2011, http://www.un.org/esa/population/publications/contraceptive-2011/wallchart_front.pdf.

[12] B. A. Oye-Adeniran, I. F. Adewole, A. V. Umoh, O. R. Fapohunda, and N. Iwere, "Characteristics of abortion care seekers in south-western Nigeria," *African Journal of Reproductive Health*, vol. 8, no. 3, pp. 81–91, 2004.

[13] F. E. Okonofua, C. Odimegwu, H. Ajabor, P. H. Daru, and A. Johnson, "Assessing the prevalence and determinants of unwanted pregnancy and induced abortion in Nigeria," *Studies in Family Planning*, vol. 30, no. 1, pp. 67–77, 1999.

[14] A. A. Fawole and A. P. Aboyeji, "Complications from unsafe abortion: presentations at Ilorin, Nigeria," *Nigerian Journal of Medicine*, vol. 11, no. 2, pp. 77–80, 2002.

[15] Nigerian Medical Association, *National Medical Directory*, 2014.

[16] S. K. Henshaw, I. Adewole, S. Singh, A. Bankole, B. Oye-Adeniran, and R. Hussain, "Severity and cost of unsafe abortion complications treated in Nigerian hospitals," *International Family Planning Perspectives*, vol. 34, no. 1, pp. 40–50, 2008.

[17] Y. Cheng, X. Gno, Y. Li, S. Li, A. Qu, and B. Kang, "Repeat induced abortions and contraceptive practices among unmarried young women seeking an abortion in China," *International Journal of Gynecology and Obstetrics*, vol. 87, no. 2, pp. 199–202, 2004.

[18] Y. Cheng, X. Xu, J. Xu et al., "The need for integrating family planning and postabortion care in China," *International Journal of Gynecology & Obstetrics*, vol. 103, no. 2, pp. 140–143, 2008.

[19] B. Ganatra and S. Hirve, "Induced abortions among adolescent women in rural Maharashtra, India," *Reproductive Health Matters*, vol. 10, no. 19, pp. 76–85, 2002.

[20] Q. Ma, M. Ono-Kihara, L. Cong et al., "Unintended pregnancy and its risk factors among university students in eastern China," *Contraception*, vol. 77, no. 2, pp. 108–113, 2008.

[21] V. Sychareun, "Meeting the contraceptive needs of unmarried young people: attitudes of formal and informal sector providers in Vientiane Municipality, Lao PDR," *Reproductive Health Matters*, vol. 12, no. 23, pp. 155–165, 2004.

[22] L. F. Adewole, B. A. Oye-Adeniran, N. Iwere, A. Oladokun, A. Gbadegesin, and L. A. Babarinsa, "Contraceptive usage among abortion seekers in Nigeria," *West African Journal of Medicine*, vol. 21, no. 2, pp. 112–114, 2002.

[23] National Population Commission, *Nigeria Demographic and Health Survey 2003*, National Population Commission and ORC Marco, Calverton, Md, USA, 2004.

[24] A. A. Olukoya, "Pregnancy termination: results of a community-based study in Lagos, Nigeria," *International Journal of Gynecology and Obstetrics*, vol. 25, no. 1, pp. 41–46, 1987.

[25] M. L. Kavanaugh, E. E. Carlin, and R. K. Jones, "Patients' attitudes and experiences related to receiving contraception during abortion care," *Contraception*, vol. 84, no. 6, pp. 585–593, 2011.

[26] UNDP, World Population Prospects: The 2012 Revision, http://esa.un.org/unpd/wpp/unpp/panel_population.htm.

Do Successive Preterm Births Increase the Risk of Postpartum Depressive Symptoms?

Timothy O. Ihongbe[1] and Saba W. Masho[1,2,3]

[1]Division of Epidemiology, Department of Family Medicine and Population Health, School of Medicine,
 Virginia Commonwealth University, Richmond, VA, USA
[2]Department of Obstetrics and Gynecology, School of Medicine, Virginia Commonwealth University, Richmond, VA, USA
[3]Institute for Women's Health, Virginia Commonwealth University, Richmond, VA, USA

Correspondence should be addressed to Timothy O. Ihongbe; ihongbeto@vcu.edu

Academic Editor: Jeffrey Keelan

Background. Postpartum depression and preterm birth (PTB) are major problems affecting women's health. PTB has been associated with increased risk of postpartum depressive symptoms (PDS). However, it is unclear if PTB in women with a prior history of PTB is associated with an incremental risk of PDS. This study aims to determine if PTB in women with a prior history of PTB is associated with an incremental risk of PDS. *Methods.* Data come from the 2009–2011 national Pregnancy Risk Assessment Monitoring System. Study sample included 55,681 multiparous women with singleton live births in the index delivery. Multiple logistic regression was used to examine the association between PTB and PDS. *Results.* The risk of PDS was 55% higher in women with PTB in both deliveries (aRR = 1.55; 95% CI = 1.28–1.88) and 74% higher in women with PTB in the index delivery only (aRR = 1.74; 95% CI = 1.49–2.05), compared to women with term deliveries. *Conclusions.* Preterm birth is a risk factor for PDS. PTB in women with a prior history of PTB is not associated with an incremental risk of PDS. Routine screening for PDS should be conducted for all women and closer monitoring should be done for high risk women with PTB.

1. Introduction

Depression is a major medical problem affecting women's perinatal health. Approximately 10% to 15% of women experience postpartum depression after childbirth [1]. Postpartum depression has a devastating impact on the mother as well as the development of the child. Postpartum depression has been linked to a wide range of adverse consequences such as impaired mother–infant interactions, infant social and emotional functioning, and disruption of cognitive development of the infant [2]. In addition, postpartum depression affects marital and personal relationships, as well as having substantial negative impact on the family [3]. It decreases relationship satisfaction, causes lack of intimacy, and can lead to sexual issues, which can disrupt and negatively impact normal functioning of the family. Furthermore, women who

suffer from postpartum depression have a twofold increased risk of experiencing future episodes of depression [4].

Poor birth outcomes such as preterm birth have been reported to increase the risk of postpartum depressive symptoms in women [5–7]. O'brien et al., in a longitudinal study on maternal depression following premature birth, reported that almost half the mothers of premature infants reported depressive symptoms during hospitalization, at discharge, and six weeks after discharge [8]. Voegtline and Stifter also reported that mothers of preterm babies had significantly higher levels of depressive symptoms within the first year after childbirth compared to mothers of children born full-term [9].

The increased risk of postpartum depressive symptoms observed in women with preterm birth may be due to stress [10–12]. Mothers of infants with preterm birth may experience increased stress related to feelings of helplessness, exclusion, and alienation and lack of sufficient knowledge regarding parenting and interacting with their infants [13]. Additionally, prolonged hospitalization and infant complications associated with preterm birth may aggravate the mother's feelings of helplessness and further increase her level of stress [13]. The increased level of stress may thus impact a woman's ability to adjust or transition to motherhood, increasing her likelihood of experiencing postpartum depressive symptoms [14]. Furthermore, infants born premature are more likely than full-term infants to have a more difficult temperament [15] and negative affect [5]. Such difficult infant temperament has been shown to be associated with postpartum depressive symptoms in the mother [16].

Previous preterm birth has been reported as one of the strongest determinants of a subsequent delivery of a preterm baby in women [17, 18]. However, it is unclear whether women with preterm births in the penultimate and index deliveries have an elevated risk of experiencing postpartum depressive symptoms relative to women with preterm birth in the index or penultimate delivery only. Though professional health organizations such as the American College of Obstetricians and Gynecologists (ACOG) [19], American Academy of Pediatrics (AAP) [20], American Psychiatric Association (APA), American Academy of Family Physicians (AAFP), and American College of Nurse Midwives (ACNM) recommend screening women at least once during the perinatal period for depression, over 50% of postpartum depression cases remain undetected [21]. A study by Psaros et al. reported that although about 61% of health care providers endorsed routine screening for postpartum depression, only 17% reported using a screening instrument [22]. One of the reasons for not screening is the lack of resources to implement universal screening and management of postpartum depression [23]. However, health care providers may be more apt to screen and provide targeted care to women with high risk conditions [24], such as a previous preterm birth. Understanding the interrelationship between successive preterm birth and postpartum depressive symptoms will enable health care providers to screen and manage this population of women more efficiently. This study, therefore, aims to examine if the delivery of a preterm baby in both the penultimate and index pregnancies increases the risk of women experiencing postpartum depressive symptoms above the risk observed in women with preterm birth in the penultimate or index delivery alone. We hypothesize that preterm birth in both the penultimate and index pregnancies will increase the risk of postpartum depressive symptoms.

2. Materials and Methods

This study utilized data from the 2009–2011 national Pregnancy Risk Assessment Monitoring System (PRAMS) and linked birth certificate data. PRAMS is a self-reported survey conducted by the Centers for Disease Control and Prevention (CDC) and state health departments. It is administered to a sample of recently delivered mothers within 2 to 6 months after delivery of a live infant and collects information on maternal behaviors, attitudes, and experiences before, during,

and immediately after pregnancy. A complex multistage sampling design was utilized and data were weighted to account for sampling design, nonresponse, and noncoverage. Data were collected using mailed questionnaires and nonrespondents were contacted by telephone. Additionally, the PRAMS survey data were linked to birth certificate data to capture birth outcome and pregnancy history data. More details on the PRAMS methodology have been previously published [25] and are also available from the PRAMS website (https://www.cdc.gov/prams). The current analysis utilized deidentifiable public-use data and was approved as exempt by the Virginia Commonwealth University's Institutional Review Board.

The study sample for this analysis included multiparous women (i.e., more than one live birth) with singleton live birth in the index delivery. Women with multifetal births (e.g., twins, triplets) or whom multifetal birth status could not be ascertained and primiparous women were excluded from the study. Women with multifetal birth were excluded from the study because multifetal birth is known to increase the risk of postpartum depressive symptoms [26]. This yielded a total of 58,224 women who were eligible for the study. Of these eligible women, those without a valid record on preterm birth in the penultimate delivery (n = 1,728; 2.9%) and those who did not provide valid responses to questions on postpartum depressive symptoms in the current postpartum period (n = 815; 1.4%) were excluded from the analysis. This yielded a total sample size of 55,681 women.

The dependent variable, postpartum depressive symptoms, was measured using three items on the PRAMS questionnaire (Cronbach's α = 0.82) based on an algorithm developed by Ohara et al. [27]. Women were asked: (1) "Since your new baby was born, how often have you felt down, depressed, or sad?," (2) "Since your new baby was born, how often have you felt hopeless?," and (3) "Since your new baby was born, how often have you felt slowed down?" Each item was measured on a scale of 1: Never to 5: Always. Scores for the three items were summed to create the postpartum depressive symptoms score. Postpartum depressive symptoms score ranged from a minimum score of 3 to a maximum score of 15. Women with scores >9 were considered to have postpartum depressive symptoms. This algorithm has been shown to have a higher specificity and positive predictive value than the Edinburgh Postnatal Depression Scale, Beck Depression Inventory, and the General Depression Scale of the Inventory of Depression and Anxiety Symptoms, when they were compared to a structured clinical interview for the Diagnostic and Statistical Manual of Mental Disorders, Fourth Edition [27]. This algorithm has also been shown to closely estimate the true prevalence of postpartum depression [27].

The independent variable, preterm birth, defined as the birth of a baby born before 37 completed weeks of gestation, was created as a mutually exclusive variable consisting of four dyadic categories based on a woman's history of preterm birth in the penultimate delivery and the gestational age at birth of the index delivery. Categories include (1) successive preterm births (preterm births in both the penultimate and index deliveries), (2) preterm birth in penultimate delivery but no preterm birth in index delivery, (3) no preterm birth in penultimate delivery but preterm birth in index delivery, and (4) no preterm birth in both penultimate and index deliveries (i.e., term births). Preterm birth in the penultimate delivery was measured using an item on the PRAMS questionnaire which asked mothers "Was the baby just before your new one born more than 3 weeks before his or her due date?" and preterm birth in the index delivery was determined using the clinical estimate of gestation at birth documented on the birth certificate. Further, preterm birth in the index delivery was categorized into very preterm (<32 weeks) and moderate-to-late (32–<37 weeks) preterm birth.

Covariates including sociodemographic factors, risky behaviors, and medical and obstetric factors were examined as potential confounders. Sociodemographic factors such as age (≤24, 25–34, and ≥35 years), education (high school or less and college or higher), income (<$20,000, $20,000–49,999, and ≥$50,000), and prenatal insurance (private, Medicaid, multiple, other, and no coverage) were assessed. Race/ethnicity was categorized as non-Hispanic (NH) White, NH Black, Hispanic, and NH other. Non-Hispanic other consisted of other Asian, American Indian, Chinese, Japanese, Filipino, Hawaiian, other non-White, Alaska Native, and mixed race. Risky behaviors such as alcohol drinking and cigarette smoking were assessed using a woman's use in the last two years prior to the index pregnancy and categorized as dichotomous variables (yes or no). Medical morbidities (gestational diabetes, prepregnancy diabetes, and hypertensive disorders of pregnancy) in the index pregnancy (yes or no) were also assessed. Pregnancy intention (intended or unintended) and intimate partner violence during the index pregnancy (yes or no) were measured as dichotomous variables. Prepregnancy body mass index (BMI) was calculated as weight in kilograms divided by height in meters squared (kg/m^2) and categorized based on the World Health Organization (WHO) classification into underweight (<18.50), normal weight (18.50–24.99), overweight (25.00–29.99), and obese (≥30.00). Stressful life events were assessed using a set of 13 questions that asked women to indicate whether they had experienced stressful events in the 12 months before giving birth (e.g., separation from partner, loss of job, bills she was unable to pay, etc.) and were categorized based on the number of stressful experiences (none, 1–2, 3–5, and ≥6). Problems with breastfeeding was measured as an abrupt termination of breastfeeding in women who commenced breastfeeding of their babies. It was categorized into 3 categories—no breastfeeding problems, breastfeeding problems, and never breastfed. Previous live births (1 and ≥2) and marital status (married and not married) were obtained from the birth certificate.

Statistical analysis was conducted using SAS-callable SUDAAN (Research Triangle Institute, Research Triangle Park, North Carolina) utilizing appropriate weights to account for the complex survey design. Descriptive analyses were conducted to assess the distribution of participants' characteristics. Prevalence of postpartum depressive symptoms was calculated and factors associated with postpartum depressive symptoms were determined. Multiple logistic regression analysis was conducted to compute the risk ratios

(RRs) and 95% confidence intervals (CIs) of the association between preterm birth and postpartum depressive symptoms using the average marginal prediction as described by Graubard and Korn [28]. Average marginal predictions allow comparisons of predicted outcomes (risk) between groups of people in the population, after controlling for differences in covariate distributions between the groups [29]. Because postpartum depressive symptoms are prevalent in the study sample, the risk ratio is more appropriate for this analysis [30]. Potential confounding factors whose inclusion in the regression model resulted in a change of 10% or more in the unadjusted risk ratio were retained in the final adjusted model [31]. The final model adjusted for maternal age, race/ethnicity, stressful life events, intimate partner violence, pregnancy intention, and medical morbidities in pregnancy. Interaction between preterm birth and race/ethnicity was tested based on extant literature and was not statistically significant (p value = 0.5217). To determine if respondents who were excluded from the analysis due to missing data (4.3%) were different than those included in the analysis, we examined the distribution of preterm birth in the index delivery (which had complete data for all respondents). Findings show that both groups were not significantly different (8.3% versus 7.8%, $p = 0.5435$). A significance level of $\alpha = 0.05$ was used for all analyses. All results presented are based on analyses of weighted data.

3. Results

Sociodemographic characteristics of the study population are shown in Table 1. Over half of the study sample were between the ages of 25 and 34 years (60.6%), NH White (56.9%), and married (66.0%) and had college education or higher (54.1%). Nearly half (46.7%) of the study sample had private insurance. Approximately 5% of women reported experiencing violence perpetrated by their partners and 42.3% reported their pregnancies as being unintended. About 10.5%, 5%, and 2.8% of the study sample reported preterm birth in the penultimate delivery only, index delivery only, and both penultimate and index deliveries, respectively. Approximately, one in nine women (11.4%) in the study population reported experiencing postpartum depressive symptoms.

The prevalence of postpartum depressive symptoms was higher in unmarried women, women who experienced stressful life events, women who were victims of intimate partner violence, those who never breastfed or had problems in breastfeeding, obese women, women who engaged in risky behaviors such as smoking cigarettes and drinking alcohol, and those whose pregnancies were unintended (Table 2). The prevalence of postpartum depressive symptoms was also greater for younger women, NH Black women, women with a household income of <$20,000, and women who were on Medicaid. Similarly, postpartum depressive symptoms were positively associated with younger maternal age, NH Blacks, unmarried women, lower household income, Medicaid and multiple insurance, overweight and obesity, medical morbidity in pregnancy, intimate partner violence victimization, unintended pregnancy, stressful life events, problems with breastfeeding, cigarette smoking, and alcohol use.

TABLE 1: Sample-weighted characteristics of study participants by preterm birth, Pregnancy Risk Assessment Monitoring System, 2009–2011.

Maternal characteristics	Total study population $N = 55,681^a$%	P–P– $n = 40,504^a$%	P+P– $n = 5,523^a$%	P–P+ $n = 6,042^a$%	P+P+ $n = 3,612^a$%	p value[b]
All participants	100	81.7	10.5	5.0	2.8	—
Maternal age (years)						<0.0001
≤24	21.3	20.8	24.0	21.6	24.6	
25–34	60.6	61.1	59.3	56.0	58.0	
≥35	18.1	18.1	16.7	22.4	17.4	
Maternal education						<0.0001
High school or less	45.9	44.6	52.1	49.9	55.0	
College or higher	54.1	55.4	47.9	50.1	45.0	
Race/ethnicity						<0.0001
Non-Hispanic White	56.9	58.6	49.8	48.4	47.5	
Non-Hispanic Black	13.5	12.5	15.5	19.6	23.3	
Hispanic	22.4	21.7	27.8	23.9	21.6	
Non-Hispanic other[c]	7.3	7.2	7.0	8.2	7.53	
Marital status						<0.0001
Married	66.0	67.8	59.3	59.1	51.8	
Not married	34.0	32.3	40.8	40.9	48.2	
Household income						<0.0001
<20,000	36.4	34.4	44.7	43.7	51.4	
20,000–49,999	29.0	29.5	27.4	25.5	26.4	
≥50,000	34.6	36.1	27.9	30.9	22.2	
Insurance						<0.0001
Private	46.7	48.2	39.9	44.0	33.4	
Medicaid	39.0	37.6	45.0	41.2	52.2	
Multiple	6.7	6.7	6.9	7.4	7.4	
Other	3.9	3.8	5.0	3.7	3.9	
No coverage	3.7	3.8	3.2	3.8	3.0	
Prepregnancy body mass index (kg/m^2)						0.0002
Underweight	3.6	3.3	4.1	5.2	6.3	
Normal weight	46.9	47.6	44.1	45.0	41.3	
Overweight	25.4	25.2	26.9	25.1	25.4	
Obese	24.1	23.9	24.8	24.8	27.0	
Medical morbidity in pregnancy[d]	20.6	18.1	29.1	32.6	41.6	<0.0001
Intimate partner violence	4.9	4.5	7.1	5.6	7.5	<0.0001
Pregnancy intention						<0.0001
Intended	57.7	58.5	54.6	54.8	50.0	
Unintended	42.3	41.5	45.4	45.2	50.0	

TABLE 1: Continued.

Maternal characteristics	Total study population N = 55,681[a]%	P–P– n = 40,504[a]%	P+P– n = 5,523[a]%	P–P+ n = 6,042[a]%	P+P+ n = 3,612[a]%	p value[b]
Stressful life events[e]						<0.0001
None	30.7	31.7	24.6	30.7	23.3	
1-2	41.1	41.4	40.8	37.5	41.7	
3–5	22.4	21.7	25.9	24.5	27.0	
≥6	5.8	5.3	8.6	7.4	8.1	
Previous live birth						0.0039
1	54.1	54.5	53.3	51.1	48.4	
≥2	45.9	45.5	46.7	48.9	51.6	
Problems with breastfeeding						<0.0001
Never breastfed	20.0	19.4	22.1	22.3	25.9	
Yes	34.1	33.1	37.5	39.7	39.8	
No	45.9	47.5	40.5	38.0	34.3	
Postpartum depressive symptoms	11.4	10.7	14.1	15.4	17.0	<0.0001
Cigarette smoking[f]	25.4	24.4	29.9	27.9	31.0	<0.0001
Alcohol use[f]	60.8	61.5	57.9	59.3	54.1	0.0006

P+P–, preterm birth in penultimate delivery but no preterm birth in index delivery; P–P+, no preterm birth in penultimate delivery but preterm birth in index delivery; P+P+, preterm birth in both penultimate and index deliveries; P–P–, no preterm birth in both penultimate and index deliveries. [a]Unweighted frequency. [b]Chi square for preterm birth. [c]American Indian, Chinese, Japanese, Filipino, Hawaiian, other non-White, Alaska native, other Asian. [d]Gestational diabetes, prepregnancy diabetes, and hypertensive disorders of pregnancy. [e]12 months before the birth of child. [f]Last two years.

TABLE 2: Factors associated with postpartum depressive symptoms, Pregnancy Risk Assessment Monitoring System, 2009–2011.

Maternal characteristics	Prevalence of postpartum depressive symptoms (%)[a]	Unadjusted RR (95% CI)
Maternal age (years)		
≤24	15.9	1.93 (1.69–2.20)*
25–34	10.9	1.32 (1.17–1.48)*
≥35	8.3	Reference
Maternal education		
High school or less	13.5	1.36 (1.26–1.48)*
College or higher	9.9	Reference
Race/ethnicity		
Non-Hispanic White	11.5	Reference
Non-Hispanic Black	13.5	1.17 (1.06–1.30)*
Hispanic	10.8	0.95 (0.83–1.07)
Non-Hispanic Other[b]	9.7	0.85 (0.74–0.97)*
Marital status		
Married	9.4	Reference
Not married	15.5	1.64 (1.52–1.78)*
Household income		
<20,000	16.4	2.30 (2.08–2.54)*
20,000–49,999	11.6	1.63 (1.46–1.83)*
≥50,000	7.1	Reference
Insurance		
Private	8.6	Reference
Medicaid	15.1	1.77 (1.62–1.93)*
Multiple	13.2	1.55 (1.33–1.80)*
Other	9.0	1.05 (0.77–1.43)
No coverage	8.0	0.94 (0.68–1.29)
Prepregnancy body mass index (kg/m^2)		
Underweight	11.0	1.06 (0.85–1.33)
Normal weight	10.3	Reference
Overweight	11.5	1.12 (1.00–1.24)*
Obese	14.4	1.39 (1.26–1.53)*
Medical morbidity in pregnancy[c]		
No	10.8	Reference
Yes	14.3	1.32 (1.20–1.44)*
Intimate partner violence		
No	10.4	Reference
Yes	31.9	3.06 (2.74–3.41)*
Pregnancy intention		
Intended	8.7	Reference
Unintended	15.4	1.77 (1.63–1.92)
Stressful life events[d]		
None	5.0	Reference
1-2	9.4	1.89 (1.64–2.17)*
3–5	18.2	3.67 (3.21–4.20)*
≥6	34.5	6.95 (6.02–8.04)*
Previous live birth		
1	11.1	0.93 (0.86–1.01)
≥2	12.0	Reference
Problems with breastfeeding		
Never breastfed	14.9	1.94 (1.74–2.16)*
Yes	13.6	1.77 (1.61–1.95)*
No	7.7	Reference

TABLE 2: Continued.

Maternal characteristics	Prevalence of postpartum depressive symptoms (%)[a]	Unadjusted RR (95% CI)
Cigarette smoking[e]		
No	9.1	Reference
Yes	18.3	2.01 (1.86–2.18)*
Alcohol use[e]		
No	9.6	Reference
Yes	12.7	1.33 (1.21–1.44)*

[a]Weighted percent. [b]American Indian, Chinese, Japanese, Filipino, Hawaiian, other non-White, Alaska native, other Asian. [c]Gestational diabetes, prepregnancy diabetes, and hypertensive disorders of pregnancy. [d]12 months before the birth of child. [e]Last two years. *$p < 0.05$.

TABLE 3: Association between preterm birth and postpartum depressive symptoms.

Preterm birth	Postpartum depressive symptoms	
	Crude RR (95% CI)	Adjusted RR (95% CI)[a]
P+P−	1.33 (1.17–1.51)*	1.14 (1.00–1.29)
P−P+		
Moderate-to-late preterm birth in current delivery	1.28 (1.08–1.53)*	1.19 (0.99–1.42)
Very preterm birth in current delivery	1.96 (1.69–2.27)*	1.74 (1.49–2.05)*
P+P+		
Moderate-to-late preterm birth in current delivery	1.45 (1.17–1.80)*	1.23 (1.00–1.52)
Very preterm birth in current delivery	2.02 (1.71–2.40)*	1.55 (1.28–1.88)*
P−P−	Ref.	Ref.

P+P−, preterm birth in penultimate delivery but no preterm birth in index delivery; P−P+, no preterm birth in penultimate delivery but preterm birth in index delivery; P+P+, preterm birth in both penultimate and index deliveries; P−P−, no preterm birth in both penultimate and index deliveries; RR, risk ratio; CI, confidence interval; [a]adjusted for maternal age, race/ethnicity, stressful live events in current pregnancy, intimate partner violence, pregnancy intention, and medical morbidity in pregnancy (gestational diabetes, prepregnancy diabetes, and hypertensive disorders of pregnancy); *p value < 0.05.

Table 3 shows the association between preterm birth and postpartum depressive symptoms. The unadjusted analyses show statistically significant associations between all categories of preterm birth and postpartum depressive symptoms. Compared to women with term births in both the penultimate and index deliveries, women with preterm birth in the penultimate delivery only, index delivery only, and both penultimate and index deliveries had significantly higher risk of postpartum depressive symptoms. However, after adjusting for maternal age, race/ethnicity, stressful live events, intimate partner violence, pregnancy intention, and medical morbidities in pregnancy, the association between preterm birth in the penultimate delivery only and postpartum depressive symptoms lost its statistical significance (aRR = 1.14; 95% CI = 1.00–1.29). On the other hand, the adjusted regression analyses show that the risk of postpartum depressive symptoms was 74% higher in women who had preterm birth in the index delivery only (aRR = 1.74; 95% CI = 1.49–2.05) and 55% higher among those with preterm births in both the penultimate and index deliveries (aRR = 1.55; 95% CI = 1.28–1.88), compared to women with term births in both deliveries. However, among women with preterm births in both the penultimate and index deliveries, as well as women with preterm birth in the index delivery only, the risk of postpartum depressive symptoms was significantly elevated only when the index delivery was very preterm (i.e., <32 weeks gestation). There was no significantly elevated risk when the index delivery was moderate-to-late preterm.

4. Discussion

The present study shows that women with preterm birth in the index delivery only and those with preterm births in both the penultimate and index deliveries have an increased risk of experiencing postpartum depressive symptoms. These findings are consistent with those from previous studies that reported increased risk of postpartum depressive symptoms in women with preterm birth [5, 7–9]. Although, no study has previously examined the effect of successive preterm birth on the risk of postpartum depressive symptoms, Bener reported that postpartum mothers of preterm infants with a history of preterm birth had higher prevalence of psychological distress [32], which may increase their risk of developing postpartum depressive symptoms [12]. The elevated risk of postpartum depressive symptoms observed in women with preterm birth in the current study may be due to an increase in maternal level of stress associated with infant illness and complications and concerns about the infant's outcome as explained by the preterm parental distress model [10].

Further, the study shows that women with preterm births in both the penultimate and index deliveries did not have greater risk of postpartum depressive symptoms than women with preterm birth in the index delivery only. A nonsignificant association between preterm birth and postpartum depressive symptoms in women with preterm birth in the penultimate delivery only, coupled with the lower risk of postpartum depressive symptoms observed in women with preterm births in both the penultimate and index deliveries than with women with preterm birth in the index delivery only, suggests that the risk of postpartum depressive symptoms may be driven by the experience of preterm birth in the index delivery. Furthermore, the risk of postpartum depressive symptoms in the index delivery was shown to only be significantly elevated in women with very preterm birth (i.e., <32 weeks of gestation) and was not significantly elevated in women with moderate-to-late preterm birth (32–<37 weeks of gestation). This may suggest that even though preterm birth in the index delivery increases the risk of postpartum depressive symptoms, the risk may only be evident in women with very preterm birth. This may be due to greater level of stress in women with very preterm birth [33], as higher maternal stress levels have been associated with greater postpartum depressive symptoms [11, 12].

Our findings were in contrast to the study hypothesis. The absence of a greater risk of postpartum depressive symptoms in women who had preterm births in both the penultimate and index deliveries over women who had preterm birth in the index delivery only may be explained by the acquisition of parenting skills and the development of self-efficacy in women with preterm birth in the penultimate delivery. Randomized controlled trials (RCTs) have demonstrated that interventions which addressed sources of maternal stress effectively reduced the level of stress in mothers [34, 35]. Melnyk et al., in an RCT that evaluated the efficacy of an educational-behavioral intervention program in women with preterm birth, reported that mothers who were educated on the appearance and behavioral characteristics of preterm infants and parenting them reported significantly less stress in the NICU and less depression and anxiety at two months' corrected infant age and were more positive in interactions with their infants than did comparison mothers [34]. In another RCT, Matricardi et al. examined the effects of a parental intervention to reduce parents' stress levels during the hospitalization of very preterm infants in a NICU [35]. They reported that parents of preterm infants admitted in the NICU who were taught how to observe and massage their infants in an effort to enhance parental engagement reported significantly lower levels of stress related to infants' appearance/behavior and parental role alteration than those of the control group, at discharge.

In keeping with the recommendations of the ACOG [19] and other professional health organizations, routine screening for postpartum depressive symptoms in the postpartum period for all women should be performed by health care providers using standardized, validated tools. However, beyond the routine screening for postpartum depressive symptoms, high risk women with preterm birth may require closer monitoring by their physicians. Furthermore, preterm birth may provide a teachable moment to educate women and their families on postpartum depressive symptoms. The AAP

recommends that women be screened for postpartum depressive symptoms at the 1-, 2-, 4-, and 6-month child visits [20]. However, some women may not present with postpartum depressive symptoms at these screening visits or may develop depressive symptoms at a later period. The knowledge and understanding of postpartum depressive symptoms obtained at the birth of a preterm baby may thus help to enhance recognition of the onset of depressive symptoms and facilitate early presentation to their primary care provider for further evaluation. Additionally, the current movement towards single-family room NICU has been reported to increase maternal involvement in the care of preterm babies and reduce maternal stress [36]. Incorporation of single-family rooms in the NICU setting may help to increase maternal self-efficacy and ultimately reduce the risk of postpartum depressive symptoms.

This study provided important evidence regarding the relationship between preterm births in the penultimate and index deliveries and postpartum depressive symptoms. Despite the cross-sectional design of the study, temporal sequence of the exposure and outcome was established and this enabled us to calculate the risk of postpartum depressive symptoms utilizing robust statistical methods. Findings of this study should, however, be viewed in the light of some limitations. First, postpartum depressive symptoms were self-reported by women in PRAMS. There is the possibility that postpartum depressive symptoms may have been underreported due to social desirability or the stigma attached to postpartum depression. Second, we were unable to measure some important factors such as prior history of depression or depression in pregnancy, social support, and quality of mother's relationship with partner, due to nonascertainment of these factors in the PRAMS survey. Third, history of previous preterm birth was self-reported and not clinically measured. There is the possibility of recall bias in women who had their previous delivery several years back. Fourth, due to limitations of the data, we could not distinguish between spontaneous and iatrogenic preterm birth, and, lastly, study findings are not nationally generalizable as not all states in the US participate in PRAMS.

5. Conclusions

This study showed that women with preterm births in the index delivery only and women with preterm births in both the penultimate and index deliveries have an increased risk of experiencing postpartum depressive symptoms. While preterm birth, particularly, very preterm birth, in the index delivery is associated with postpartum depressive symptoms, a prior history of preterm birth does not present an incremental risk in postpartum depressive symptoms. Routine screening for postpartum depressive symptoms should be conducted for all women using standardized, validated tools, and closer monitoring should be done for high risk women with preterm birth. Further, the birth of a preterm baby could serve as a teachable moment to educate women about preterm birth, appropriate maternal-infant interactions that can reduce the level of stress experienced by the mother, and identification of postpartum depressive symptoms. This will enable mothers of preterm babies to develop self-efficacy in the care of their babies, as well as recognize and seek immediate care for symptoms of postpartum depression.

Conflicts of Interest

The authors declare that they have no conflicts of interest.

Acknowledgments

The authors acknowledge PRAMS Working Group: Alabama—Izza Afgan, MPH; Alaska—Kathy Perham-Hester, MS, MPH; Arkansas—Mary McGehee, Ph.D.; Colorado—Alyson Shupe, Ph.D.; Connecticut—Jennifer Morin, MPH; Delaware—George Yocher, MS; Florida—Alisa Simon; Georgia—Qun Zheng, MS; Hawaii—Jihae Goo; Illinois—Patricia Kloppenburg, MT (ASCP), MPH; Iowa—Sarah Mauch, MPH; Louisiana—Megan O'Connor, MPH; Maine—Tom Patenaude, MPH; Maryland—vacant; Massachusetts—Emily Lu, MPH; Michigan—Peterson Haak; Minnesota—Mira Grice Sheff, Ph.D.; Mississippi—Brenda Hughes, MPPA; Missouri—David McBride, Ph.D.; Montana—JoAnn Dotson; Nebraska—Brenda Coufal; New Hampshire—David J. Laflamme, Ph.D., MPH; New Jersey—Lakota Kruse, MD; New Mexico—Oralia Flores; New York State—Anne Radigan; New York City—Candace Mulready-Ward, MPH; North Carolina—Kathleen Jones-Vessey, MS; North Dakota—Sandra Anseth; Ohio—Connie Geidenberger, Ph.D.; Oklahoma—Alicia Lincoln, MSW, MSPH; Oregon—Claudia W. Bingham, MPH; Pennsylvania—Tony Norwood; Rhode Island—Karine Tolentino Monteiro, MPH; South Carolina—Mike Smith, MSPH; Texas—Tanya Guthrie, Ph.D.; Tennessee—Ramona Lainhart, Ph.D.; Utah—Nicole Stone; Vermont—Peggy Brozicevic; Virginia—Christopher Hill, MPH, CPH; Washington—Linda Lohdefinck; West Virginia—Melissa Baker, MA; Wisconsin—Christopher Huard; Wyoming—Amy Spieker, MPH; and CDC PRAMS Team, Applied Sciences Branch, Division of Reproductive Health.

References

[1] T. L. Liberto, "Screening for depression and help-seeking in postpartum women during well-baby pediatric visits: an integrated review," *Journal of Pediatric Health Care*, vol. 26, no. 2, pp. 109–117, 2012.

[2] L. Murray, S. Halligan, and P. Cooper, "Effects of postnatal depression on mother-infant interactions and child development," in *The Wiley-Blackwell Handbook of Infant Development*, vol. 2, pp. 192–220, 2nd edition, 2010.

[3] N. L. Letourneau, C.-L. Dennis, K. Benzies et al., "Postpartum depression is a family affair: addressing the impact on mothers, fathers, and children," *Issues in Mental Health Nursing*, vol. 33, no. 7, pp. 445–457, 2012.

[4] M. W. O'hara and A. M. Swain, "Rates and risk of postpartum degression—a meta-analysis," *International Review of Psychiatry*, vol. 8, no. 1, pp. 37–54, 1996.

[5] N. E. Barroso, C. M. Hartley, D. M. Bagner, and J. W. Pettit, "The effect of preterm birth on infant negative affect and maternal postpartum depressive symptoms: a preliminary examination in an underrepresented minority sample," *Infant Behavior & Development*, vol. 39, pp. 159–165, 2015.

[6] R. Drewett, P. Blair, P. Emmett, and A. Emond, "Failure to thrive in the term and preterm infants of mothers depressed in the postnatal period: a population-based birth cohort study," *Journal of Child Psychology and Psychiatry*, vol. 45, no. 2, pp. 359–366, 2004.

[7] S. N. Vigod, L. Villegas, C. Dennis, and L. E. Ross, "Prevalence and risk factors for postpartum depression among women with preterm and low-birth-weight infants: a systematic review," *BJOG: An International Journal of Obstetrics and Gynaecology*, vol. 117, no. 5, pp. 540–550, 2010.

[8] M. O'brien, J. H. Asay, and K. McCluskey-Fawcett, "Family functioning and maternal depression following premature birth," *Journal of Reproductive and Infant Psychology*, vol. 17, no. 2, pp. 175–188, 1999.

[9] K. M. Voegtline and C. A. Stifter, "Family life project investigators, late-preterm birth, maternal symptomatology, and infant negativity," *Infant Behavior and Development*, vol. 33, no. 4, pp. 545–554, 2010.

[10] D. Holditch-Davis and M. Shandor Miles, "Mothers' stories about their experiences in the neonatal intensive care unit," *Neonatal Network*, vol. 19, no. 3, pp. 13–21, 2000.

[11] A. Alkozei, E. McMahon, and A. Lahav, "Stress levels and depressive symptoms in NICU mothers in the early postpartum period," *The Journal of Maternal-Fetal & Neonatal Medicine*, vol. 27, no. 17, pp. 1738–1743, 2014.

[12] K. M. Reid and M. G. Taylor, "Stress and maternal postpartum depression: the importance of stress type and timing," *Population Research and Policy Review*, vol. 34, no. 6, pp. 851–875, 2015.

[13] I. R. Chertok, S. McCrone, D. Parker, and N. Leslie, "Review of interventions to reduce stress among mothers of infants in the NICU," *Advances in Neonatal Care*, vol. 14, no. 1, pp. 30–37, 2014.

[14] S. S. Gulamani, S. S. Premji, Z. Kanji, and S. I. Azam, "A review of postpartum depression, preterm birth, and culture," *The Journal of Perinatal and Neonatal Nursing*, vol. 27, no. 1, pp. 52–61, 2013.

[15] M. B. Hughes, J. Shults, J. McGrath, and B. Medoff-Cooper, "Temperament characteristics of premature infants in the first year of life," *Journal of Developmental & Behavioral Pediatrics*, vol. 23, no. 6, pp. 430–435, 2002.

[16] J. R. Britton, "Infant temperament and maternal anxiety and depressed mood in the early postpartum period," *Women & Health*, vol. 51, no. 1, pp. 55–71, 2011.

[17] C. Y. Spong, "Prediction and prevention of recurrent spontaneous preterm birth," *Obstetrics & Gynecology*, vol. 110, no. 2, part 1, pp. 405–415, 2007.

[18] J. M. Schaaf, M. H. Hof, B. W. J. Mol, A. Abu-Hanna, and A. C. Ravelli, "Recurrence risk of preterm birth in subsequent twin pregnancy after preterm singleton delivery," *BJOG: An International Journal of Obstetrics & Gynaecology*, vol. 119, no. 13, pp. 1624–1629, 2012.

[19] "The American College of Obstetricians And Gynecologists, Screening for Perinatal Depression. Committee Opinion No. 630," *Obstetrics and Gynecology*, vol. 125, pp. 1268–1271, 2015.

[20] M. Earls, "Committee on Psychosocial Aspects of Child and Family Health American Academy of Pediatrics. Incorporating Recognition and Management of Perinatal and Postpartum Depression into Pediatric Practice," *Pediatrics*, vol. 126, no. 5, pp. 1032–1039, 2010.

[21] S. Thurgood, D. M. Avery, and L. Williamson, "Postpartum depression (PPD)," *American Journal of Clinical Medicine*, vol. 6, no. 2, pp. 17–22, 2009.

[22] C. Psaros, P. A. Geller, A. C. Sciscione, and A. Bonacquisti, "Screening practices for postpartum depression among various health care providers," *Journal of Reproductive Medicine*, vol. 55, no. 11-12, pp. 477–484, 2010.

[23] M. G. Evans, S. Phillippi, and R. E. Gee, "Examining the screening practices of physicians for postpartum depression: implications for improving health outcomes," *Women's Health Issues*, vol. 25, no. 6, pp. 703–710, 2015.

[24] N. Byatt, K. Hicks-Courant, A. Davidson et al., "Depression and anxiety among high-risk obstetric inpatients," *General Hospital Psychiatry*, vol. 36, no. 6, pp. 644–649, 2014.

[25] H. B. Shulman, B. C. Gilbert, C. G. Msphbrenda, and A. Lansky, "The Pregnancy Risk Assessment Monitoring System (PRAMS): current methods and evaluation of 2001 response rates," *Public Health Reports*, vol. 121, no. 1, pp. 74–83, 2006.

[26] Y. Choi, D. Bishai, and C. S. Minkovitz, "Multiple births are a risk factor for postpartum maternal depressive symptoms," *Pediatrics*, vol. 123, no. 4, pp. 1147–1154, 2009.

[27] M. W. Ohara, S. Stuart, D. Watson, P. M. Dietz, S. L. Farr, and D. D'angelo, "Brief scales to detect postpartum depression and anxiety symptoms," *Journal of Women's Health*, vol. 21, no. 12, pp. 1237–1243, 2012.

[28] B. I. Graubard and E. L. Korn, "Predictive margins with survey data," *Biometrics*, vol. 55, no. 2, pp. 652–659, 1999.

[29] G. S. Bieler, G. G. Brown, R. L. Williams, and D. J. Brogan, "Estimating model-adjusted risks, risk differences, and risk ratios from complex survey data," *American Journal of Epidemiology*, vol. 171, no. 5, pp. 618–623, 2010.

[30] L. J. Mayberry, J. A. Horowitz, and E. Declercq, "Depression symptom prevalence and demographic risk factors among US women during the first 2 years postpartum," *Journal of Obstetric, Gynecologic, & Neonatal Nursing*, vol. 36, no. 6, pp. 542–549, 2007.

[31] G. Maldonado and S. Greenland, "Simulation study of confounder-selection strategies," *The American Journal of Epidemiology*, vol. 138, no. 11, pp. 923–936, 1993.

[32] A. Bener, "Psychological distress among postpartum mothers of preterm infants and associated factors: a neglected public health problem," *Revista Brasileira de Psiquiatria*, vol. 35, no. 3, pp. 231–236, 2013.

[33] L. J. Woodward, S. Bora, C. A. Clark et al., "Very preterm birth: maternal experiences of the neonatal intensive care environment," *Journal of Perinatology*, vol. 34, no. 7, pp. 555–561, 2014.

[34] B. M. Melnyk, N. F. Feinstein, L. Alpert-Gillis et al., "Reducing premature infants' length of stay and improving parents' mental health outcomes with the Creating Opportunities for Parent Empowerment (COPE) neonatal intensive care unit program: a randomized, controlled trial," *Pediatrics*, vol. 118, no. 5, pp. e1414–e1427, 2006.

[35] S. Matricardi, R. Agostino, C. Fedeli, and R. Montirosso, "Mothers are not fathers: differences between parents in the reduction of stress levels after a parental intervention in a NICU," *Acta Paediatrica*, vol. 102, no. 1, pp. 8–14, 2013.

[36] B. M. Lester, K. Hawes, B. Abar, and et al, "Single-family room care and neurobehavioral and medical outcomes in preterm infants," *Pediatrics*, vol. 134, no. 4, pp. 754–760, 2014.

11-Year Trends in Pregnancy-Related Health Indicators in Maine, 2000–2010

**David E. Harris,[1] AbouEl-Makarim Aboueissa,[2] Nancy Baugh,[1]
Cheryl Sarton,[1] and Erika Lichter[3]**

[1] *School of Nursing, University of Southern Maine, Portland, ME 04104, USA*
[2] *Department of Mathematics and Statistics, University of Southern Maine, Portland, ME 04104, USA*
[3] *Department of Applied Medical Sciences, University of Southern Maine, Portland, ME 04104, USA*

Correspondence should be addressed to David E. Harris; deharris@usm.maine.edu

Academic Editor: Fabio Facchinetti

The objective of this study is to understand health and demographic trends among mothers and infants in Maine relative to the goals of *Healthy People 2020*. Pregnancy risk assessment monitoring system (PRAMS) data from Maine for 2000–2010 were used to determine yearly values of pregnancy-related variables. Means (for continuous variables) and percentages (for categorical variables) were calculated using the survey procedures in SAS. Linear trend analysis was applied with study year as the independent variable. The slope and significance of the trend were then calculated. Over the study period, new mothers in Maine became better educated but the fraction of households with incomes <$20,000/year remained stagnant. Maternal prepregnancy BMI increased. Average pregnancy weight gain decreased but the number of women whose pregnancy weight gain was within the recommended range was unchanged. The rates of smoking and alcohol consumption (before and during pregnancy) increased. The Caesarean section rate rose and the fraction of infants born premature (<37 wks gestation) or underweight (<2500 gms) remained unchanged. The fraction of infants who were breast-fed increased. These results suggest that, despite some positive trends, Maine faces significant challenges in meeting *Healthy People 2020* goals.

1. Introduction

Women's health and health behaviors before, during, and after pregnancy can impact the course and outcome of their pregnancy as well as the health of the children born from those pregnancies. Maternal smoking before [1], during [2, 3], and after [4] pregnancy is a risk to children's health and development. Maternal smoking [5] and even moderate drinking [6] during pregnancy increase the risk of having a small for gestational age infant which could prolong hospital stays, require admission to a neonatal intensive care unit, increase mortality during infancy [7], and produce developmental problems as the child grows [8]. Maternal prepregnancy obesity and excessive weight gain during pregnancy are associated with increased risk of pregnancy complications and childhood health challenges [9–11] while inadequate gestational weight gain is associated with low birth weight [10].

The presence of two parents in a family unit and adequate family income can also impact child health. Poverty is associated with health challenges while families with incomes near or below the federal poverty level and single-parent households are at risk for food insecurity [12] which is, in turn, a health risk for children [13, 14]. There are also maternal behaviors that can improve infant health. Seeking early prenatal care is associated with reduced risk of having a low birth weight infant and of infant death [15]. Breast-feeding an infant is associated with reduced rates of childhood illnesses [16], improved cognitive development at school age, and health benefits that last into adulthood [17].

When the US Department of Health and Human Services led an interagency workgroup known as *Healthy People 2020* in the development of national health objectives, they specified multiple maternal and infant health objectives. These include the objectives of reducing the number of women who smoke and drink alcohol (before, during, and after pregnancy), increasing the number of women who enter pregnancy at a healthy weight and have a healthy level of weight gain during pregnancy, increasing the number of women who receive early prenatal care, decreasing the number of infants who are born by Caesarean section, premature, or at low birth weight, and increasing the number of infants who are breast-fed [18]. *Healthy People 2020* also recognizes the negative impact that poverty can have on the health, as well as the high rate of poverty for children nationwide [18].

This study analyzes 11 years of data (2000–2010) from the pregnancy risk assessment monitoring system (PRAMS) [19] for the state of Maine. PRAMS, a joint effort of the US Center for Disease Control and Prevention and Individual State Departments of Health, is a public health survey that uses standardized collection techniques to gather information from women who have recently delivered live babies. PRAMS data provide a powerful tool for analyzing either a small number of pregnancy-related variables across broad geographical regions or a broad range of pregnancy-related variables with a more limited geographical context. By focusing on the state of Maine, this study takes the second approach.

The objective of this study is to define the year-to-year trends in health variables for women giving birth in Maine and for their infants. These results will indicate if Maine is likely to meet *Healthy People 2020* maternal and infant health objectives. This information is important because, while Maine has relatively low rates of infant mortality and low birth weight compared to national averages, it is a state where these important indicators are not improving [20]. The results of this study may suggest interventions for improving maternal-child health in Maine. Maine is also a state with communities distributed across the rural-urban continuum and where rurality impacts health [21]. Thus, the results of this study may also be of interest to those who work in similar areas. Finally, these results will also be of interest to anyone who wishes to use PRAMS data to analyze trends in their own area relative to Maine or to *Healthy People 2020* guidelines [18].

2. Methods

PRAMS identifies women who gave birth to a live infant within the previous 2–4 months from birth certificate data. It then uses mailed questionnaires and telephone follow-up to obtain information from a stratified representative sample of these women, with members of high-risk groups oversampled, and links questionnaire answers to birth certificate data [21]. In Maine, as elsewhere, women with low birth weight infants are oversampled. PRAMS data for Maine from 2000 to 2010 were obtained from the Maine Center for Disease Control and Prevention [22].

For this study, variables from multiple categories were analyzed.

(i) Maternal demographic and prepregnancy health indicator variables analyzed included (1) age, (2) marital status as a dichotomous variable, (3) household income (converted to a dichotomous variable of <$20,000 or >$20,000/year because PRAMS used multiple questionnaire formats with different income cut points during the study period but all versions had a cut point at $20,000/year), (4) education as a dichotomous variable (≤12 yrs or >12 yrs), (5) race as a dichotomous variable (white versus "other") reflecting the low level of racial diversity in Maine, and (6) age and % of women with no previous live births.

(ii) Maternal weight and pregnancy weight gain variables analyzed included (1) maternal prepregnancy height and weight (used to calculate BMI) and (2) weight gain during pregnancy as a continuous variable, as a categorical variable (<15 lbs, 15–45 lbs, and >45 lbs), and as a categorical variable relative to current weight gain recommendations (< recommended range, within recommended range, and > recommended range).

(iii) Prenatal care variables analyzed included (1) gestational age at earliest prenatal care in weeks as a continuous variable and (2) the fraction of women who received their first prenatal care within the first trimester (≤12 weeks).

(iv) Maternal tobacco and alcohol consumption variables analyzed included (1) alcohol consumption in the 3 months before pregnancy and in the last 3 months of pregnancy as dichotomous variables and (2) smoking in the 3 months before pregnancy, in the last 3 months of pregnancy, and at the time the questionnaire was administered, all as dichotomous variables.

(v) Variables related to Caesarean section birth analyzed included (1) the total rate of Caesarean section birth as well as (2) the rate of first-time and (3) the rate of repeat Caesarean section birth.

(vi) Infant outcomes variables analyzed included (1) the rate of plural births, (2) the fraction of infants born at gestational age <37 weeks, (3) the fraction of infants admitted to an intensive care unit, (4) the length of hospital stay as a categorical variable (1-2 days, 3–5 days, and ≥6 days), and (5) birth weights both as a continuous variable and as a categorical variable (<2500 gms, 2500–3999 gms, and ≥4000 gms).

(vii) Variables related to breast-feeding analyzed included the fraction of women who (1) never breast-fed their infants, (2) breast-fed for <8 weeks, and (3) breast-fed for ≥8 weeks.

Infant birth weight was obtained from the birth certificate; all other variables were self-reported. All results reflect values only among those who took the PRAMS survey.

Three different forms of the PRAMS questionnaire were used during the time period covered by this study (2000–2010). The Phase 4 questionnaire was in use until 2003, the Phase 5 questionnaire was used from 2004 to 2008, and the Phase 6 questionnaire was used from 2009 onward. It is important to note that there were minor changes in the format of PRAMS questions about smoking and drinking

TABLE 1: Prepregnancy demographics for women giving birth in Maine, 2000–2010.

Variable	N	Grand mean	95% CI		P trend	Slope
Maternal age (yrs)	12561	28.1	28.0	28.3	0.351	
Maternal age 1st birth (yrs)	6124	26.1	26.0	26.3	0.804	
Maternal BMI	12561	25.8	25.6	25.9	**<0.0001**	0.153
No previous live birth (%)	12460	45.7	44.7	46.8	**0.042**	0.014
Married (%)	12561	63.6	62.5	64.6	**<0.0001**	−0.062
Maternal education ≤12 yrs (%)	12514	45.2	44.2	46.2	**0.0009**	−0.023
Household income <$20 k/yr (%)	11981	31.8	30.8	32.8	0.210	
Maternal race not white (%)	12270	3.1	2.7	3.5	**0.020**	0.049

over the time covered by this study. For smoking, PRAMS asks a screening question to determine if a study participant smoked cigarettes and follows up with specific questions about smoking before, during, and after pregnancy only if the subject answers the screening question in the affirmative. However, PRAMS Phases 4 and 5 used "Have you smoked at least 100 cigarettes in the past 2 years?" as a screening question while Phase 6 uses "Have you smoked any cigarettes in the past 2 years?" [23]. In the case of the amount of alcohol consumption in the 3 months before pregnancy, the Phase 4 questionnaire allowed a response of "I don't know" while Phases 5 and 6 did not [23]. This necessitates that temporal trends in preconception smoking and alcohol consumption variables be interpreted with caution.

Results were analyzed using the survey procedures in SAS to adjust for the complex sampling strategy of the PRAMS dataset. The PRAMS dataset contains weighting variables, including the weighting stratum and the weighting coefficient, for each entry. This allows the statistical analysis software package used (SAS) to adjust for the complex sampling strategy of PRAMS (oversampling) and effectively "undo" the impact of oversampling. This produces results that accurately reflect the full population from which the PRAMS dataset was obtained and still take advantage of the reduced "noise" that oversampling is designed to produce.

Means (for continuous variables) and percentages (for categorical variables) were calculated for the overall study period and for each study year, along with 95% confidence intervals. Significant differences between years were tested for using F-tests (for continuous variables) and Chi-square tests (for dichotomous variables). If significant differences between years existed, linear trend analysis was applied with study year as the independent variable. The slope and significance of the trend were then calculated. Significance was accepted at $P < 0.05$.

3. Results

During the 11-year study period, Maine PRAMS questionnaires were obtained from 12,600 women, an average of 1,145.5/year. The PRAMS methodology has a minimum overall response rate threshold policy for the release of data of 70% for data prior to 2007 and 65% for data from 2007 on. The questionnaire response rate in Maine is consistently well above 70% but did not vary significantly over the study

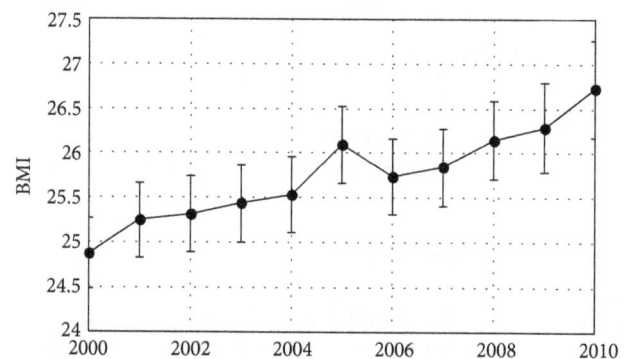

FIGURE 1: Maternal prepregnancy BMI ± 95% CI of women giving birth in Maine shown by year. Mean BMI increased at an average rate of 0.15 BMI units/year. *Healthy People 2020* objectives include a 10% increase in the proportion of women who had a healthy weight prior to pregnancy. Given that BMI > 25 is currently defined as overweight while BMI > 30 is currently defined as obese, Maine is not moving toward this goal.

period. We excluded 29 participants for whom infant birth weight was unknown, leaving 12,571 possible respondents to any question. For each question, all the responses that were available were analyzed. The number of responses for each variable was consistently >95% of the possible respondents.

The average age of women giving birth in Maine during the study period was 28.1 years and the average age of women giving birth to their first child was 26.1 years. Over the study period, 31.8% of new mothers were in households with incomes less than $20,000 per year. There were no significant trends over time in these variables (Table 1). There were significant trends in other prepregnancy health and demographic variables. Average maternal BMI was 24.9 in 2000 and increased by 0.15 BMI units/year during the study period (Table 1, Figure 1). In 2000, 69.9% of women giving birth in Maine were married (decreasing by 0.06%/year during the study period), 45.9% were having their first child (increasing by 0.01% per year during the study period), 49.9% had no education past high school (decreasing at 0.02% per year), and 2.8% reported a race other than white (increasing at 0.05% per year) (Table 1).

Average maternal weight gain during pregnancy was 31.3 lbs in 2000 and fell by 0.24 lbs/year during the study period. This change resulted from an increase in the fraction

TABLE 2: Pregnancy weight gain and prenatal care for women giving birth in Maine, 2000–2010.

Variable	Grand mean	95% CI		P trend	Slope
Weight gain (lbs)	29.7	29.4	30.0	**<0.0001**	**−0.24**
<15 lbs (%)	11.2	10.5	11.8	**<0.0001**	**0.07**
15–45 lbs (%)	77.9	77.0	78.8	**<0.0001**	**−0.04**
>45 lbs (%)	10.9	10.3	11.6	0.83	
<recommended range (%)	21.1	20.3	22.0	**<0.0001**	**0.04**
Within recommended range (%)	36.4	35.4	37.4	0.07	
>recommended range (%)	42.5	41.5	43.5	0.07	
1st prenatal care (weeks)	8.6	8.5	8.7	0.65	
Prenatal care 1st trimester (%)	92.8	92.2	93.4	0.47	

TABLE 3: Alcohol consumption and smoking by women giving birth in Maine, 2000–2010.

Variable	N	Grand mean	95% CI		P trend	Slope
Drank 3 mths before pregnancy (%)	12311	63.1	62.1	64.1	**<0.0001**	0.031
Drank last 3 mths of pregnancy (%)	12388	6.7	6.2	7.2	**0.02**	0.03
Smoked 3 mths before pregnancy (%)	12371	31.6	30.6	32.6	**0.002**	0.024
Smoked last 3 mths of pregnancy (%)	12429	18.1	17.3	19.0	**0.01**	0.02
Mother currently smokes (%)	12440	23.4	22.5	24.3	0.06	

of women who gained <15 lbs and a decrease in the number of women who gained 15–45 lbs. The fraction who gained >45 lbs did not change. The Institute of Medicine (IOM) defines healthy levels of maternal weight gain inversely with obesity status. For instance, the IOM recommends that women who have a normal prepregnancy weight gain 25–35 lbs during pregnancy while those who are overweight prior to conception gain only 15–25 lbs [24]. By IOM definitions, 36.4% of pregnant Maine women had gestational weight gain within the recommended range, 21.1% gained less than the recommended amount, and 42.4% gained more than the recommended amount of weight. Only the percent gaining less than the recommended amount showed a significant temporal trend; it increased by 0.4%/year over the study period.

The mean time at which women received their first prenatal care was 8.6 weeks and the average fraction who received prenatal care in the first trimester was 92.8%. There were no significant trends in either of these variables during the study period (Figure 2, Table 2).

In 2000, 31.3% of women in this study smoked cigarettes in the 3 months prior to pregnancy (increasing by 0.02% per year during the study period), and 60.1% drank alcohol in the 3 months prior to pregnancy (increasing by 0.03% per year during the study period). The fractions of pregnant women who smoked and drank during the last 3 months of pregnancy also increased during the study period at similar rates but the fraction who smoked at the time of the questionnaire did not change (Figures 3 and 4, Table 3). The overall rate of Caesarean section deliveries was 22.2% in 2000 and increased at an average rate of 0.04%/year during the study period. This increase was the result of an increase in first-time Caesarean sections which started at 12.7% in 2000 and also increased by an average of 0.04%/year. The rate of repeat Caesarean sections did not change (Figure 5, Table 4).

TABLE 4: Caesarean section rates for women giving birth in Maine, 2000–2010.

Variable	Grand mean	95% CI		P trend	Slope
All C-sections (%)	28.2	27.3	29.1	<0.0001	0.035
First-time C-sections (%)	17.5	16.7	18.3	<0.0001	0.038
Repeat C-sections (%)	10.7	10.1	11.4	0.12	

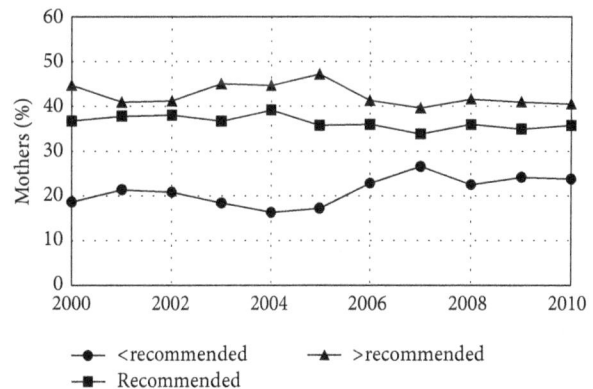

FIGURE 2: Gestational weight gain for women giving birth in Maine by year. The fraction of women gaining less than the recommended amount of weight increased while the fraction gaining an amount of weight that was within the recommended range or above that range remained unchanged. *Healthy People 2020* objectives include an increase in the proportion of women who achieved recommended levels of weight gain during pregnancy (numerical goal under development). Maine is not moving toward this goal.

There were no significant trends during the study period in a range of infant outcome variables including the fraction of plural births (1.5%), the fraction of births that were premature (<37 weeks gestation) (8.1%), and the fraction of infants

TABLE 5: Infant outcomes for newborns in Maine, 2000–2010.

Variable	N	Grand mean	95% CI		P trend	Slope
Plural births (%)	12561	1.5	1.3	1.7	0.60	
Gestational age <37 wks (%)	12556	8.1	7.6	8.5	0.37	
Infant admitted to ICU (%)	12479	9.3	8.8	9.8	0.05	

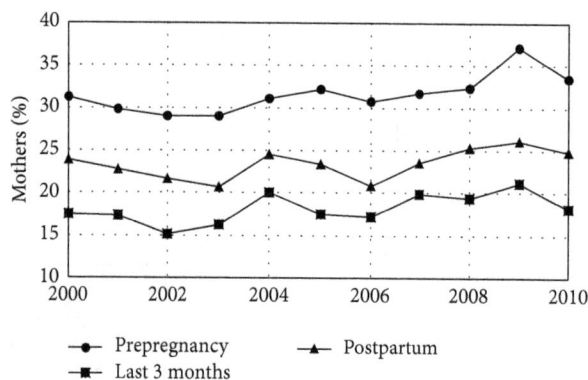

FIGURE 3: Maternal smoking by year. Fraction of mothers who smoked cigarettes in the last 3 months before pregnancy, the last 3 months of pregnancy, and postpartum (at the time of the questionnaire) for women giving birth in Maine by year. *Healthy People 2020* has objectives of a 10% increase in the percent of women who did not smoke cigarettes prior to pregnancy as well as a 10% increase in abstinence from cigarettes among pregnant women. Maine is not moving toward this goal.

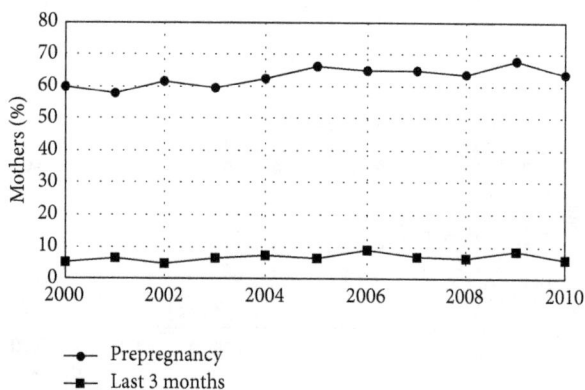

FIGURE 5: Caesarean section rate by year. Fraction of mothers giving birth in Maine who delivered by Caesarean section by year. The overall Caesarean section rate increased as a result of an increase in the rate of first-time Caesarean sections. The rate of repeat Caesarean sections remained unchanged. *Healthy People 2020* has the objective of a 10% reduction in the rate of births by first-time Caesarean section. Maine is not moving toward this goal.

TABLE 6: Length of hospital stay for infants born in Maine hospitals, 2000–2010.

Variable	Grand mean	95% CI		P trend	Slope
1–2 days (%)	59.6	58.6	60.6	**<0.0001**	**−0.03**
3–5 days (%)	32.2	31.2	33.2	**0.004**	**0.02**
≥6 days (%)	8.2	7.7	8.7	**0.002**	**0.03**

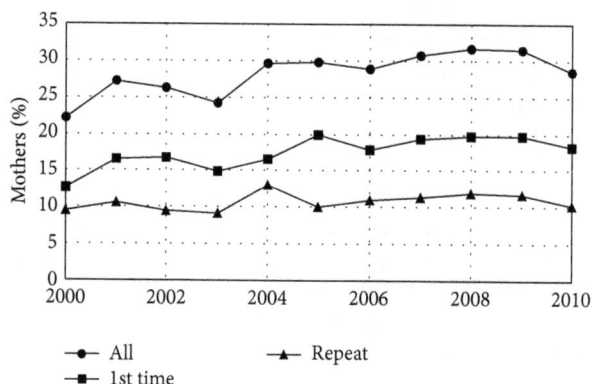

FIGURE 4: Maternal alcohol consumption by year. Fraction of mothers who drank alcohol in the last 3 months before pregnancy and the last 3 months of pregnancy for women giving birth in Maine by year. *Healthy People 2020* has objectives of a 10% increase in the percent of women who did not drink alcohol prior to pregnancy as well as a 10% increase in abstinence from alcohol among pregnant women. Maine is not moving toward this goal.

This decline resulted from fewer infants with birth weights >4000 (a cutoff that has been used for newborn macrosomia [25]) with no change in the fraction born <2500 grams (a weight well below the 3rd percentile for both male and female infants [26]) (Figure 7, Table 7). There were also significant trends in breast-feeding. The fraction of infants who were never breast-fed declined by 0.04%/year while the fraction who were breast-fed for <8 weeks increased by 0.02%/year and the fraction who were breast-fed for ≥8 weeks increased by 0.01%/year. Overall, 78.2% of infants born during the study period were breast-fed at least some and 56.7% were breast-fed for ≥8 weeks (Figure 8, Table 8).

4. Discussion

4.1. Demographics. The demographic results reported in Table 1 show increases during the study period in the fraction of women giving birth in Maine who had education past high school, the fraction who reported a race other than white, the fraction who were unmarried, the fraction who were giving birth to their first baby, and the age of first-time (but not

admitted to an intensive care unit (9.3%) (Table 5). However, there were significant trends in the length of time infants spent in the hospital after birth with fewer staying 1-2 days and more staying either 3–5 days or longer (Figure 6, Table 6). There were also significant trends in infant weight. Average infant weight was 3416 gms in 2000 and fell by 4.4 gms/year.

TABLE 7: Birth weight distribution for infants born in Maine, 2000–2010.

Variable	Grand mean	95% CI		P trend	Slope
Infant birth weight (gms)	3409.1	3399.3	3418.8	**0.01**	−4.4
Birth wt <2500 gms (%)	5.7	5.6	5.7	0.27	
Birth wt 2500–3999 gms (%)	81.1	80.4	81.8	0.05	
Birth wt ≥4000 gms (%)	13.2	13.5	13.9	**0.02**	−0.02

TABLE 8: Breast-feeding by women giving birth in Maine, 2000–2010.

Variable	Grand mean	95% CI		P trend	Slope
Never breast-fed (%)	21.9	21.0	22.8	**<0.0001**	−0.04
Breast-fed <8 wks (%)	21.5	20.6	22.3	**0.02**	0.02
Breast-fed ≥8 wks (%)	56.7	55.6	57.7	**0.04**	0.01

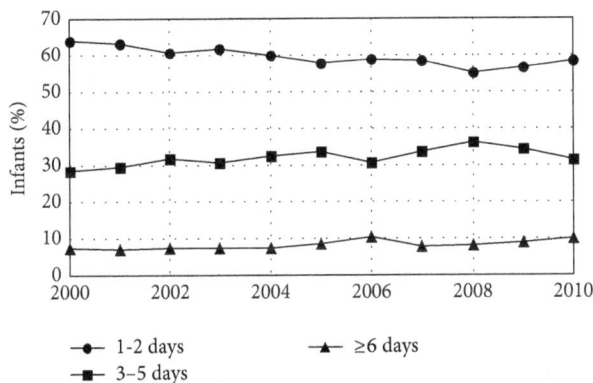

FIGURE 6: Hospital length of stay for infants born in Maine hospitals by year. The fraction of infants who were hospitalized for 1-2 days after birth declined while the fraction hospitalized in both of the two longer stay categories increased.

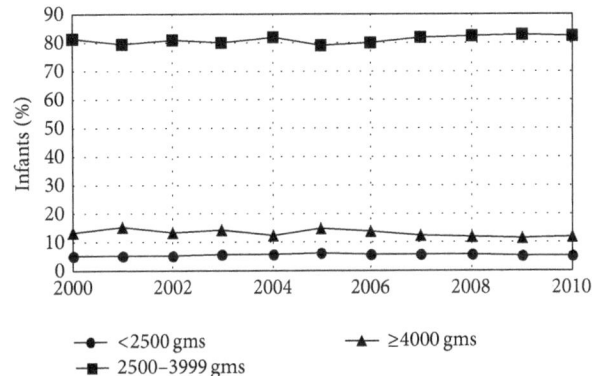

FIGURE 7: Birth weights for infants born in Maine by year. The fraction of infants who weighed ≥4000 gms at birth declined over time. *Healthy People 2020* has the objective of a reduction in low birth weight births to 7.8% of total births. Maine currently meets this goal.

all) mothers. The educational trend is not unexpected. Maine high school graduation rates are rising [27], so more Mainers are eligible to pursue postsecondary education. This trend toward better educated mothers is positive. More extensive education is associated with improved health [28] although the effect may be via the increased income that comes with more education [29].

The declining marriage rate found in this study follows national trends at work since the 1960s [30]. However, it too has health implications. Being unmarried is generally associated with poorer health [31] and parental health has an impact on children's health [32]. Furthermore, children born to unmarried women are at higher risk of adverse birth outcomes including low birth weight, preterm birth, and infant mortality than are children born to married women [33], probably because being an unmarried mother is a marker for having a low income and a risk factor for a range of measures of social disadvantage including food insecurity [12]. The rise in the number of women giving birth to their first child and the increasing age of first time mothers may suggest delayed childbearing, also a nationwide trend [34], while the increase in racial diversity reported here suggests

that Maine, like the country as a whole, is becoming more racially diverse.

One troubling finding reported here is that the fraction of women giving birth in Maine with annual household incomes less than $20,000 has remained constant over the 11-year study period (Table 1) even as income poverty thresholds have risen. A $20,000/year income represented 141% of the federal poverty limit for a family of 3 in 2000 but only 109% of the poverty level in 2010 and 102% of the federal poverty limit for a family of 3 in 2013 [35]. This suggests that more Maine children may have been born into households challenged by poverty as the study period progressed, although more work is needed to determine this. This may represent a health challenge because low income is correlated with higher rates of prepregnancy smoking, obesity, and chronic health challenges [36] and because poverty is associated with increased risk of complications during pregnancy [37]. *Healthy People 2020* recognizes the negative impact of childhood poverty on health but sets no specific objectives in the area of childhood poverty [18].

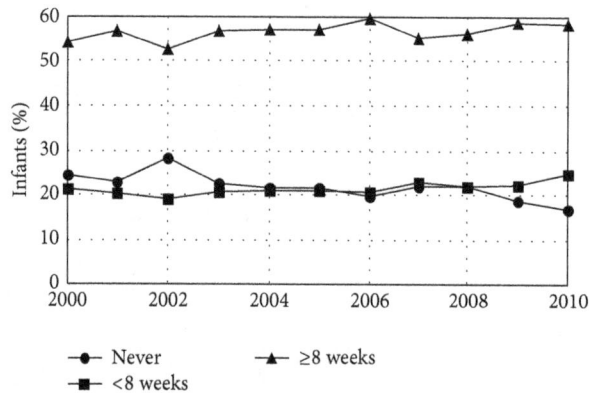

FIGURE 8: Fraction of infants breast-fed in Maine by year. The fraction never breast-fed declined while the fractions beast-fed for <8 wks and ≥8 wks increased. *Healthy People 2020* has the objective of increasing the number of infants ever breast-fed to 81.9%. Maine does not currently meet this goal but is moving toward it.

4.2. Obesity and Gestational Weight Gain.

4.2. Obesity and Gestational Weight Gain. Prepregnancy obesity is associated with an increased incidence of gestational diabetes, gestational hypertension, preeclampsia, Caesarean section [11, 38], macrosomia, postpartum hemorrhage, congenital defects, miscarriage, stillbirth, maternal mortality [39], and childhood obesity [11]. These impacts are generally exacerbated by excessive weight gain during pregnancy [9, 10] while inadequate gestational weight gain is associated with low birth weight [10]. As a result, *Healthy People 2020* objectives include a 10% increase in the proportion of women who had a healthy weight prior to pregnancy and an increase in the proportion of women who achieved recommended levels of weight gain during pregnancy (numerical goal under development) [18]. Evidence from the National Health and Nutrition Examination Survey (NHANES) show that obesity rates among US adults may have plateaued, although at an unacceptably high level [40]. However, PRAMS results suggest that preconception obesity rates continued to increase nationally, at least through 2009, and that the number of women who had a healthy weight prior to pregnancy was just over 50%. Although obesity rates are similar in Maine to national levels, the trends in obesity in Maine are less clear, with preconception obesity rates increasing significantly only for those with BMI ≥40 in a comparison of 2003 versus 2006 versus 2009 [41].

This study found that the average preconception BMI of Maine mothers for the entire study period (25.8) was in the overweight range (25–29.9) [42] and that the yearly average BMI increased steadily from 2000 to 2010, reaching 26.7 by 2010 (Table 1, Figure 1). Because this study used a continuous variable (BMI) rather than a categorical variable with somewhat arbitrary cut points [42] that can change over time [43] and for which age may need to be considered in younger women [41] (obesity rates), these results give a clear picture of increasing preconception weight in Maine. This study also found that while gestational weight gain is declining in Maine, this change results from an increase in the fraction of women who gained less than the IOM

recommended amount of weight with no change in the number whose weight gain was within the recommended range (Figure 2, Table 2).

Helping women achieve a healthy level of weight gain during pregnancy is not easy but it is possible. Simply having a practitioner give pregnant women advice about healthy weight gain during a standard prenatal visit has little impact on whether or not a women actually achieves healthy weight gain [44]. However, a light to moderate intensity exercise program for pregnant women can prevent excessive gestational weight gain [45]. Postpartum weight retention is also a health issue. One face-to-face meeting during pregnancy with a designated interventionist with telephonic and mail follow-up focusing on healthy diet, increased exercise, and self-monitoring of eating, exercise, and weight gain was found to decrease weight retention 12 months postpartum but not to increase the number of women who regained their prepregnancy weight [46]. Thus, interventions that go beyond what is possible at a prenatal visit and include active participation by the patients are probably needed for Maine to reverse current trends of increasing prepregnancy BMI with no increase in the number of women who achieved healthy weight gain during pregnancy as will be necessary if Maine is to meet *Healthy People 2020* goals around prepregnancy weight and gestational weight gain [18].

4.3. Tobacco and Alcohol. The high rates of smoking and drinking reported here also have negative health implications. Smoking during pregnancy increases the risks of pregnancy complications including spontaneous abortions, ectopic pregnancies, and placenta previa. It may also increase the risk that the child born from that pregnancy will experience behavioral disorders [47]. Heavy smoking before pregnancy is associated with children having lower cognitive abilities even if the mother has quit smoking before she conceives [1]. Alcohol consumption in the months prior to pregnancy is also generally considered a risk to the child born from the subsequent pregnancy. Heavy drinking in the 3 months prior to conception is associated with low birth weight [6] and alcohol consumption prior to pregnancy may interact with smoking during that same period to produce a particularly high risk of cardiac defect [48]. However, not all studies find an association between moderate alcohol consumption early in pregnancy and negative outcomes such as low birth weight, preeclampsia, and preterm birth [49].

Following the belief that both maternal smoking and drinking are health risks to a developing fetus, *Healthy People 2020* has objectives of a 10% increase in the percent of women who did not smoke cigarettes or drink alcohol prior to pregnancy as well as a 10% increase in abstinence from alcohol and cigarettes among pregnant women [18]. For the entire study period, the results reported here show a preconception nonsmoking rate for Maine of 68.4% and a preconception nondrinking rate of 36.9%. During pregnancy, 81.9% of expectant women did not smoke and 93.3% did not drink (Figures 3 and 4, Table 3). The smoking results extend previous reports for shorter time periods [50, 51].

Because of minor changes in the PRAMS questions around smoking and drinking during the study period, the significant increases in preconception smoking and drinking found here may reflect the change in PRAMS methodology rather than an actual increase and must be interpreted with caution. A multisite study of smoking that included Maine included the change in smoking question in its analysis and found no significant increase in smoking prior to pregnancy [52]. However, smoking levels in Maine reported here are more than double *Health People 2020* goals prior to pregnancy and over 15 times national goals during pregnancy. Drinking levels in Maine are 40% higher than national goals prior to pregnancy and are nearly 4 times the *Healthy People 2020* goals during pregnancy. (compare Table 3 to [18].) Furthermore, there is no sign, either in the results reported here or in previously reported results, that smoking and drinking before or during pregnancy are declining in Maine as would be necessary to meet *Healthy People 2020* goals.

As with weight gain, a single intervention during a prenatal visit may not be enough to positively impact smoking and drinking behavior. A brief computer-based intervention during a prenatal visit failed to reduce drinking during pregnancy [53] but counselling combined with incentives, feedback, and peer support did prove effective at getting pregnant women who smoked to quit [54]. Even prepregnancy behavior is amenable to change through robust interventions. Motivational interviewing and feedback have been shown to reduce alcohol-exposed pregnancy risk among nonpregnant college students [55]. Clearly, major efforts will be necessary for Maine to reach the goals of *Healthy People 2020* for reducing pregnancy-related smoking and alcohol consumption. As is the case with weight gain, interventions that go beyond what is possible at a prenatal visit and include active participation by the patients are probably needed.

4.4. Prenatal Care. Seeking prenatal care is associated with reduced risk of delivering a low birth weight infant and of infant death [56] and *Healthy People 2020* has an objective of increasing the percent of women who received prenatal care beginning in the first trimester by 10%. The results reported here show that 92.8% of pregnant women in Maine obtain prenatal care within the first trimmest. However, they here fail to show any change in the fraction of women who access early prenatal care (Table 2). Community outreach and education may be necessary to reverse this trend.

4.5. Birth and Postpartum. Preterm birth (birth prior to 37 weeks gestation) is a leading cause of respiratory and neurological disability in infants and infant death [57, 58]. Low birth weight/small for gestational age infants (generally those <2500 gms in weight) are also at risk for increased mortality [59] as well as problems around thermoregulation, hypoglycemia, and sepsis [60, 61]. Birth by Caesarean section subjects the mother to major abdominal surgery and is a risk for reduced subsequent fertility [62]. Although randomized controlled studies are lacking, Caesarean section birth may also place infants at risk for several health challenges including obesity, metabolic syndrome, hypertension, type 1 diabetes, asthma, and inflammatory bowel disease [63] probably because babies born by Caesarean section do not experience the physiological stress of labor and vaginal birth [64].

Healthy People 2020 has multiple specific objectives for improved birth and postpartum outcomes including 10% reductions in preterm birth rate and the rate of births by first-time Caesarean section and a reduction in low birth weight births to 7.8% of total births [18]. The results reported here show that the rate of first-time Caesarean sections in Maine is increasing (Figure 5, Table 4) and show no decrease in the rate of preterm births (Table 5). Low weight (<2500 gms) births in Maine were within the *Healthy People 2020* objectives but were not decreasing (Figure 7, Table 7). Caesarean section rates, at least, may be amendable to nonclinical intervention. Both a nurse-led relaxation program and guideline implementation programs with mandatory second opinion have been shown to reduce Caesarean section rates [65].

Breast-feeding an infant is associated with a reduction in the risk of ear, respiratory, and skin diseases; GI diseases of infancy including nonspecific gastroenteritis and necrotizing enterocolitis; metabolic diseases including obesity, type 1 diabetes, and type 2 diabetes; childhood leukemia; and sudden infant death syndrome (SIDS) [16]. It is also associated with improved cognitive development at school age; lower blood pressure persisting into adulthood; and lower risk of hypercholesterolemia, obesity, and type 2 diabetes mellitus among adults who were breast-fed as infants [17].

The fraction of Maine babies ever breast-fed was 78.1%, 3.8% below *Healthy People 2020* objectives [18], but rate of breast-feeding was increasing (Figure 8, Table 8). It may be possible to further improve this rate by some simple interventions. A brief questionnaire that explores a baby's nursing behavior as a neonate has proven effective at predicting successful nursing behavior at 3 to 6 months of age [66]. This raises the possibility that infants who may not succeed at longer-term breast-feeding can be identified early and their mothers provided extra support. There is also evidence that home visits which combine education and patient-specific advice beginning before a new mother returns to work and continuing after she begins working reduce anxiety and increase the frequency of breast-feeding among working mothers in Turkey [67]. Once a mother has returned to work, policies that encourage women to nurse and/or pump breast milk in the workplace combined with coworker encouragement are associated with breast-feeding past 6 months after return to work in Taiwan [68]. These findings highlight the importance of policies and interventions that continue to support new mothers in breast feeding after birth.

5. Limitation and Conclusions

The PRAMS dataset is a rich source of information but working with it comes with limitations. First, as discussed in the matter of smoking and drinking variables, changes in the question format were introduced during the study period. Although minor, these changes probably account for the increasing trend we found in prepregnancy smoking (compare Tong et al., 2013 [52], to Table 3). Nonetheless, there is no indication that prepregnancy smoking rates are declining in Maine, so the conclusion presented here that much more needs to be done in this area to meet *Healthy People 2020* objectives is valid.

Second, *Healthy People 2020* does not use PRAMS as a data source, so it can be difficult to compare absolute measures from PRAMS data in this study to *Healthy People 2020* objectives. For instance, in the matter of breastfeeding, *Healthy People 2020* uses results from the National Immunization Survey (NIS) which uses telephone interviews generated from a randomized list of phone numbers to locate households with young children [69] rather than the PRAMS approach of beginning with birth certificate contact information. Thus, the most meaningful comparisons between the results reported here and *Healthy People 2020* objectives may be in trends, and that has been the main focus of the analysis presented here. Fortunately, many of the objectives of *Healthy People 2020* are presented as % changes. There are some examples, however, such as smoking rates and drinking rates, where Maine PRAMS results are far below *Healthy People 2020* objectives. These almost certainly represent areas where Maine needs to improve.

In summary, this study identifies prepregnancy, prenatal, and postpartum demographic, behavioral, and health trends for women having children in Maine from 2000 to 2010 and for their babies which may challenge Maine's efforts to meet *Healthy People 2020* objectives. These results may suggest specific health priorities and interventions for Maine and areas of important inquiry for those in other states.

Conflict of Interests

The authors declare that there is no conflict of interests regarding the publication of this paper.

Acknowledgments

The authors acknowledge the PRAMS Working Group, the US CDC, and the Maine CDC. Particular thanks are due to Tom Patenaude, MPH, the Maine member of the PRAMS Working Group. This protocol was approved by the University of Southern Maine Institutional Review Board and vetted before the Maine Center for Disease Control and Prevention.

References

[1] K. Heinonen, K. Räikkönen, A.-K. Pesonen et al., "Longitudinal study of smoking cessation before pregnancy and children's cognitive abilities at 56 months of age," *Early Human Development*, vol. 87, no. 5, pp. 353–359, 2011.

[2] A. Agrawal, J. F. Scherrer, J. D. Grant et al., "The effects of maternal smoking during pregnancy on offspring outcomes," *Preventive Medicine*, vol. 50, no. 1-2, pp. 13–18, 2010.

[3] B. Durmuş, C. J. Kruithof, M. H. Gillman et al., "Parental smoking during pregnancy, early growth, and risk of obesity in preschool children: the Generation R Study," *The American Journal of Clinical Nutrition*, vol. 94, no. 1, pp. 164–171, 2011.

[4] D. E. Levy, J. P. Winickoff, and N. A. Rigotti, "School absenteeism among children living with Smokers," *Pediatrics*, 2011.

[5] M. Terada, Y. Matsuda, M. Ogawa, H. Matsui, and S. Satoh, "Effects of maternal factors on birth weight in Japan," *Journal of Pregnancy*, vol. 2013, Article ID 172395, 5 pages, 2013.

[6] N. Whitehead and L. Lipscomb, "Patterns of alcohol use before and during pregnancy and the risk of small-for-gestational-age birth," *American Journal of Epidemiology*, vol. 158, no. 7, pp. 654–662, 2003.

[7] M. J. Teune, S. Bakhuizen, C. G. Bannerman et al., "A systematic review of severe morbidity in infants born late preterm," *American Journal of Obstetrics & Gynecology*, vol. 205, no. 4, pp. e1–e9, 2011.

[8] E. Arpi and F. Ferrari, "Preterm birth and behaviour problems in infants and preschool-age children: a review of the recent literature," *Developmental Medicine and Child Neurology*, vol. 55, no. 9, pp. 788–796, 2013.

[9] J. E. Norman and R. Reynolds, "Consequences of obesity and overweight during pregnancy: the consequences of obesity and excess weight gain in pregnancy," *Proceedings of the Nutrition Society*, vol. 70, no. 4, pp. 450–456, 2011.

[10] L. Poston, "Gestational weight gain: influences on the long-term health of the child," *Current Opinion in Clinical Nutrition & Metabolic Care*, vol. 15, no. 3, pp. 252–257, 2012.

[11] R. Gaillard, B. Durmuş, A. Hofman, J. P. MacKenbach, E. A. P. Steegers, and V. W. V. Jaddoe, "Risk factors and outcomes of maternal obesity and excessive weight gain during pregnancy," *Obesity*, vol. 21, no. 5, pp. 1046–1055, 2013.

[12] A. Coleman-Jensen, M. Nord, and A. Singh, "Household food security in the United States in 2012," USDA Economic Research Report no. (ERR-155), 2014, http://www.ers.usda.gov/publications/err-economic-research-report/err155.aspx#.UnOuYFOmUSU.

[13] J. T. Cook, D. A. Frank, C. Berkowitz et al., "Food insecurity is associated with adverse health outcomes among human infants and toddlers," *The Journal of Nutrition*, vol. 134, no. 6, pp. 1432–1438, 2004.

[14] A. Skalicky, A. F. Meyers, W. G. Adams, Z. Yang, J. T. Cook, and D. A. Frank, "Child food insecurity and iron deficiency anemia in low-income infants and toddlers in the United States," *Maternal and Child Health Journal*, vol. 10, no. 2, pp. 177–185, 2006.

[15] Health Resources and Services Administration Maternal and Child Health, "Prenatal Services," 2014, http://mchb.hrsa.gov/programs/womeninfants/prenatal.html.

[16] S. Ip, M. Chung, G. Raman et al., "Breastfeeding and maternal and infant health outcomes in developed countries," Evidence Report/Technology Assessment 153, AHRQ Publication no. 07-E007, Agency for Healthcare Research and Quality, 2007.

[17] B. L. Horta, R. Bahl, J. C. Martines, and C. G. Victora, *Evidence on the Long-Term Effects of Breastfeeding*, Department of Child and Adolescent Health and Development, World Health Organization, 2007, http://www.quenoosseparen.info/documentos/LMlargoplazo.pdf.

[18] Healthy People 2020, "Maternal, infant, and child health," 2014, http://www.healthypeople.gov/2020/topicsobjectives2020/objectiveslist.aspx?topicId=26.

[19] Centers for Disease Control & Prevention, "What is PRAMS?" 2014, http://www.cdc.gov/prams/.

[20] Division of Public Health Systems, Maine Center for Disease Control & Prevention Data Research, and Vital Statistics,

"Pregnancy Risk Assessment Monitoring System (PRAMS)," 2014, http://www.maine.gov/dhhs/mecdc/public-health-systems/data-research/prams/index.shtml.

[21] D. E. Harris, A. Aboueissa, and D. Hartley, "Myocardial infarction and heart failure hospitalization rates in Maine, USA—variability along the urban-rural continuum," *Rural and Remote Health*, vol. 8, no. 2, p. 980, 2008, http://www.rrh.org.au/articles/subviewnew.asp?ArticleID=980.

[22] Maine Center for Disease Control & Prevention, "Maine CDC Home," 2014, http://www.maine.gov/dhhs/mecdc/.

[23] Centers for Disease Control & Prevention, "PRAMS questionnaires," 2014, http://www.cdc.gov/prams/Questionnaire.htm.

[24] Institute of Medicine, "Weight gain during pregnancy: reexamining the guidelines," 2009, http://iom.edu/~/media/Files/Report%20Files/2009/Weight-Gain-During-Pregnancy-Reexamining-the-Guidelines/Report%20Brief%20-%20Weight%20Gain%20During%20Pregnancy.pdf.

[25] T. Henriksen, "The macrosomic fetus: a challenge in current obstetrics," *Acta Obstetricia et Gynecologica Scandinavica*, vol. 87, no. 2, pp. 134–145, 2008.

[26] American Academy of Pediatrics, "Intrauterine growth curves," 2014, https://www2.aap.org/sections/perinatal/PDF/GrowthCurves.pdf.

[27] Department of Education State of Maine, "Maine high school graduation rates," 2014, http://www.maine.gov/education/gradrates/.

[28] D. M. Cutler and A. Lleras-Muney, "Education and health: evaluating theories and evidence," NBER Working Paper Series, Working Paper 12352, 2006, http://www.nber.org/papers/w12352.pdf?new_window=1.

[29] L. Picker, "The effects of education on health," The National Bureau of Economic Research, 2014, http://www.nber.org/digest/mar07/w12352.html.

[30] S. J. Ventura, "Changing patterns of nonmarital childbearing in the United States," NCHS Data Brief 18, National Center for Health Statistics, Hyattsville, Md, USA, 2009.

[31] C. A. Schoenborn, *Marital Status and Health: United States, 1999–2002*, Advance Data from Vital and Health Statistics, no. 351, National Center for Health Statistics, Hyattsville, Md, USA, 2004.

[32] C. S. Weisman, D. P. Misra, M. M. Hillemeier et al., "Preconception predictors of birth outcomes: prospective findings from the central Pennsylvania women's health study," *Maternal and Child Health Journal*, vol. 15, no. 7, pp. 829–835, 2011.

[33] T. J. Mathews and M. F. MacDorman, "Infant mortality statistics from the 2008 period linked birth/infant death data set," *National Vital Statistics Reports*, vol. 60, no. 5, 2012.

[34] T. J. Mathews and B. E. Hamilton, "Delayed childbearing: more women are having their first child later in life," NCHS Data Brief 21, National Center for Health Statistics, Hyattsville, Md, USA, 2009.

[35] US Department of Health & Human Services, *Poverty Guidelines, Research, and Measurement*, 2014, http://aspe.hhs.gov/poverty/index.cfm.

[36] J. M. Bombard, P. M. Dietz, C. Galavotti et al., "Chronic diseases and related risk factors among low-income mothers," *Maternal and Child Health Journal*, vol. 16, no. 1, pp. 60–71, 2012.

[37] N. S. Whitehead, W. Callaghan, C. Johnson, and L. Williams, "Racial, ethnic, and economic disparities in the prevalence of pregnancy complications," *Maternal and Child Health Journal*, vol. 13, no. 2, pp. 198–205, 2009.

[38] J. H. Chung, K. A. Melsop, W. M. Gilbert, A. B. Caughey, C. K. Walker, and E. K. Main, "Increasing pre-pregnancy body mass index is predictive of a progressive escalation in adverse pregnancy outcomes," *Journal of Maternal-Fetal and Neonatal Medicine*, vol. 25, no. 9, pp. 1635–1639, 2012.

[39] N. E. Marshall and C. Y. Spong, "Obesity, pregnancy complications, and birth outcomes," *Seminars in Reproductive Medicine*, vol. 30, no. 6, pp. 465–471, 2012.

[40] K. M. Flegal, D. Carroll, B. K. Kit, and C. L. Ogden, "Prevalence of obesity and trends in the distribution of body mass index among US adults, 1999-2010," *Journal of the American Medical Association*, vol. 307, no. 5, pp. 491–497, 2012.

[41] S. C. Fisher, S. Y. Kim, A. J. Sharma, R. Rochat, and B. Morrow, "Is obesity still increasing among pregnant women? Prepregnancy obesity trends in 20 states, 2003–2009," *Preventive Medicine*, vol. 56, no. 6, pp. 372–378, 2013.

[42] National Institutes of Health, "NHLBI obesity education initiative expert panel on the identification, evaluation, and treatment of overweight and obesity in adults," The Evidence Report NIH no. 98-4083, National Institutes of Health, 1998.

[43] R. J. Kuczmarski and K. M. Flegal, "Criteria for definition of overweight in transition: background and recommendations for the United States," *The American Journal of Clinical Nutrition*, vol. 72, no. 5, pp. 1074–1081, 2000.

[44] R. M. Ferrari and A. M. Siega-Riz, "Provider advice about pregnancy weight gain and adequacy of weight gain," *Maternal and Child Health Journal*, vol. 17, no. 2, pp. 256–264, 2013.

[45] J. R. Ruiz, M. Perales, M. Pelaez, C. Lopez, A. Lucia, and R. Barakat, "Supervised exercise-based intervention to prevent excessive gestational weight gain: a randomized controlled trial," *Mayo Clinic Proceedings*, vol. 88, no. 12, pp. 1388–1397, 2013.

[46] S. Phelan, M. G. Phipps, B. Abrams et al., "Does behavioral intervention in pregnancy reduce postpartum weight retention? Twelve-month outcomes of the Fit for Delivery randomized trial1-3," *American Journal of Clinical Nutrition*, vol. 99, no. 2, pp. 302–311, 2014.

[47] S. Cnattingius, "The epidemiology of smoking during pregnancy: smoking prevalence, maternal characteristics, and pregnancy outcomes," *Nicotine and Tobacco Research*, vol. 6, supplement 2, pp. S125–S140, 2004.

[48] W. A. Mateja, D. B. Nelson, C. D. Kroelinger, S. Ruzek, and J. Segal, "The association between maternal alcohol use and smoking in early pregnancy and congenital cardiac defects," *Journal of Women's Health*, vol. 21, no. 1, pp. 26–34, 2012.

[49] F. P. McCarthy, L. M. O'keeffe, A. S. Khashan et al., "Association between maternal alcohol consumption in early pregnancy and pregnancy outcomes," *Obstetrics and Gynecology*, vol. 122, no. 4, pp. 830–837, 2013.

[50] D. DAngelo, L. Williams, B. Morrow et al., "Preconception and interconception health status of women who recently gave birth to a live-born infant—Pregnancy Risk Assessment Monitoring System (PRAMS), United States, 26 reporting areas, 2004," *Morbidity and Mortality Weekly Report*, vol. 56, no. SS10, pp. 1–35, 2007.

[51] V. T. Tong, J. R. Jones, P. M. Dietz, D. D'Angelo, and J. M. Bombard, "Trends in smoking before, during, and after pregnancy—pregnancy risk assessment monitoring system (PRAMS), United States, 31 sites, 2000–2005," *Morbidity and Mortality Weekly Report*, vol. 58, no. 4, pp. 1–29, 2009.

[52] V. T. Tong, P. M. Dietz, B. Morrow et al., "Trends in smoking before, during, and after pregnancy—pregnancy risk assessment monitoring system, United States, 40 Sites, 2000–2010," *MMWR*, vol. 62, no. 6, 2013.

[53] G. K. Tzilos, R. J. Sokol, and S. J. Ondersma, "A Randomized phase i trial of a brief computer-delivered intervention for alcohol use during pregnancy," *Journal of Women's Health*, vol. 20, no. 10, pp. 1517–1524, 2011.

[54] C. Chamberlain, A. O'Mara-Eves, S. Oliver et al., "Psychosocial interventions for supporting women to stop smoking in pregnancy (Review)," *Cochrane Database of Systematic Reviews*, vol. 10, pp. 1–354, 2013.

[55] S. D. Ceperich and K. S. Ingersoll, "Motivational interviewing + feedback intervention to reduce alcohol-exposed pregnancy risk among college binge drinkers: determinants and patterns of response," *Journal of Behavioral Medicine*, vol. 34, no. 5, pp. 381–395, 2011.

[56] US Department of Health & Human Services, *Prenatal Services*, 2014, http://mchb.hrsa.gov/programs/womeninfants/prenatal.html.

[57] A. Kugelman and A. A. Colin, "Late preterm infants: near term but still in a critical developmental time period," *Pediatrics*, vol. 132, no. 4, pp. 741–751, 2013.

[58] Centers for Disease Control and Prevention, *Preterm Birth*, 2014, http://www.cdc.gov/reproductivehealth/maternalinfanthealth/pretermbirth.htm.

[59] M. R. Battin, D. B. Knight, C. A. Kuschel, and R. N. Howie, "Improvement in mortality of very low birthweight infants and the changing pattern of neonatal mortality: the 50-year experience of one perinatal centre," *Journal of Paediatrics and Child Health*, vol. 48, no. 7, pp. 596–599, 2012.

[60] S. S. Miller, H. C. Lee, and J. B. Gould, "Hypothermia in very low birth weight infants: distribution, risk factors and outcomes," *Journal of Perinatology*, vol. 31, pp. S49–S56, 2011.

[61] Barbara Bush Children's Hospital, *Small for Gestational Age (SGA) Clinical Practice Guideline—Newborn Nursery*, 2009, http://www.bbch.org/clinicians/Documents/small_for_gestational_age.pdf.

[62] I. Gurol-Urganci, S. Bou-Antoun, C. P. Lim et al., "Impact of Caesarean section on subsequent fertility: a systematic review and meta-analysis," *Human Reproduction*, vol. 28, no. 7, pp. 1943–1952, 2013.

[63] M. J. Hyde and N. Modi, "The long-term effects of birth by caesarean section: the case for a randomised controlled trial," *Early Human Development*, vol. 88, no. 12, pp. 943–949, 2012.

[64] M. J. Hyde, A. Mostyn, N. Modi, and P. R. Kemp, "The health implications of birth by Caesarean section," *Biological Reviews*, vol. 87, no. 1, pp. 229–243, 2012.

[65] S. Khunpradit, E. Tavender, P. Lumbiganon, M. Laopaiboon, J. Wasiak, and R. L. Gruen, "Non-clinical interventions for reducing unnecessary caesarean section (review)," *Cochrane Library*, no. 6, pp. 1–63, 2011.

[66] K. Mizuno, K. Fujimaki, and M. Sawada, "Sucking behavior at breast during the early newborn period affects later breast-feeding rate and duration of breast-feeding," *Pediatrics International*, vol. 46, no. 1, pp. 15–20, 2004.

[67] E. K. Çiftçi and D. Arikan, "The effect of training administered to working mothers on maternal anxiety levels and breastfeeding habits," *Journal of Clinical Nursing*, vol. 21, no. 15-16, pp. 2170–2178, 2012.

[68] S. Y. Tsai, "Impact of a breastfeeding-friendly workplace on an employed mother's intention to continue breastfeeding after returning to work," *Breastfeeding Medicine*, vol. 8, no. 2, pp. 210–216, 2013.

[69] Healthy People 2020, *National Immunization Survey (NIS)*, 2014, http://www.healthypeople.gov/2020/Data/datasource.aspx?id=96.

4

Knowledge of Pregnant Women on Mother-to-Child Transmission of HIV in Meket District, Northeast Ethiopia

Tesfaye Birhane,[1] Gizachew Assefa Tessema,[2] Kefyalew Addis Alene,[3] and Abel Fekadu Dadi[3]

[1]Meket District Health Office, Meket, Ethiopia
[2]Department of Reproductive Health, Institute of Public Health, University of Gondar, P.O. Box 196, Gondar, Ethiopia
[3]Department of Epidemiology and Biostatistics, Institute of Public Health, University of Gondar, P.O. Box 196, Gondar, Ethiopia

Correspondence should be addressed to Gizachew Assefa Tessema; agizachew@gmail.com

Academic Editor: Sinuhe Hahn

Knowledge of pregnant women on the three periods of mother-to-child transmission (MTCT) of HIV has implication for child HIV acquisition. This study aims to assess the knowledge of pregnant women on mother-to-child transmission of HIV and to identify associated factors in Meket district, northeast Ethiopia. Logistic regression models were fitted to identify associated factors. Adjusted odds ratios (AOR) with 95% confidence intervals (CI) were used to determine the presence and strength of association. About one-fifth (19%) of women were knowledgeable on mother-to-child transmission of HIV (95% CI: 15.5%, 22.4%). Being urban resident (AOR: 2.69, 95% CI: 1.48, 4.87), having primary education (AOR: 2.41, 95% CI: 1.03, 5.60), reporting receiving information on HIV from health care providers (AOR: 3.24, 95% CI: 1.53, 6.83), having discussion with partner about mother-to-child transmission of HIV (AOR: 2.64, 95% CI: 1.59, 4.39), and attending antenatal care (AOR: 5.80, 95% CI: 2.63, 12.77) were positively associated with increased maternal knowledge of mother-to-child transmission of HIV. Knowledge of mother-to-child transmission of HIV among pregnant women was low. Providing information, especially for rural women and their partners, is highly recommended.

1. Background

Vertical transmission of Human Immunodeficiency Virus (HIV) is still a major challenge in the world, especially in developing countries [1]. A report in 2012 reported about 35.3 million people are living with HIV of which 2.3 million are new infections whereas an estimated 3.3 million infected people are less than 15 years of age. Worldwide, there are about 6,300 new infections and 700 HIV-related deaths daily in 2012. Sub-Saharan Africa remains the region most heavily affected by HIV [2].

Without any intervention, the risk of a baby getting HIV infection from an infected mother ranges from 15% to 25% in the developed nations and from 25% to 35% in developing countries. HIV transmission rate and timing are estimated to be 5% to 10% during pregnancy, 10% to 15% during delivery and 5% to 20% through breast-feeding. In general mother to child transmission contributes 15-45% of HIV acquisition for children [3].

The national adult HIV prevalence in Ethiopia is 1.2% [4]. The national accelerated emergency plan includes three targeted objectives, that is, reaching 90% of pregnant women with access to antenatal care services, ensuring that all pregnant women have access to delivery by a skilled attendant, and providing antiretroviral prophylaxis to at least 80% of HIV-positive pregnant women [5].

It is estimated that 138,906 children less than 15 years are living with HIV in 2014. There are an estimated 3,886 new infections each year due to mother-to-child transmission [4]. However, timely interventions can reduce mother-to-child transmission to 2–5% [3, 6, 7]. A global target has also been established to be achieved by the year 2015, that is, elimination of new HIV infections among children and prolonging the lives of the mothers with HIV [1].

According to Ethiopian Demographic and Health Survey (EDHS) report, about three-quarters of reproductive aged women know that HIV can be transmitted to a baby through breastfeeding [8].

The prevention of Mother-To—Child-Transmission (MTCT) of HIV is dependent on the knowledge of the mothers of the timing of possible transmission periods. However, knowledge of women on transmission periods of HIV from mother to child varies from country to country and has not been measured in Ethiopia at community level.

Different studies reported that sociodemographic factors like age [9], urban living [10], higher educational level [11], and being house wife [12] as factors that affect mothers' knowledge of MTCT of HIV. Studies conducted in southern and northwest Ethiopia [10, 12, 13] reported that gravidity, parity, antenatal care (ANC) visits, and male partner discussion are factors associated with good knowledge of mothers on MTCT of HIV.

Maternal knowledge on MTCT is a corner stone of effective implementation of the World Health Organization (WHO) recommendation of the four-pronged approach to reduce mother-to-child transmission of HIV [1].

Despite the large challenge of vertical transmission of HIV, there were also limited community-based studies on women knowledge on mother-to-child transmission of HIV. Hence, this study attempts to fill the gap through assessing the level of knowledge of MTCT of HIV and its associated factors at Meket district, Northeast Ethiopia.

2. Methods

2.1. Study Design, Population, and Setting. A community-based cross-sectional study design was conducted in Meket district, northeast Ethiopia, from March 8 to 21, 2014. Meket district is located 665 km north of Addis Ababa, the Ethiopian capital city. The district has an estimated population size of 254,520 of which 59,939 are reproductive aged women, and an estimated 8,246 were pregnant women. Those pregnant women are living in Meket district were constituted our study population.

2.2. Sample Size and Sampling Procedure. Sample size was determined using single population proportion formula with the assumptions of 95% level of confidence, 12% proportion of knowledgeable women on MTCT of HIV [12], 4% of margin of error, and design effect of two. Finally, considering a non-response rate of 10%, the total sample size was calculated to be 556. Multistage stratified sampling technique was used to select the study participants. In the district, there are two urban and 46 rural kebeles. Hence, in the first step, eight rural kebeles were randomly selected; however, since they are few, all the urban kebeles were included. On the second stage, 79 pregnant women from urban kebeles and 477 pregnant women from rural kebeles were randomly selected.

2.3. Operational Definitions. In the present study, pregnant woman was regarded as being knowledgeable on MTCT if she correctly identified the three different modes/periods of MTCT of HIV; otherwise she was classified as non-knowledgeable. Comprehensive knowledge of HIV was also measured if a pregnant woman correctly identified three modes of transmission of HIV (unsafe sexual practice, blood transfusion, and MTCT) and recognized two common misconceptions.

Comprehensive knowledge about HIV/AIDS was measured after posing the following questions: (1) knowing that condom use and limiting sex partners to one uninfected partner are HIV prevention methods, (2) being aware that a healthy-looking person can have HIV, and (3) rejecting the two most common local misconceptions, that is, HIV/AIDS can be transmitted through mosquito bites and by supernatural means in Ethiopia [8].

2.4. Data Collection Procedures. Data were collected using pretested, structured, and interviewer administered questionnaire. The questionnaire was prepared after reviewing relevant literatures. Five female nurses supervised by two BSc health professionals collected the data. For eligible women who were not at home during our first attempt, the interviewers revisited the participant's home at least two times before excluding the participant.

Training was given to the data collectors about informed consent, techniques of interviewing, data collection procedures, and different sections of the questionnaire. Supervisors and principal investigators checked the questionnaire on its completeness and consistency on the daily basis.

2.5. Data Processing and Analysis. The data were entered into EPI info version 3.5.3 statistical software and then sorted, cleaned, and analyzed by using SPSS version 20 statistical package. Descriptive statistics were done to describe the study participants in relation to relevant variables. Both bivariate and multiple logistic regression analyses were carried out to see the effect of sociodemographic factors, maternal condition factors, and other factors on the knowledge of MTCT of HIV and to control cofounding. Odds ratios with 95% CI were computed to identify factors associated with mothers' MTCT knowledge.

2.6. Ethical Consideration. Ethical clearance was obtained from the Research and Ethical Review Committee (REC) at the Institute of Public Health, College of Medicine and Health Science of University of Gondar. Permission letter was secured from Meket District Health Office. Written informed consent was taken from each study participant after reading the consent form. The purpose and benefit of the study and their right to withdraw at any time were also delivered to each participant prior to the interview. Confidentiality of the information was maintained throughout by using anonymity identifiers, keeping their privacy by interviewing them individually.

3. Results

3.1. Sociodemographic Characteristics of Pregnant Women. Five hundred forty-two pregnant women participated in the study (97.5% response rate). The majority (85.4%) were rural dwellers. The mean age of the study participants was 29.45 years (SD = 5.4). Four hundred and sixty (84.9%) were married, 196 (36.2%) were able to read and write, and nearly four-fifths (80.1%) were homemaker (Table 1).

TABLE 1: Selected sociodemographic characteristics of respondents, Meket district, northeast Ethiopia, 2014 (*n* = 542).

Variables	Frequency	Percent
Age (years)		
15–24	99	18.3
25–34	326	60.1
35–49	117	21.6
Residence		
Urban	79	14.6
Rural	463	85.4
Marital status		
Married	460	84.9
Single	27	5
Divorced	55	10.1
Educational status		
Unable to read and write	176	32.5
Able to read and write only	196	36.2
Primary	127	23.4
Secondary and above	43	7.9
Occupation		
Housewife	434	80.1
Student	26	4.8
Merchant	55	10.1
Government employee	27	5.0
Income (ETB)		
≤450	458	84.5
451–999	77	14.2
≥1000	7	1.3

TABLE 2: Reproductive health related characteristics and information received from health care providers, Meket district, northeast Ethiopia, 2014 (*n* = 542).

Variables	Frequency	Percent
Number of pregnancies		
1	161	29.7
2-3	276	50.9
4+	105	19.4
Gestational age		
≤16	10	1.9
17–24	134	24.7
25–35	333	61.4
≥36	65	12.0
Antenatal visit		
Yes	312	57.6
No	230	42.4
Number of ANC visit (*n* = 312)		
1	122	39.1
2-3	176	56.4
4+	14	4.5
Received information from health care providers		
On HIV		
Yes	346	63.8
No	196	36.2
On antenatal care		
Yes	304	56.1
No	238	43.9
On MTCT		
Yes	284	52.4
No	258	47.6
On infant feeding		
Yes	181	33.4
No	361	66.6
Comprehensive knowledge of HIV/AIDS		
Yes	346	63.8
No	196	36.2
Heard of PITC		
Yes	345	63.7
No	197	36.3
Heard about MTCT		
Yes	458	84.5
No	84	15.5
Know the means of transmission on MTCT (*n* = 458)		
During pregnancy	309	67.5
During labor/delivery	324	70.7
During breast feeding	251	54.8
Exact timing of MTCT answered by women		
None	84	15.5
One	130	24.0
Two	225	41.5
Three	103	19.0

3.2. Reproductive Health Related Characteristics and MTCT of HIV Knowledge. One hundred sixty-one (19.7%) were pregnant for the first time. More than half (57.6%) had ANC during their current pregnancy. Nearly two-thirds (63.8%) had received information about HIV/AIDS from health care providers.

Half (51.8%) of the respondents received information about HIV, antenatal care (65.7%), mother-to-child transmission of HIV (40.6%), and infant feeding with their partners (21.4%) (Table 2).

3.3. Knowledge of Pregnant Women on MTCT. One hundred three (19%) (95% CI: 15.5%, 22.4%) were knowledgeable on MTCT of HIV. Most (84.5%) heard about mother to child transmission of HIV. Among those who heard MTCT, more than two-thirds (70.7%) mentioned labor/delivery as a time of HIV transition from mother to child. 225 (41.5%) pregnant women identified at least two periods of mother-to-child transmission of HIV. Nearly two-thirds (63.8%) had comprehensive knowledge on HIV/AIDS, and another equivalent proportion of women heard about PITC (Table 2).

3.4. Factors Associated with Knowledge of Pregnant Women on MTCT of HIV. In multivariable analysis, higher levels of maternal education status, having received information about HIV from health professionals, and reported discussion of

TABLE 3: Crude and adjusted odds ratios (OR) and 95% confidence intervals (CI) of factors associated with knowledge of mothers on MTCT of HIV among pregnant women, Meket district, 2014 ($n = 542$).

Variables	Knowledge on MTCT		COR (95% CI)	AOR (95% CI)
	Yes	No		
Residence				
Urban	31	48	3.51 (2.01, 5.88)	**2.69 (1.48, 4.87)** **
Rural	72	391	1.0	1.0
Age				
15–24	34	65	1.0	
25–34	56	270	0.40 (0.23, 0.65)	
35–49	13	104	0.24 (0.11, 0.48)	
Education				
Unable to read and write	13	163	1.0	1.0
Able to read and write	49	147	4.18 (2.18, 8.01)	**3.25 (1.55, 6.79)** **
Primary	31	96	4.05 (2.02, 8.11)	**2.41 (1.03, 5.60)** **
Secondary and above	10	33	3.80 (1.53, 9.39)	2.05 (0.71, 5.88)
ANC information from HP				
Yes	84	220	4.40 (2.58, 7.49)	
No	19	219	1.0	
HIV information from HP				
Yes	92	254	6.09 (3.16, 11.70)	**3.24 (1.53, 6.83)** **
No	11	185	1.0	1.0
MTCT discussion with husband				
Yes	67	153	3.48 (2.21, 5.45)	**2.64 (1.59, 4.39)** **
No	36	286	1.0	1.0
ANC discussion with husband				
Yes	95	261	8.10 (3.84, 17.08)	**5.80 (2.63, 12.77)** **
No	8	178	1.0	1.0

** Statistically significant at P value <0.05.

MTCT and ANC with their partners were positively associated with knowledge of mother-to-child transmission of HIV. Those women who live in the urban settings were about three more like to be knowledgeable than their rural counterparts (AOR: 2.69, CI (1.48, 4.87)). Those literate mothers were about three times more likely to be knowledgeable than who did not read and write (AOR: 3.25, CI (1.55, 6.78)). Likewise, a woman was 2.41 times more likely to be knowledgeable if she had completed primary school as compared to those who did not read and write (AOR: 2.41, CI (1.04, 5.60)).

Pregnant women who received information on HIV from health care providers were about three times more likely to be knowledgeable than women who had not received information (AOR: 3.24, CI (1.54, 6.83)). Women who had discussions with their partner were more likely to be knowledgeable than those who had not (AOR: 5.80, CI (2.63, 12.78)). Correspondingly, mothers who discussed MTCT with their partners were more likely to be knowledgeable than those who had not (AOR: 2.64, CI (1.59, 4.39)) (Table 3).

4. Discussion

Being knowledgeable on MTCT of HIV and the fact that the risk of transmission can be reduced by using antiretroviral drugs are critical in reducing MTCT of HIV. This can contribute greatly towards the achievement of the Millennium Development Goals related to HIV.

This study revealed that 19% (95% CI: 15.5%, 22.4%) of respondents were knowledgeable on MTCT of HIV. This result is in line with a cross-sectional study conducted at Temeke District Hospital, Dar Es Salaam (15.7%) [14]. However, it is higher than that of studies done in southern Ethiopia (11.5%) and Gondar town (8.5%) [10, 13] but lower than a health institution based study in Debre Markos town, Ethiopia (42.3%) [15]. This could be due to the difference in the study setting and accessibility of health facilities.

In the present study, nearly two-thirds of pregnant women had comprehensive knowledge on HIV/AIDS which is higher than studies in Yaoundé (23%) [16], the Ethiopian Demographic and Health Survey (19%) [8], and a study in Gondar town (59.8%) [10].

Knowledge of pregnant women on MTCT of HIV among pregnant women was significantly varied based on their place of residence. Those pregnant women residing in urban areas were more likely to be knowledgeable when compared to the rural residents. This finding is in line with studies conducted at Gondar and Hawassa towns in Ethiopia [10, 13]. It might be due to the rural location and geographical inaccessibility and poor availability of nearby health services, compared with urban areas. This could also be partly explained due to the presence of media exposure amongst urbanites.

Educated pregnant women who were able to read and write were more likely to be knowledgeable than those who were unable to read and write. This supports the government attempt to address adult informal education. Pregnant women with primary education were also more likely to be knowledgeable than those who were unable to read and write. This result is in line with a previous study conducted in southern Ethiopia [12]. This could be because when the women become educated their access to information is also increased. With this regard, they might have access to print media exposure.

In this study, pregnant women who discussed and received information about HIV/AIDS from health care providers were more knowledgeable. They were found to be three times more likely to be knowledgeable than those who had not.

Spouse discussion on antenatal care follow-up was also positively associated with knowledge of MTCT. Those pregnant women who had discussions with their partners were six times more likely to be knowledgeable than those who had not discussed the issue. This is similar to reports from other studies [12, 17]. This might be explained due to male partners possessing better knowledge on HIV transmission and eventually transfer this information to these pregnant women if discussion is triggered.

Pregnant women may receive information from a variety of sources about health services. Spouses having delivered information and participated in discussions about MTCT of HIV with their wives (40.6%) were associated with good knowledge of the subject. Accordingly, pregnant women who had discussion with their partners were more than two times more likely to have good knowledge of MTCT. This might be because partner discussion in this regard could enhance their knowledge.

This study tried to assess pregnant women who did not attend health care facilities for ANC and HIV concerning their knowledge about MTCT of HIV. However, because of financial and time constraints, this study did not include the knowledge part of prevention of mother-to-child transmission of HIV.

5. Conclusions

Despite many efforts, the knowledge of pregnant women on mother-to-child transmission of HIV is low. If pregnant woman resides in urban environment, she attends school, if she receives information on HIV from health care providers, and if she attends antenatal care, she is more likely to be knowledgeable on MTCT of HIV. Strengthening women education and by reaching previously inaccessible parts of the community, integration of HIV, prevention of MTCT, and ANC service, is highly recommended. Moreover, strengthening discussion of MTCT with spouses is important.

Conflict of Interests

The authors declare that they have no competing interests.

Authors' Contribution

Tesfaye Birhane originated and wrote the proposal, participated in data collection, analyzed the data, and drafted the paper. Gizachew Assefa Tessema and Kefyalew Addis Alene approved the proposal with some revisions and participated in data analysis. Tesfaye Birhane, Gizachew Assefa Tessema, Kefyalew Addis Alene, and Abel Fekadu Dadi drafted the paper and sent for the journal for publication. All the authors read the paper.

Acknowledgments

The authors would like to acknowledge University of Gondar and Meket Health Office for technical and financial support, respectively. They are also grateful to the study participants for their time and data collectors for their commitment.

References

[1] UNAIDS, *Global Plan Powards the Elimination of New HIV Infections among Children by 2015 and Keeping Their Mothers Alive, 2011–2015*, Joint United Nations Programme on HIV/AIDS, Geneva, Switzerland, 2011.

[2] UNAIDS, *Global Report: UNAIDS Report on the Global AIDS Epidemic 2013*, United Nations Programme on HIV/AIDS, Geneva, Switzerland, 2013.

[3] World Health Organization, *Mother to Child Transmission of HIV*, World Health Organization, 2011.

[4] Federal HIV/AIDS Prevention and control Office, *HIV/AIDS Estimates and Projections in Ethiopia, 2011–2016*, Federal HIV/AIDS Prevention and control Office, Addis Ababa, Ethiopia, 2014.

[5] Ethiopia launches national plan to prevent new HIV infections among children, http://www.unaids.org/sites/default/files/en/media/unaids/contentassets/documents/pressrelease/2011/12/20111204_PR_EthiopiaPMTCT_en.pdf.

[6] UNAIDS WHO, *Technical Guidance Note for Global Fund HIV Proposals Prevention of Mother-to-Child Transmission of HIV*, WHO/UNAIDS Global-Plan-Elimination-HIV-Children, 2011.

[7] Federal Ministry of Health, *Manual for the Implementation of Prevention of Mother-to-Child Transmission of HIV in Ethiopia*, Federal Ministry of Health, Addis Ababa, Ethiopia, 2011.

[8] CSA [Ethiopia] and ICF International, *Ethiopian Demographic and Health Survey Report 2011*, Central Statistical Agency, Addis Ababa, Ethiopia; ICF International, Calverton, Md, USA, 2012.

[9] O. E. Amoran, O. F. Salami, and F. A. Oluwole, "A comparative analysis of teenagers and older pregnant women in the utilization of prevention of mother to child transmission [PMTCT] services in, Western Nigeria," *BMC International Health and Human Rights*, vol. 12, article 13, 2012.

[10] M. T. Malaju and G. D. Alene, "Determinant factors of pregnant mothers' knowledge on mother to child transmission of HIV and its prevention in Gondar town, North West Ethiopia," *BMC Pregnancy and Childbirth*, vol. 12, article 73, 2012.

[11] Y. Luo and G.-P. He, "Pregnant women's awareness and knowledge of mother-to-child transmission of HIV in South Central China," *Acta Obstetricia et Gynecologica Scandinavica*, vol. 87, no. 8, pp. 831–836, 2008.

[12] A. Asefa and H. Beyene, "Awareness and knowledge on timing of mother-to-child transmission of HIV among antenatal care

attending women in Southern Ethiopia: a cross sectional study," *BMC Reproductive Health*, vol. 10, no. 1, article 66, 2013.

[13] A. A. Abajobir and A. B. Zeleke, "Knowledge, attitude, practice and factors associated with prevention of mother-to-child transmission of HIV/AIDS among pregnant mothers attending antenatal clinic in Hawassa referral hospital, South Ethiopia," *Journal of AIDS and Clinical Research*, vol. 4, no. 6, 2013.

[14] N. Mujumali, *Knowledge and attitude on prevention of mother to child transmission of hiv among pregnant women attending reproductive and child health clinic at Temeke district*, Muhimbili University of Health and Allied Sciences, 2011.

[15] Z. Moges and A. Amberbir, "Factors associated with readiness to VCT service utilization among pregnant women attending antenatal clinics in Northwestern Ethiopia: a health belief model approach," *Ethiopian Journal of Health Sciences*, vol. 21, supplement 1, pp. 107–115, 2011.

[16] A.-C. Zoung-Kanyi Bissek, I. E. Yakana, F. Monebenimp et al., "Knowledge of pregnant women on mother-to-child transmission of HIV in Yaoundé," *The Open AIDS Journal*, vol. 5, no. 1, pp. 25–28, 2011.

[17] A. I. Olugbenga-Bello, E. A. Oladele, A. A. Adeomi, and A. Ajala, "Perception about HIV testing among women attending antenatal clinics at Primary Health Centres in Osogbo, Southwest, Nigeria," *Journal of AIDS and HIV Research*, vol. 4, no. 4, pp. 105–112, 2012.

5

Impact of the Implementation of New WHO Diagnostic Criteria for Gestational Diabetes Mellitus on Prevalence and Perinatal Outcomes

Katja Erjavec,[1] Tamara Poljičanin,[2] and Ratko Matijević[1,3]

[1]Department of Obstetrics and Gynecology, University Hospital Merkur, Zajčeva 19, 10 000 Zagreb, Croatia
[2]Department of Medical Informatics and Biostatistics, Croatian Institute of Public Health, Rockefellerova 7, 10 000 Zagreb, Croatia
[3]Department of Obstetrics and Gynecology, School of Medicine, University of Zagreb, Šalata 3, 10 000 Zagreb, Croatia

Correspondence should be addressed to Katja Erjavec; katya.erjavec@gmail.com

Academic Editor: Jeffrey Keelan

Objectives. To determine the impact of the implementation of new WHO diagnostic criteria for gestational diabetes mellitus (GDM) on prevalence, predictors, and perinatal outcomes in Croatian population. *Methods*. A cross-sectional study was performed using data from medical birth certificates collected in 2010 and 2014. Data collected include age, height, and weight before and at the end of pregnancy, while perinatal outcome was assessed by onset of labor, mode of delivery, and Apgar score. *Results*. A total of 81.748 deliveries and 83.198 newborns were analysed. Prevalence of GDM increased from 2.2% in 2010 to 4.7% in 2014. GDM was a significant predictor of low Apgar score (OR 1.656), labor induction (OR 2.068), and caesarean section (OR 1.567) in 2010, while in 2014 GD was predictive for labor induction (OR 1.715) and caesarean section (OR 1.458) only. Age was predictive for labor induction only in 2014 and for caesarean section in both years, while BMI before pregnancy was predictive for all observed perinatal outcomes in both years. *Conclusions*. Despite implementation of new guidelines, GDM remains burdened with increased risk of labor induction and caesarean section, but no longer with low Apgar score, while BMI remains an important predictor for all three perinatal outcomes.

1. Introduction

Gestational diabetes mellitus (GDM) significantly contributes to perinatal mortality and morbidity. It has increasing prevalence worldwide [1] and imposes a significant economic burden with important short-term and long-term consequences for the mother and her baby [2]. Women with GDM have 3 to 4 times higher risk of metabolic syndrome later in life [3] and a two times higher risk of developing type 2 diabetes [4]. Children born from pregnancies complicated with GDM also seem to have an increased risk of obesity, altered carbohydrate metabolism, and abdominal adiposity during childhood and adolescence [5–7], although evidence might still be inconsistent [8].

GDM is defined as carbohydrate intolerance of variable severity with onset or first recognition during pregnancy that does not meet the diagnostic criteria of overt diabetes [9]. Present national guidelines in Croatia for diagnosis and management of GDM are based on the recommendation of the International Association of the Diabetes in Pregnancy Study Group (IADPSG) and are in use since 2011 [10]. The same criteria for GDM diagnosis have been used worldwide ever since publication of the HAPO study in 2008 [11], culminating with publication of new WHO guidelines for diagnosis of GDM in 2013 [12]. Before that period, Croatian national guidelines for GDM diagnosis and management were using the 1999 WHO criteria [13]. Those two guidelines have not been compared regarding their efficacy, but a recently published report estimated that new criteria will increase two- to threefold the number of women diagnosed with GDM during pregnancy, with unclear benefits [14].

In order to assess the current situation regarding GDM in Croatia and the potential impact of new diagnostic GDM criteria on perinatal outcome, a retrospective study was conducted and women diagnosed with GDM in 2010 with the 1999 WHO diagnostic criteria were compared to GDM women in 2015 diagnosed using the new WHO criteria of 2013.

2. Materials and Methods

This cross-sectional study was performed using data from medical birth certificates (MBC) collected in 2010 and 2014 by Croatian Institute of Public Health (CIPH) as a part of mandatory national perinatal statistics data reporting.

Named years were selected because we believe that they present two different populations of pregnant women concerning diagnosis and management of GDM. GDM care throughout the country is defined by national guidelines published by the perinatal society and it is presumed to be the same regarding diagnosis and management in all centers. GDM screening is suggested for all pregnant women in second trimester by glucose tolerance test in a one-step manner.

The first group delivered in 2010 was selected as representative of pregnant women diagnosed and managed for GDM using the 1999 WHO criteria where cut-off values after intake of the 75 g OGTT were fasting glucose value ≤ 6.1 mmol/L and 2-hour glucose value ≤ 7.8 mmol/L [13]. These criteria were used in Croatia until 2011 when they were changed with current national guidelines. For comparison group we opted for year 2014 when all perinatal units changed their guidelines to those defined by the HAPO study and the International Association of Diabetes and Pregnancy Study Group (IADPSG) [10], recommending one-step 75 g OGTT test at 24–28 weeks for women not previously diagnosed with overt diabetes. GDM is diagnosed if plasma glucose values meet or exceed fasting value ≤ 5.1 mmol/L, 1-hour value ≤10.0 mmol/L, and 2-hour value of ≤8.5 mmol/L [15, 16].

Data from MBC used in this study consists of maternal data (age, height, and weight before and at the end of pregnancy), antenatal and perinatal issues (presence of GDM, onset of delivery, and mode of delivery), and neonatal data (birth weight and five-minute Apgar score). In order to compare two periods and consequently two diagnostic GDM policies we also assessed selected data concerning GDM incidence.

Primary objective of this study was to determine the incidence of GDM in Croatian population before and after implementation of new guidelines. Secondary objectives assessed the influence of GDM on labor outcome (birth weight and proportion of newborns in three weight categories: <2500 g, between 2500 and 4000 g, and >4000 g, incidence of 5-minute Apgar score <7, induction of labor, and caesarean section rate) and maternal risk factors for GDM (age, prepregnancy BMI, and weight gain during pregnancy) again, before and after implementation of new guidelines.

All statistical analyses were performed using STATIS-TICA ver. 12.0. Normality of distribution was tested using Shapiro-Wilks test, while homogeneity of variance was tested using Levene test. Differences between groups of independent continuous variables were analysed using Kruskal-Wallis test and test of multiple comparison for post hoc comparison,

while differences in the occurrence of individual conditions were compared using the chi²-test. Logistic regression (LR) analysis was performed for prediction of the probability of low Apgar score, induction of labor, and caesarean section rate. The predictors included in the regression analyses were age, body mass index (BMI) before pregnancy, and diagnosis of GD. An error threshold of $\alpha = 0.05$ was used in the interpretation of the results.

Ethical approval for the study was obtained from CIPH Ethical Committee for Public Health Researches grant number 80-437/1-16. Informed consent was not needed for the study.

3. Results

A total of 81.826 deliveries with 84.537 newborns in years 2010 and 2014 together had been reported through MBC to CIPH. If one or more piece of data analysed in this study were missing for some individual, they were excluded from further assessment leaving 81.748 deliveries and 83.198 newborns analysed in this study.

The number of deliveries decreased by 8.3% from year 2010 to 2014. The incidence of GDM was more than double from 2.2% in 2010 to 4.7% in 2014.

Associated factors for GDM are presented in Table 1. In general, women with GDM were significantly older, being more overweight before pregnancy, but gained less weight during pregnancy in both years compared to the rest of the pregnant population in Croatia (Table 1).

Differences in age, BMI, and weight gain between women with and without GDM in 2010 and in 2014 were statistically significant (all p's < 0.001, Kruskal-Wallis test). However, results of multiple comparison showed no difference in those parameters between women with GDM in 2010 and 2014 (test of multiple comparison). Also, differences in rates of newborns with birthweight < 2500 g or above 4000 g were statistically significant between women with and without GDM in 2010 and in 2014 (all p's < 0.001), but no difference was shown in these parameters between women with GDM in 2010 and 2014 ($p = 0.230$, chi²-test).

In order to compare the influence of GDM and diagnostic criteria used on labor outcome multivariate logistic regression (MVLR) models with low Apgar score, induction of labor and caesarean section rate were built. MVLR model revealed that the risk for low Apgar score after 5 minutes did not differ significantly between 2010 and 2014. When years were analysed separately, MVLR models suggested that GDM was a significant predictor of low Apgar score in 2010 ($p = 0.047$), but not in 2014 ($p = 0.330$), meaning that the risk of low Apgar score was significantly higher among newborns of women with GDM compared to newborns of women without GDM in 2010 but not in 2014. BMI before pregnancy was a significant predictor of low Apgar score in both years ($p < 0.001$ in 2010 and $p = 0.001$ in 2014) while maternal age was not ($p = 0.419$ in 2010 and $p = 0.337$ in 2014). Children of women with higher BMI had a significantly higher chance to have low Apgar score compared to children of women with lower BMI in both years. By rise of BMI of 1 kg/m² the chance of having low Apgar score increased for 1.5–6%. The chance of

TABLE 1: Maternal and newborn characteristics of women with and without GDM in Croatia in 2010 and 2014.

	Without GDM 2010	With GDM 2010	Without GDM 2014	With GDM 2014
Pregnant women	$n = 41703$	$n = 953$	$n = 37263$	$n = 1829$
Age (years)*	28.77 ± 5.23 (28.72–28.82)	30.88 ± 5.23 (30.55–31.20)	29.49 ± 5.33 (29.44–29.55)	31.34 ± 5.19 (31.10–31.57)
BMI (kg/m²)*	23.38 ± 3.99 (23.34–23.41)	25.84 ± 528 (25.51–26.18)	23.38 ± 4.11 (23.33–23.42)	26.03 ± 5.64 (25.77–26.29)
Weight gain (kg)*	14.51 ± 5.29 (14.46–14.56)	12.57 ± 5.62 (12.21–12.92)	14.19 ± 5.71 (14.14–14.25)	12.50 ± 5.76 (12.24–12.77)
Excessive weight gain (BMI)°				
Underweight (<18.5)	535 (24.6)	6 (26.1)	434 (20.3)	7 (15.9)
Normal weight (18.5–24.99)	9201 (32.8)	112 (23.8)	7401 (30.5)	225 (25.6)
Overweight (25.0–29.9)	5135 (66.1)	147 (55.9)	4468 (63.5)	228 (49.5)
Obese (≥30)	1851 (66.1)	92 (48.7)	1719 (64.7)	185 (47.4)
Obesity class (BMI)°*				
I (≥30 kg/m²)	2101 (5.0)	127 (13.3)	2021 (5.4)	248 (13.6)
II (≥35 kg/m²)	541 (1.3)	49 (5.1)	483 (1.3)	105 (5.7)
III (≥40 kg/m²)	156 (0.4)	13 (1.4)	151 (0.4)	37 (2.0)
Newborns	$n = 42438$	$n = 981$	$n = 37904$	$n = 1875$
Birth weight (g)*	3401 ± 555 (3396–3407)	3439 ± 621 (3400–3478)	3386 ± 564 (3381–3392)	3455 ± 619 (3427–3483)
Birth weight categories°				
<2500	2019 (4.8)	66 (6.7)	2024 (5.3)	98 (5.2)
2500–4000	35371 (83.4)	746 (76.0)	31625 (83.5)	1463 (78.0)
>4000	5048 (11.9)	169 (17.2)	4245 (11.2)	314 (16.8)

* Data are presented as mean ± SD (95 −CI–95 +CI)
° Data are presented as number (%)
* Obesity classes are defined according to The International Classification of adult underweight, overweight, and obesity according to BMI. Available at http://www.who.int/mediacentre/factsheets/fs311/en/.

low Apgar score did not differ among women in different age groups in neither year. There was no difference concerning number of newborns with low Apgar score and women's age in general population comparing 2010 and 2014.

MVLR models also suggest that GDM and BMI before pregnancy were significant predictors for induction of labor in both years (all p's < 0.001) while maternal age was a significant predictor only in 2014 but not in 2010 ($p = 0.057$ in 2010 and $p = 0.008$ in 2014), meaning that labor was induced more often among women with GDM or higher BMI compared to the rest of Croatian pregnant population in both years, but for older women only in 2014, not in 2010. Assessed year was not a significant predictor for induction of labor ($p = 0.111$) as the induction of labor incidence was similar in 2010 and 2014.

By MVLR models, all three assessed parameters (age, GDM, and BMI before pregnancy) were found to be predictors of caesarean section delivery in both 2010 and 2014 (all p's < 0.001), meaning that women with GDM, higher BMI, and older age had a significantly higher risk of having a caesarean section compared to the rest of the pregnant population. Assessed year again was not a significant predictor of caesarean section ($p = 0.396$), meaning that despite significantly higher GDM prevalence in 2014 compared to 2010, there was no increase of caesarean section risk in GDM group. Results of multivariate logistic regression analysis for low Apgar score, induction of labor, and caesarean section as outcomes are presented in Table 2.

4. Discussion

Perinatal data reporting through MBC organized and collected by CIPH has a long history in Croatia giving us an opportunity to assess and analyse national perinatal statistics. It is mandatory that every single birth in the country is recorded in this registry from all delivery units both in 2010 and in 2014. Therefore, all birth centers included in the data from 2010 are also included in the data from 2014, since it is mandatory for each center in the country to report to the CIPH through MBC.

To the best of our knowledge, the diagnosis and management of GDM should be the same in all centers around the country and are defined by national recommendations [15, 16]. Possible avoidance of universal screening, underreporting, and minor variabilities in local policies of GDM management (i.e., induction of labor, etc.) represent the weaknesses of our study. However, all these factors were present in both analysed years and were not significantly

TABLE 2: Multivariate LR models for low Apgar score, induction of labor, and caesarean section as an outcome.

Year	Risk factors	Odds ratio	95% CI	p
		Low Apgar score		
2010	GDM	1.656	1.008–2.720	0.047
	Age	1.008	0.989–1.028	0.419
	BMI before pregnancy	1.050	1.028–1.073	<0.001
2014	GDM	1.246	0.800–1.939	0.330
	Age	0.991	0.971–1.911	0.337
	BMI before pregnancy	1.038	1.015–1.062	0.001
		Induction of labor		
2010	GDM	2.068	1.761–2.427	<0.001
	Age	0.994	0.988–1.000	0.057
	BMI before pregnancy	1.042	1.035–1.050	<0.001
2014	GDM	1.715	1.515–1.940	<0.001
	Age	1.008	1.002–1.014	0.008
	BMI before pregnancy	1.039	1.031–1.046	<0.001
		Caesarean section		
2010	GDM	1.567	1.360–1.806	<0.001
	Age	1.040	1.035–1.045	<0.001
	BMI before pregnancy	1.049	1.043–1.055	<0.001
2014	GDM	1.458	1.310–1.622	<0.001
	Age	1.040	1.035–1.045	<0.001
	BMI before pregnancy	1.045	1.039–1.051	<0.001

altered during the period between 2010 and 2014 and we would not consider them to significantly interfere with the validity of our results.

Prevalence of GDM in Croatia has risen more than two times from year 2010 to 2014. However, it is still lower compared to other developed countries but comparable to some retrospective studies such as the one of Meek at al. [17] Furthermore, a tertiary referral center in Croatia GDM prevalence is reported to be above 20% [18].

Rising prevalence of GDM is a well-known trend observed in the majority of countries worldwide. There are several possible reasons for that. Rise in incidence of obesity [19] as well as older maternal age [20] observed in recent years, being main risk factors associated with GDM [21], gives one possible explanation for increasing numbers of pregnancies being burdened with GDM. Our results confirm this observation as we demonstrated that women with GDM are older and have higher BMIs but gain less weight during pregnancy no matter which criterion is used for diagnosis and management of GDM. However, new GDM guidelines and lower glucose cut-off values surely also influenced GDM prevalence as by new criteria, a substantial number of women were classified to have GDM that would be considered normal according to old criteria.

It was noted that GDM significantly influenced the incidence of low Apgar score after 5 minutes in 2010 but not in 2014. This finding can be interpreted in two ways. One explanation is that, by lowering the threshold for diagnosis of GDM with new criteria, more women were classified to have GDM that were otherwise considered without GDM, so "less severe cases" with better prognosis in 2014 affected the

results and presented better overall outcome. On the other hand, rise of awareness of GDM in the past few years leads to better diagnosis, management and appropriate timing, and mode of delivery of women with GDM that may consequently influenced the incidence of low Apgar score in 2014. Still, there was no difference in perinatal mortality between years, being 4.7/1000 in 2010 [22] and 4.2/1000 in 2014 [23].

To support that, GDM was found to influence both induction of labor and caesarean section rate in both years. This was not influenced by diagnostic criteria used and was independent of age and prepregnancy BMI of women included in this study. Women with GDM had a 50% higher risk of having a caesarean section and a more than double risk of labor being induced compared to women without GDM in both years. However, the chance for both outcomes previously listed was higher in 2010 than in 2014. GDM is traditionally associated with increased rate of caesarean deliveries [24], but only according to data reported before results of HAPO study in 2010 and before new WHO guidelines for GDM in 2013, while studies on perinatal outcomes after implementation of new GDM guidelines are scarce. This suggests that despite significant increase in prevalence of GDM, the prevalence of GDM related induction of labor and caesarean section has decreased, highlighting improvements in management of GDM in recent years. Also, comparing years 2010 and 2014 it is clear that overall incidence of caesarean section and induction of labor rose in Croatian pregnant population [22, 23]. Therefore, introduction of new guidelines defined by the HAPO study and the International Association of Diabetes and Pregnancy Study Group (IADPSG) [10] had positive influence on induction of labor and caesarean section rate in

Croatian GDM population. Children of women with GDM had less often normal birth weight (2500–4000 g) and more often low (<2500 g) or high birth weight (>4000 g) compared to children of women without GDM in both years. The rate of macrosomia (newborns born with more than 4000 g) among women with GDM was similar in both years (17.23% in 2010 and 16.75% in 2014); hence we do not consider macrosomia to have significantly influenced the results presented in this study.

Absence of difference in age, BMI, and weight gain between women with GDM in 2010 and 2014 (test of multiple comparison) means that the population of pregnant women with GDM is so strongly associated with these risk factors that even more strict glucose cut-off criteria did not change this association. BMI before pregnancy is an important predictor for all three perinatal outcomes analysed in this study. Higher incidence of low Apgar score might be explained by increased chance of pregnancy complications for overweight and obese women including preeclampsia, gestational hypertension, gestational diabetes, and macrosomia [25, 26], as an indirect cause of adverse neonatal morbidities. Also, neonates born to obese women have an increased risk of birth defects and neonatal hypoglycemia [27]. However, newborns of women with GDM had significantly lower Apgar score in 2010 compared to 2014. This might be influenced, among others, not only by improvement of perinatal care but also by diagnostic criteria used for selecting GDM population. By more intensive surveillance, closer follow-up, and appropriate timing of induction of labor, it is possible that we reduced incidence of low Apgar score as adverse perinatal outcome in GDM population.

Increased induction of labor and caesarean section rate among women with higher BMI have already been reported in certain studies [28] and a recent meta-analysis has estimated the risk of caesarean section to be double for obese women and triple for women with severe obesity with BMI > 35 kg/m^2 [29]. The myometrium of obese women is considered to be less responsive to oxytocin and obese women more often give birth to macrosomic babies potentially being responsible for caesarean section as mode of delivery [30, 31]. By MVLR models women with higher BMI as well as women with GDM had a significantly higher risk of induction of labor and delivery by caesarean section. However, none of these two outcomes were influenced by GDM criteria used in different years. The only difference found comparing two analysed periods was higher proportion of older women with GDM having induction of labor in 2014 compared to 2010, but we were unable to relate this observation to the GDM diagnostic criteria used.

5. Conclusions

GDM remains burdened with increased risk of induction of labor and caesarean section rate as well as the incidence of low Apgar score despite implementation of new diagnostic criteria and management guidelines. However, we found GDM to be associated with lower incidence of low 5 min Apgar score in 2014 compared to 2010. This may be influenced by several parameters, but more precise and more strict

diagnostic guidelines as well as management adjusted to these guidelines may be indirectly responsible for this observation. Ideally, well-designed randomised controlled trials comparing present and new diagnostic GDM criteria will give us an answer to entirely understand the significance and impact of new diagnostic guidelines on pregnancy outcome.

Competing Interests

The authors declare that there is no conflict of interests regarding the publication of this paper.

Acknowledgments

The authors thank Urelija Rodin, M.D. and Ph.D., from the Croatian Institute of Public Health for providing data from Medical Birth Certificates that were analysed in this study.

References

[1] International Diabetes Federation, Gestational diabetes.

[2] T. M. Dall, W. Yang, P. Halder et al., "The economic burden of elevated blood glucose levels in 2012: diagnosed and undiagnosed diabetes, gestational diabetes mellitus, and prediabetes," *Diabetes Care*, vol. 37, no. 12, pp. 3172–3179, 2014.

[3] Y. Xu, S. Shen, L. Sun, H. Yang, B. Jin, and X. Cao, "Metabolic syndrome risk after gestational diabetes: a systematic review and meta-analysis," *PLoS ONE*, vol. 9, no. 1, Article ID e87863, 2014.

[4] G. Rayanagoudar, A. A. Hashi, J. Zamora, K. S. Khan, G. A. Hitman, and S. Thangaratinam, "Quantification of the type 2 diabetes risk in women with gestational diabetes: a systematic review and meta-analysis of 95,750 women," *Diabetologia*, vol. 59, no. 7, pp. 1403–1411, 2016.

[5] I. Nehring, A. Chmitorz, H. Reulen, R. von Kries, and R. Ensenauer, "Gestational diabetes predicts the risk of childhood overweight and abdominal circumference independent of maternal obesity," *Diabetic Medicine*, vol. 30, no. 12, pp. 1449–1456, 2013.

[6] B. E. Metzger, "Long-term outcomes in mothers diagnosed with gestational diabetes mellitus and their offspring," *Clinical Obstetrics and Gynecology*, vol. 50, no. 4, pp. 972–979, 2007.

[7] K. Wroblewska-Seniuk, E. Wender-Ozegowska, and J. Szczapa, "Long-term effects of diabetes during pregnancy on the offspring," *Pediatric Diabetes*, vol. 10, no. 7, pp. 432–440, 2009.

[8] S. Y. Kim, J. L. England, J. A. Sharma, and T. Njoroge, "Gestational diabetes mellitus and risk of childhood overweight and obesity in offspring: a systematic review," *Experimental Diabetes Research*, vol. 2011, Article ID 541308, 9 pages, 2011.

[9] Committee on Practice Bulletins—Obstetrics, "Practice Bulletin No. 137: gestational diabetes mellitus," *Obstetrics and Gynecology*, vol. 122, no. 2, part 1, pp. 406–416, 2013.

[10] International Association of Diabetes and Pregnancy Study Group, "International Association of Diabetes and Pregnancy Study Groups recommendations on the diagnosis and classification of hyperglycemia in pregnancy," *Diabetes Care*, vol. 33, no. 3, pp. 676–682, 2010.

[11] HAPO Study Cooperative Research Group, B. E. Metzger, L. P. Lowe et al., "Hyperglycemia and adverse pregnancy outcomes," *The New England Journal of Medicine*, vol. 358, no. 19, pp. 1991–2002, 2008.

[12] World Health Organization, *Diagnostic Criteria and Classification of Hyperglycaemia First Detected in Pregnancy*, WHO, 2013.

[13] World Health Organization, *Definition, Diagnosis and Classification of Diabetes Mellitus and Its Complications. Part 1: Diagnosis and Classification of Diabetes Mellitus*, WHO, 1999.

[14] T. Cundy, "Proposed new diagnostic criteria for gestational diabetes—a pause for thought?" *Diabetic Medicine*, vol. 29, no. 2, pp. 176–180, 2012.

[15] Croatian Society for Gynecology and Obstetrics, "Diagnosis of hyperglycemia in pregnancy," Croatian Society for Gynaecology and Obstetrics, http://www.hdgo.hr/Pages/Print.aspx?sifraStranica=171&kultura=hr.

[16] J. Djelmis, M. Ivanisevic, J. Juras, and M. Herman, "Dijagnoza hiperglikemijeu trudnoci," *Gynecologia at Perinatologia*, vol. 19, pp. 86–89, 2010.

[17] C. L. Meek, H. B. Lewis, C. Patient, H. R. Murphy, and D. Simmons, "Diagnosis of gestational diabetes mellitus: falling through the net," *Diabetologia*, vol. 58, no. 9, pp. 2003–2012, 2015.

[18] J. Djelmis, M. Pavić, V. Mulliqi Kotori, I. Pavlić Renar, M. Ivanisevic, and S. Oreskovic, "Prevalence of gestational diabetes mellitus according to IADPSG and NICE criteria," *International Journal of Gynecology & Obstetrics*, vol. 135, no. 3, pp. 250–254, 2016.

[19] World Health Organisation, Global Health Observatiry Data. Obestiy.

[20] Eurostat. Births and fertility data, http://ec.europa.eu/eurostat/web/population-demography-migration-projections/births-fertitily-data.

[21] L. Jovanovic and D. J. Pettitt, "Gestational diabetes mellitus," *The Journal of the American Medical Association*, vol. 286, no. 20, pp. 2516–2518, 2001.

[22] J. Djelmis, J. Juras, and U. Rodin, "Perinatal mortality in Republic of Croatia in the year 2012," *Gynaecologia et Perinatologia*, vol. 22, no. 1, pp. 47–62, 2013.

[23] Croatian Institute of Public Health, *Croatian Health Service Yearbook 2014*, CIPH, Zagreb, Croatia, 2015.

[24] H. M. Ehrenberg, C. P. Durnwald, P. Catalano, and B. M. Mercer, "The influence of obesity and diabetes on the risk of cesarean delivery," *American Journal of Obstetrics and Gynecology*, vol. 191, no. 3, pp. 969–974, 2004.

[25] C. Athukorala, A. R. Rumbold, K. J. Willson, and C. A. Crowther, "The risk of adverse pregnancy outcomes in women who are overweight or obese," *BMC Pregnancy and Childbirth*, vol. 10, article no. 56, 2010.

[26] A. S. Khashan and L. C. Kenny, "The effects of maternal body mass index on pregnancy outcome," *European Journal of Epidemiology*, vol. 24, no. 11, pp. 697–705, 2009.

[27] L. K. Callaway, J. B. Prins, A. M. Chang, and H. D. McIntyre, "The prevalence and impact of overweight and obesity in an Australian obstetric population," *Medical Journal of Australia*, vol. 184, no. 2, pp. 56–59, 2006.

[28] F. Yousuf, T. Naru, and S. Sheikh, "Effect of body mass index on outcome of labour induction," *Journal of the Pakistan Medical Association*, vol. 66, no. 5, pp. 598–601, 2016.

[29] S. Y. Chu, S. Y. Kim, C. H. Schmid et al., "Maternal obesity and risk of cesarean delivery: a meta-analysis," *Obesity Reviews*, vol. 8, no. 5, pp. 385–394, 2007.

[30] J. Zhang, L. Bricker, S. Wray, and S. Quenby, "Poor uterine contractility in obese women," *BJOG: An International Journal of Obstetrics and Gynaecology*, vol. 114, no. 3, pp. 343–348, 2007.

[31] N. Kobayashi and B. H. Lim, "Induction of labour and intrapartum care in obese women," *Best Practice and Research: Clinical Obstetrics and Gynaecology*, vol. 29, no. 3, pp. 394–405, 2016.

6

Early Detection of Fetal Malformation, a Long Distance Yet to Cover: Present Status and Potential of First Trimester Ultrasonography in Detection of Fetal Congenital Malformation in a Developing Country

Namrata Kashyap, Mandakini Pradhan, Neeta Singh, and Sangeeta Yadav

Department of Maternal and Reproductive Health, Sanjay Gandhi Post Graduate Institute of Medical Sciences (SGPGIMS), Lucknow 226 014, India

Correspondence should be addressed to Namrata Kashyap; dr.nmrata@gmail.com

Academic Editor: R. L. Deter

Background. Early detection of malformation is tremendously improved with improvement in imaging technology. Yet in a developing country like India majority of pregnant women are not privileged to get timely diagnosis. *Aims and Objectives.* To assess the present status and potential of first trimester ultrasonography in detection of fetal congenital structural malformations. *Methodology.* This was a retrospective observational study conducted at Sanjay Gandhi Postgraduate Institute of Medical Sciences. All pregnant women had anomaly scan and women with fetal structural malformations were included. *Results.* Out of 4080 pregnant women undergoing ultrasound, 312 (7.6%) had fetal structural malformation. Out of 139 patients who were diagnosed after 20 weeks, 47 (33.8%) had fetal structural anomalies which could have been diagnosed before 12 weeks and 92 (66.1%) had fetal malformations which could have been diagnosed between 12 and 20 weeks. *Conclusion.* The first trimester ultrasonography could have identified 50% of major structural defects compared to 1.6% in the present scenario. This focuses on the immense need of the hour to gear up for early diagnosis and timely intervention in the field of prenatal detection of congenital malformation.

1. Introduction

Fetal structural malformations are seen in 3 to 5% of all pregnancies [1]. Detection of malformation is tremendously improved with improvement in imaging technology. In majority of countries worldwide, second trimester scan between 18 and 22 weeks remains the standard of care for fetal anatomical assessment; however, most recent literature shows a significant improvement in detection of fetal abnormalities in first trimester of pregnancy [2]. Besides nuchal abnormalities a wide range of central nervous system, heart, anterior abdominal wall, urinary tract, and skeletal abnormalities can be diagnosed between 11 and 14 weeks of scan. The clear benefits of first trimester ultrasound are early detection and exclusion of major congenital anomalies (not compatible with life or followed by severe handicap),

reassurance, and relatively easier pregnancy termination if required.

Currently, the review of recent literature suggests classification of fetal abnormalities as always detectable, potentially detectable, and undetectable till first trimester and anomaly scan. The diagnostic efficacy of first trimester anomaly scan and echocardiography between 11 and 14 weeks has been assessed in medium risk population by Becker and Wegner [3]. The prevalence of major anomalies in their study group was 2.8%. The overall detection rate of fetal anomalies including cardiac defects was 84% and increased with raised nuchal thickness particularly more than 2.5 mm. This highlights the scope of first trimester scan apart from its conventional role in detection of chromosomal abnormality.

First trimester screening is now no more limited to detection of raised nuchal thickness (NT). Becker [4] et al.

analysed 6879 cases to assess the prevalence and detection rate of major anomalies by applying first trimester anomaly scan and fetal echocardiography. They concluded that a significant number of fetal anomalies occur with normal NT and more than half of them could be detected in first trimester. Hence, even fetuses with normal NT should be offered first trimester anomaly scan and fetal echocardiography considering the ethical principles of nonmaleficence, justice, and respect for autonomy of pregnant women. Even in this era the benefits of this established technology are not in the reach of all. A vast majority of patients in India are not yet undergoing anomaly scan. We frequently encounter malformations always or potentially detectable during first trimester scan at third trimester or in postnatal period. It depends on both the expertise and resources available along with the awareness and sensitization in general population. This fact of diagnosis is particularly more important in countries like India where medical termination of pregnancy [5] is legally allowed up to 20 weeks of gestation irrespective of malformation being lethal. We see a fair number of patients who are diagnosed with fetal malformation beyond 20 weeks and in that situation they are forced to seek termination services at small substandard centres since they get refusals from all relatively good hospitals due to legal issues associated with termination. Many of such patients get deteriorated due to septic abortion and unnecessary hysterotomy and so forth. Question then arises that where lies the fault, the awareness of the patients or the expertise of the sonologist.

Henceforth, the study was planned to assess the prevalence of fetal malformation in a tertiary care referral centre and to assess the present status of first trimester ultrasonography in the detection of fetal malformations in a tertiary care centre in India.

2. Materials and Methods

This was a retrospective observational study conducted at Sanjay Gandhi Postgraduate Institute of Medical Sciences. All pregnant women attending Department of Maternal and Reproductive Health, OPD, from August 2009 till October 2013 were enrolled in the study. All pregnant women underwent ultrasound (General electrical Voluson S8) and those with fetal structural malformations were evaluated. Malformations were classified according to gestational age of diagnosis, system involved, and type of malformation. Descriptive proportions and frequencies have been used to depict the data.

3. Results

A total number of 4080 pregnant women underwent USG and amongst them 312 (7.6%) patients had fetal structural malformation. The malformations were classified according to gestational age as shown in Table 1. Malformations were classified according to various systems as shown in Table 2.

3.1. Malformations Detected prior to 20 Weeks. Out of total malformed fetuses, 103 (33%) were detected prior to 20 weeks of gestational age and 209 (66.9%) were detected after

TABLE 1: Number of malformations at different gestational age.

Gestational age	Number
<12 weeks	5
12–20 weeks	98
>20 weeks	209

20 weeks of gestational age. Out of 103 women who were diagnosed with fetal malformations before 20 weeks, only 5 (1.6%) were detected prior to 12 weeks of gestational age and the remaining 98 (31.4%) were diagnosed between 12 and 20 weeks. Six patients amongst them presented before 12 weeks but malformations were missed and diagnosed later between 12 and 20 weeks. These cases were omphalocele, osteogenesis imperfecta, harlequin ichthyosis, Stickler syndrome, Fraser syndrome, and Dandy-Walker malformation. These conditions, however, are known to present late.

Out of 103 patients diagnosed to have malformation prior to 20 weeks, 80 patients willingly underwent termination of pregnancy in view of malformation being lethal like a fetus with occipital encephalocoele terminated at 20 weeks of gestational age (Figure 1). We had prescribed protocol of oral mifepristone (200 mg) followed by misoprostol induction after 48 hours of mifepristone. Three patients were lost to follow-up. Ten patients had nonlethal malformation and were willing to continue pregnancy. All of them had postpartum neonatal intervention in the Department of Pediatric Surgery, Neonatology and Plastic Surgery, respectively (for posterior urethral valve, extra lobar sequestration, tracheoesophageal fistula, anorectal malformation, congenital diaphragmatic hernia with good LH ratio, meningocele, polycystic kidneys, megacystis, vesicoureteral reflux, and cleft lip palate).

Ten patients refused to continue pregnancy despite malformation being lethal. They had obstetrical procedure at their convenient places. Four amongst them had preterm still birth and six babies died in neonatal period. Biggest agony is that two amongst those continuing pregnancies with known lethal malformations had hysterotomy and two had cesarean section for anomalous fetus which could have been avoided.

We found that with the present available technology majority of malformation could be diagnosed before 20 weeks (Box 1).

First trimester sonography has huge potential of diagnosing fetal anomalies. We found that there are few malformations which could be easily diagnosed before 12 weeks (Box 2).

Five patients were diagnosed prior to 12 weeks for neural tube defect, holoprosencephaly, gastroschisis, cystic hygroma, and anencephaly. All of them had easy termination of pregnancy.

3.2. Malformations Detected after 20 Weeks. Out of 312 pregnant women with malformations, 209 (66.9%) were diagnosed after 20 weeks. 109 had their first USG after 20 weeks and 100 had USG prior to 20 weeks but malformations were missed.

Out of those 100 patients, 6 patients presented to our institute before 20 weeks and malformations were not confirmed

TABLE 2: Classification of malformation according to the system involved.

CNS, brain	Number	Skeletal	Number
Neural tube defects	30	Achondroplasia	2
Porencephaly	1	Hypochondroplasia	2
Anencephaly	11	Osteogenesis imperfecta	3
Occipital encephalocoele	8	Short rib polydactyly	6
Iniencephaly	2	Thanatophoric dysplasia	1
Ventriculomegaly	14	Single forearm bone	1
Arachnoid cyst	2	Cooks syndrome	1
Holoprosencephaly	8	*Respiratory*	
Agenesis of corpus callosum	8	CCAM	7
Dandy-Walker malformation	16	Pleural effusion	1
Diastematomyelia	2	Congenital high airway obstruction	3
Vermian agenesis	2	Extralobar pulmonary sequestration	2
Genitourinary		*Heart*	
ADPKD	3	Structural cardiac malformations	44
ARPKD	1	Congenital heart blocks	8
Megacystis	1	Pericardial effusion	2
Gonadal cyst	2	Structural and rhythmic	1
Hydronephrosis	12	*AV malformation*	
Lower urinary tract obstruction	9	Vein of Galen malformation	1
Horseshoe kidney	1	Klippel-Trenaunay-Weber syndrome	1
Unilateral multicystic kidney	17	*Others*	
Bilateral cystic kidney disease	9	Fetal goitre	1
Gastrointestinal		Cystic hygroma	6
Fetal ascites	1	*Multiple*	
Meconium peritonitis	2	Limb body wall complex	2
Gastroschisis	3	VACTERL	1
Mesenteric cyst	1	Meckel-Gruber syndrome	6
Enteric duplication cyst	1	Multiple malformations	20
Hirschsprung disease	1	*Fetal tumors*	
Tracheoesophageal fistula	2	Adrenal neuroblastoma	1
Congenital diaphragmatic hernia	3	Teratoma	3
Duodenal atresia	4	Sacrococcygeal teratoma	1
Isolated fetal ascites	2		
Omphalocele	6		

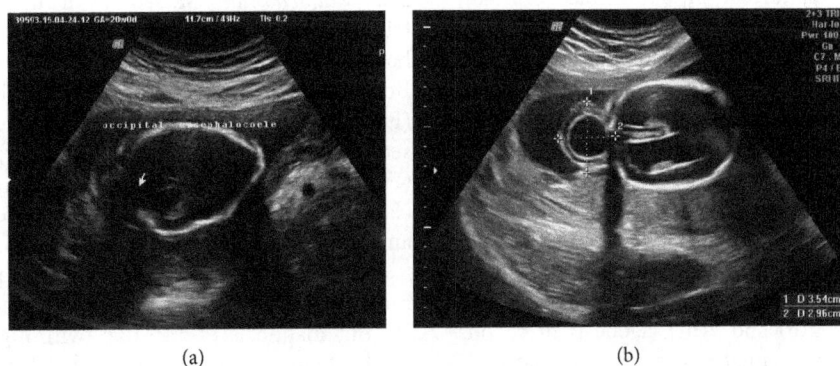

(a)   (b)

FIGURE 1: Occipital encephalocoele diagnosed at 20 weeks which was terminated.

Skeletal dysplasia (achondrogenesis, thantophoric dysplasia, osteogenesis imperfecta), *frequently continued as wrong dates*
Limb body wall complex
Renal agenesis, *frequently continued as severeoligohydramnious*
Agenesis of corpus callosum,
Occipital encephalocoele
Porencephaly, Posterior fossa cyst
Spinal defects like diastematomelia, hemivertebrae, iniencephaly
Ventriculomegaly
Multiple malformations (Meckel grcuber, VACTREL, Kleipell Trenaunay Weber, Cooks)
Hydronephrosis, VUR, PUJ Obstruction
Congenital Diaphragmatic Hernia
Congenital Cystic Adenomatoid Malformation
Hypoplastic left and right heart
Lower urinary tract obsruction
Bilateral multicystic dysplastic kidney
Megacystis
Tracheoesophageal fistula
Meconium peritonitis
Congenital high airway obstruction
Urorectal septal malformations
Teratomas,
Isolated pleural effusion and
Extralobar pulmonary sequestration
TRAP sequence
Cystic hygroma

Box 1: List of common malformations detected before 20 weeks.

Acrania, anencephaly, encephaocoele, etopia cordis (100% detectable)
Spina bifida, hydrocephalous, holoprosencephaly
Cystic hygroma,
Hypoplastic left heart syndrome, atrioventricular septal defect
Limb reduction defects
Megacystis
Skeletal dysplasia

Box 2: List of common malformations we found usually detectable before 12 weeks.

until 24 weeks. In 94 women, they went for USG prior to 20 weeks at some other centre and malformation was missed. Amongst those six patients who presented to SGPGI prior to 20 weeks but were missed, there were one case each of Dandy-Walker malformation, autosomal dominant polycystic kidneys, late onset hydrocephalus, and tetralogy of Fallot. All of these tend to be diagnosed late. Two fetuses, one with cleft lip and one with neural tube defect, could have been diagnosed but were missed. There exists a group of malformation which lies in the grey zone of diagnosis before 20 weeks (Box 3).

Out of 209 detected cases after 20 weeks, 70 (33.4%) patients had malformations which were detected after 20 weeks and are acceptable because these include conditions which tend to be diagnosed late in gestation like hydrocephalus (Figures 2(a) and 2(b)), agenesis of corpus callosum (Figure 2(c)), congenital cystic adenomatoid malformation (Figure 2(d)), various cardiac structural malformations, cystic kidney diseases, horseshoe kidney, Dandy-Walker malformations and variants, vein of Galen aneurysm,

duodenal atresia, fetal goitre, intra-abdominal tumours, gonadal cyst, Hirschsprung disease, and isolated fetal ascites.

3.3. Malformation Missed. Even though missed in first trimester, in 139 (66.5%) patients, fetal malformations could have been diagnosed between 12 and 20 weeks as shown in Box 1. These included malformations like neural tube defect (Figures 3(a) and 3(b)), acrania-exencephaly-anencephaly sequence (Figures 4(a), 4(b), and 4(c)), skeletal dysplasia (Figures 5(a), 5(b), and 5(c)), multicystic dysplastic kidneys (Figure 5(d)), and limb body wall complex (Figures 6(a), 6(b), and 6(c)).

Prenatal interventions in very unique complications of monochorionic twins have become the treatment of choice [6] but diagnosis of acardiac twinning was delayed till 24 weeks (Figure 6(d)). This delayed pick-up of these potentially salvageable conditions leads to high likelihood of adverse pregnancy outcome. The patient had demise of normal cotwin also at 28 weeks.

Agenesis of corpus callosum
Cystic congenital adenomatoid malformation, extralobar sequestration
Dandywalker malformation and variants
Duodenal atresia
Hydronephrosis, renal agenesis, duplex kidney
Bowel obstruction

Box 3: List of malformations we found undetectable before 12 weeks and difficult between 12–20 weeks.

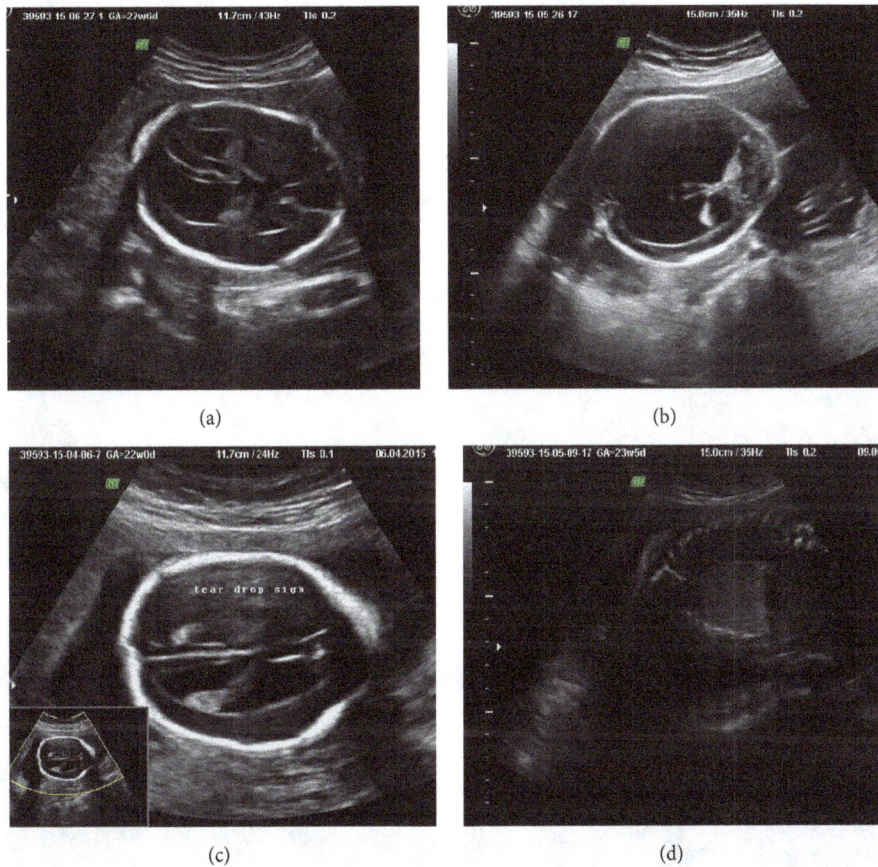

(a)   (b)

(c)   (d)

FIGURE 2: (a and b) show late onset hydrocephalus diagnosed at 27 weeks and 32 weeks, noted to occur late as a part of MASA syndrome (patient had history of X-linked hydrocephalus). (c) shows agenesis of corpus callosum which is known to be said with confirmation at later gestation. (d) shows fetal micro cystic congenital cystic adenomatoid malformation (CCAM) which is notorious to be missed early.

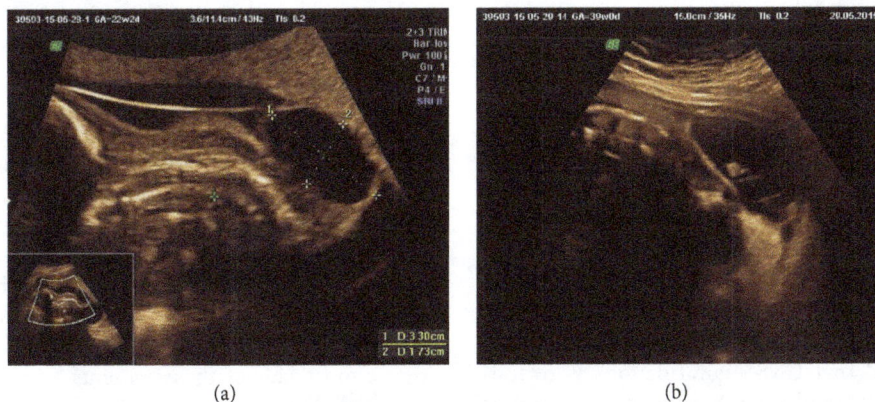

(a)   (b)

FIGURE 3: (a and b) show two cases of neural tube defect diagnosed at advanced gestational ages of 22 weeks and 39 weeks.

(a)   (b)   (c)

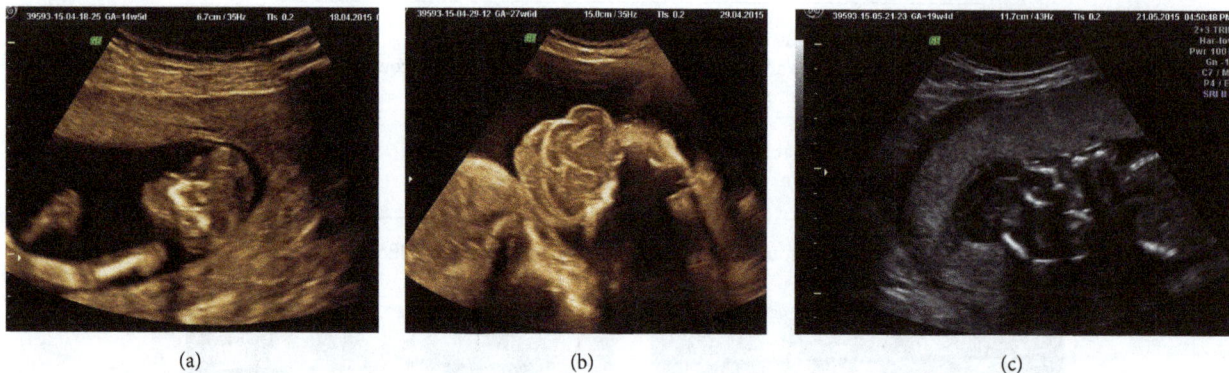

FIGURE 4: (a, b, and c) show fetal exencephaly that could be diagnosed at 14 weeks but was missed and diagnosed at 19 weeks and as late as 27 weeks.

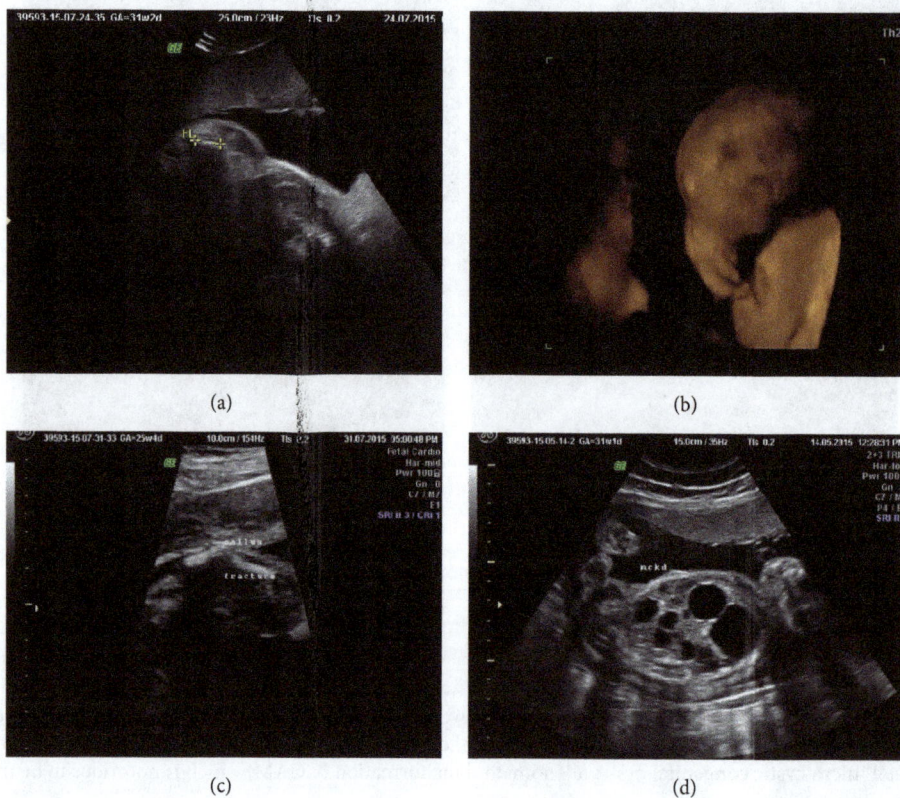

(a)   (b)

(c)   (d)

FIGURE 5: (a, b, and c) show skeletal malformation achondrogenesis (3D), thanatophoric dysplasia, and osteogenesis imperfecta. All of them potentially diagnosable before 12 weeks and usually before 20 weeks were missed and were diagnosed late. (d) shows bilateral multicystic dysplastic kidney diagnosed at 31 weeks, with fetus being continued as oligohydramnios.

4. Discussion

The overall prevalence of severe and lethal fetal structural malformation in our study was 7.6% which was higher than that reported in the literature for general population (3–5%), possibly because it was a referral centre for high risk pregnancy and fetal medicine; there is overreporting of cases. Our study calculated that CNS malformations were most common in our study population. As such, preconceptional folic acid is not commonly practiced in our study population. We realize that almost half (52.1%) of our patients had their

first USG for anomaly detection after 20 weeks. It reflects the existing darkness of unawareness and vacuum of knowledge in patients and also in basic health care that are first to encounter pregnant women.

We found that, out of the total number of women with diagnosed fetal malformation, 203 (65%) presented before 20 weeks. Hence, equally important is the fact to realize that almost half of these patients who had malformations detected after 20 weeks had their obstetrical sonography before 20 weeks and were missed. This missing out of an anomaly may be because of scarcity of good resolution

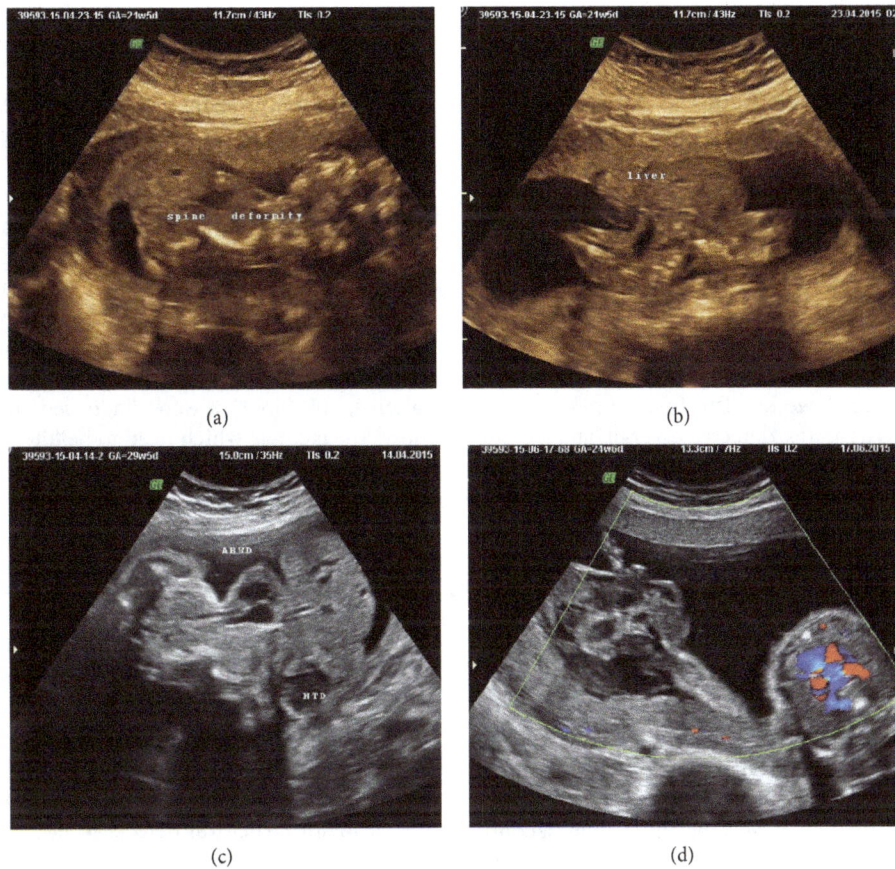

FIGURE 6: (a, b, and c) show gross fetal deformity limb body wall complex, diagnosis delayed till 21 weeks in one fetus (Figures 6(a) and 6(b)) and 29 weeks in other fetuses (Figure 6(c)). (d) shows acardiac twin (twin reverse arterial perfusion sequence) diagnosed at 25 weeks when the normal twin had already decompensated making any intervention difficult.

machines, busy schedules, and lack of expertise as well. For years together, there have been substantial advances in magnification imaging and signal processing which increased the ability to visualize fetal anatomy; there has been great concern on the possibility to diagnose a wide range of fetal anomalies at the time of nuchal translucency scan by transvaginal and transabdominal sonography [7–9].

Almost half of malformations in our study were amenable to be diagnosed in first trimester as reported in current literature. These fetuses were having malformations like neural tube defects, anencephaly, holoprosencephaly, and gastroschisis (Box 2). Castro-Aragon and Levine [10] reported that 60–67% of malformations could have been diagnosed prior to 12 weeks. This is far away from our scenario where we found that only 1.6% (5/312) were diagnosed prior to 12 weeks. This is possibly due to the lack of awareness and lack of expertise as well. Fong et al. [11] in their study scanned 8,537 women between 11 and 14 weeks of gestation (crown rump length, 45–84 mm); there were 175 fetuses with an increased NT. Besides nuchal abnormalities, a wide range of other congenital anomalies can be diagnosed with US at 11–14 weeks of gestation, including defects of the central nervous system, heart, anterior abdominal wall, urinary tract, and skeleton. Oztekin et al. [12] analyzed 1085 pregnancies; 21 (1.93%) fetuses had

at least one major structural defect considered detectable by routine ultrasound screening. 14 (1.29%) were identified at early (first trimester) screening and an additional 5 (0.47%) were identified at late (second trimester) USG. They found that majority of fetal structural abnormalities can be detected by sonographic screening at 11–14 weeks, but detailed fetal anatomic survey performed at 18–22 weeks should not be abandoned.

Rossi and Prefumo [13] also laid stress that first trimester ultrasound can detect half of fetal malformations. They included nineteen studies on 78,002 fetuses, with 996 with malformations that were confirmed by postnatal or postmortem examinations. USG at 11 to 14 weeks detected malformation in 472 of the malformed fetuses (51%). Detection rate was highest for neck anomalies (92%) and lowest for limbs, face, and genitourinary anomalies (34% for each). The presence of associated anomalies appears to increase the accuracy of early ultrasonography. Multiple defects were more likely to be identified than isolated malformations (60% versus 44%). Detection rates ranged from 1% to 49% for spina bifida or hydrocephalus, ranged from 50% to 99% for valvular disease and septal defects, were 100% for acrania and anencephaly, and were 0% for corpus callosum agenesis and bladder exstrophy. Combination of transabdominal and transvaginal techniques resulted in a 62% detection rate versus 51% for transabdominal technique only and 34% for transvaginal technique only.

Although first trimester ultrasound can detect about 50% of fetal malformations, it cannot replace second trimester ultrasound because several malformations develop later than the first trimester. Also to be kept in mind is the fact that accuracy of early ultrasonography can be compromised by transient findings like midgut herniation, small septal defects, and hydronephrosis which might get resolved during intrauterine life.

Iliescu et al. [14] did a prospective two-centre 2-year study of 5472 consecutive unselected pregnant women examined at 12 to 13 + 6 gestational weeks. The first trimester scan identified 40.6% of the cases detected overall and 76.3% of major structural defects. Major congenital heart disease (either isolated or associated with extracardiac abnormalities) was 90%. Major central nervous system anomalies were 69.5%. Fetuses with increased nuchal translucency (NT), the first trimester DR for major anomalies, were 96% compared to 66.7% amongst those with normal NT.

There have been several studies seeing application for an extended protocol in which first trimester sonography is supported by a second anomaly scan. The obvious advantage of an extended protocol is that parents are offered the option of earlier and safer termination of pregnancy for the large majority of severe/lethal abnormalities.

Early ultrasound might be more accurate than second trimester ultrasonography for detection of malformations associated with oligohydramnios and anhydramnios which lead to poor visualization at later gestation necessitating amnioinfusion.

We have applied this kind of protocol at our centre particularly in high risk women. First trimester sonography with targeted imaging for fetal malformation appeared particularly more helpful in high risk women with previous history of fetus/neonates with malformations, known risk factors, for example, type 2 diabetes, patients prone for teratogenicity, for example, thromboembolic and valve replacement patients on warfarin, methotrexate intake for connective tissue disorders, and so forth, antiepileptic, chemotherapeutic drugs, and history of infection exposure like rubella. We diagnosed and terminated patients before 16 weeks with rubella exposure and subsequent pulmonary stenosis, severe bony stippling and craniofacial malformation associated with high doses warfarin, VSD associated with type 2 diabetes, neural tube defect with antiepileptic and tetraphocomelia with chemotherapeutic agents, renal agenesis in previous history of Fraser's syndrome, encephalocoele in previous Meckel-Gruber syndrome, ARPKD and ADPKD, and so forth.

However, a detailed first trimester examination protocol involves supplementary resources: additional examination time and specialized personnel for the abnormal suspected/detected cases. Healthcare systems are yet to determine whether early first trimester diagnosis of most major structural abnormalities is cost-effective. Previous research, albeit using inferior ultrasound technology and a less extended protocol, found that the first trimester anomaly scan was cost-efficient in terms of medical and economic expenses, although they obtained lower detection rates [15, 16].

The present research about the effectiveness of early ultrasonography in the diagnosis of structural defects does have some conflicts, which made it a challenge that to what extent structural congenital abnormalities could be detected by the routine scanning of fetal anatomy combined with nuchal translucency measurement [17]. Few other basic prerequisites associated with early prenatal diagnosis consist of the high experience required and high costs in terms of time and equipment [18]. Even with all these circumstances, the situation in our country is such that a huge number of patients, 209 (66.9%), were diagnosed after 20 weeks which shows the lacunae which need to be filled.

5. Conclusion

In our study we realized that even in a tertiary care centre only 1.6% fetuses with malformation are identified in first trimester. In a way, it throws light on the importance of screening as well as an immense need for early diagnosis and timely intervention in the field of prenatal detection of congenital malformation.

A detailed examination of fetal anatomy during the routine 11–14 weeks of gestation scan provides a comprehensive assessment of fetal anatomy and can detect approximately half of major structural defects in both low-risk and high-risk pregnancies. Detection rate increases markedly beyond 13 weeks of gestation compared with 11 weeks of gestation. We have seen to be better convinced to diagnose holoprosencephaly, achondrogenesis, osteogenesis imperfecta, and spondylocostal dysostosis at 14 weeks compared to 12 weeks. It is also expected that because of the late development of some organ systems and the delayed onset of a significant number of major anomalies in the second and third trimester it is very unlikely that the early scan may replace second trimester ultrasonography.

We need to identify structural malformations before 20 weeks except those conditions which are said to appear further late or reported with confirmation at a later gestational age like few posterior fossa abnormalities, duodenal atresia, and few renal abnormalities. The most important implication is safe termination and avoiding maternal threat to life by forced termination at resourceless and substandard centres. There could be an option of incorporating anomaly scan between 18 and 20 weeks in our health plans and guides at well registered centres with expertise at reasonable cost.

Focus and emphasis should aim at detection of malformation earlier than 12 weeks owing to the very unique and clear facts that first trimester detection leads to easy termination of pregnancy and lessening of women's mental, physical, and psychological trauma.

Conflict of Interests

The authors declare that there is no conflict of interests regarding the publication of this paper.

References

[1] E. Garne, H. Dolk, M. Loane, and P. A. Boyd, "EUROCAT website data on prenatal detection rates of congenital anomalies," *Journal of Medical Screening*, vol. 17, no. 2, pp. 97–98, 2010.

[2] A. Syngelaki, T. Chelemen, T. Dagklis, L. Allan, and K. H. Nicolaides, "Challenges in the diagnosis of fetal non-chromosomal abnormalities at 11–13 weeks," *Prenatal Diagnosis*, vol. 31, no. 1, pp. 90–102, 2011.

[3] R. Becker and R.-D. Wegner, "Detailed screening for fetal anomalies and cardiac defects at the 11–13-week scan," *Ultrasound in Obstetrics and Gynecology*, vol. 27, no. 6, pp. 613–618, 2006.

[4] R. Becker, L. Schmitz, S. Kilavuz, M. Stumm, R.-D. Wegner, and U. Bittner, "'Normal' nuchal translucency: a justification to refrain from detailed scan? Analysis of 6858 cases with special reference to ethical aspects," *Prenatal Diagnosis*, vol. 32, no. 6, pp. 550–556, 2012.

[5] Medical termination of pregnancy act, 2002, Ministry of Health and Family Welfare, Government of India, http://mohfw.nic.in/index1.php?lang=1&level=3&sublinkid=3613&lid=2597.

[6] G. Pagani, F. D'Antonio, A. Khalil, A. Papageorghiou, A. Bhide, and B. Thilaganathan, "Intrafetal laser treatment for twin reversed arterial perfusion sequence: cohort study and meta-analysis," *Ultrasound in Obstetrics and Gynecology*, vol. 42, no. 1, pp. 6–14, 2013.

[7] A. P. Souka and K. H. Nicolaides, "Diagnosis of fetal abnormalities at the 10–14-week scan," *Ultrasound in Obstetrics and Gynecology*, vol. 10, no. 6, pp. 429–442, 1997.

[8] L. Dugoff, "Ultrasound diagnosis of structural abnormalities in the first trimester," *Prenatal Diagnosis*, vol. 22, no. 4, pp. 316–320, 2002.

[9] B. J. Whitlow and D. L. Economides, "The optimal gestational age to examine fetal anatomy and measure nuchal translucency in the first trimester," *Ultrasound in Obstetrics and Gynecology*, vol. 11, no. 4, pp. 258–261, 1998.

[10] I. Castro-Aragon and D. Levine, "Ultrasound detection of first trimester malformations: a pictorial essay," *Radiologic Clinics of North America*, vol. 41, no. 4, pp. 681–693, 2003.

[11] K. W. Fong, A. Toi, S. Salem et al., "Detection of fetal structural abnormalities with US during early pregnancy," *Radiographics*, vol. 24, no. 1, pp. 157–174, 2004.

[12] O. Oztekin, D. Oztekin, S. Tınar, and Z. Adıbelli, "Ultrasonographic diagnosis of fetal structural abnormalities in prenatal screening at 11–14 weeks," *Diagnostic and Interventional Radiology*, vol. 15, pp. 221–225, 2009.

[13] A. C. Rossi and F. Prefumo, "Accuracy of ultrasonography at 11–14 weeks of gestation for detection of fetal structural anomalies: a systematic review," *Obstetrics and Gynecology*, vol. 122, no. 6, pp. 1160–1167, 2013.

[14] D. Iliescu, S. Tudorache, A. Comanescu et al., "Improved detection rate of structural abnormalities in the first trimester using an extended examination protocol," *Ultrasound in Obstetrics and Gynecology*, vol. 42, no. 3, pp. 300–309, 2013.

[15] B. J. Whitlow, I. K. Chatzipapas, M. L. Lazanakis, R. A. Kadir, and D. L. Economides, "The value of sonography in early pregnancy for the detection of fetal abnormalities in an unselected population," *British Journal of Obstetrics and Gynaecology*, vol. 106, no. 9, pp. 929–936, 1999.

[16] L. A. Dolkart and F. T. Reimers, "Transvaginal fetal echocardiography in early pregnancy: normative data," *American Journal of Obstetrics and Gynecology*, vol. 165, no. 3, pp. 688–691, 1991.

[17] S. Saltvedt, H. Almström, M. Kublickas, L. Valentin, and C. Grunewald, "Detection of malformations in chromosomally normal fetuses by routine ultrasound at 12 or 18 weeks of gestation—a randomised controlled trial in 39 572 pregnancies," *BJOG*, vol. 113, no. 6, pp. 664–674, 2006.

[18] M. A. Rustico, A. Benettoni, G. D'Ottavio et al., "Early screening for fetal cardiac anomalies by transvaginal echocardiography in an unselected population: the role of operator experience," *Ultrasound in Obstetrics and Gynecology*, vol. 16, no. 7, pp. 614–619, 2000.

7

Maternal Nutritional Deficiencies and Small-for-Gestational-Age Neonates at Birth of Women Who Have Undergone Bariatric Surgery

J. Hazart,[1] D. Le Guennec,[1] M. Accoceberry,[2] D. Lemery,[2] A. Mulliez,[3] N. Farigon,[1] C. Lahaye,[1] M. Miolanne-Debouit,[1] and Y. Boirie[1,4]

[1]*CHU Clermont-Ferrand, Service de Nutrition Clinique, CRNH Auvergne, Université Clermont Auvergne, 63000 Clermont-Ferrand, France*
[2]*CHU Clermont-Ferrand, Service de Gynécologie-Obstétrique, Université Clermont Auvergne, 63000 Clermont-Ferrand, France*
[3]*CHU Clermont-Ferrand, Délégation Recherche Clinique & Innovation, 63000 Clermont-Ferrand, France*
[4]*INRA, Unité de Nutrition Humaine (UNH), CRNH Auvergne, Université Clermont Auvergne, 63000 Clermont-Ferrand, France*

Correspondence should be addressed to J. Hazart; jhazart@chu-clermontferrand.fr

Academic Editor: Rosa Corcoy

The aim is to compare the prevalence of maternal deficiencies in micronutrients, the obstetrical and neonatal complications after bariatric surgery according to surgical techniques, the time between surgery and conception, and BMI at the onset of pregnancy. A retrospective cohort study concerned 57 singleton pregnancies between 2011 and 2016 of 48 adult women who have undergone bariatric surgery. Small-for-gestational-age neonates were identified in 36.0% of pregnancies. With supplements intake (periconceptional period: 56.8%, trimester 1 (T1): 77.8%, T2: 96.3%, and T3: 100.0%), nutritional deficiencies involved vitamins A (T1: 36.4%, T2: 21.1%, and T3: 40.0%), D (T1: 33.3%, T2: 26.3%, and T3: 8.3%), C (T1: 66.7%, T2: 41.2%, and T3: 83.3%), B1 (T1: 45.5%, T2: 15.4%, and T3: 20.0%), and B9 (T1: 14.3%, T2: 0%, and T3: 9.1%) and selenium (T1: 77.8%, T2: 22.2%, and T3: 50.0%). There was no significant difference in the prevalence of nutritional deficiencies and complications according to surgery procedures and in the prevalence of pregnancy issues according to BMI at the beginning of the pregnancy and time between surgery and pregnancy. Prevalence of micronutritional deficiencies and small-for-gestational-age neonates is high in pregnant women following bariatric surgery. Specific nutritional programmes should be recommended for these women.

1. Introduction

The last ten years have seen a significant increase in the number of treatments involving bariatric surgery, particularly in women of reproductive age. Women of reproductive age are especially affected by obesity (6.0% of the 18–24-year age group, 11.1% of the 25–34-year age group, and 15.5% of the 35–44-year age group in 2012) [1]. The prevalence of moderate to severe obesity among women during the periconceptional period increased by 6.0% in 1998 to reach 9.9% in 2010 [2]. Periconceptional obesity is a well-established risk factor in the short and long term with respect to maternal, fetal, neonatal, and infantile complications such as miscarriage, gestational diabetes, preeclampsia, pregnancy-induced hypertension, induction of labour, caesarean deliveries, congenital malformations, prematurity, perinatal mortality, large-for-gestational-age neonates, transfer of newborns to intensive care units, juvenile obesity, and type 2 diabetes in mothers [3–5]. Multidisciplinary care combined with therapeutic lifestyle changes forms the first-line treatment for obesity [6]. Should this approach fail, defined by unsatisfactory weight loss over time, bariatric surgery is considered the most effective treatment available in terms of weight loss, the improvement or remission of comorbid conditions, and an increase in survival rates and quality of life in the long term [7–11]. This technique is indicated to treat patients presenting with morbid (BMI $\geq$ 40 kg/m^2) or severe (BMI $\geq$ 35 kg/m^2) obesity associated with at least one comorbid condition that is likely to improve after surgery (high blood pressure, obstructive sleep apnoea hypopnea syndrome, and other severe respiratory disorders, severe metabolic disorders, particularly type 2 diabetes, disabling bone and joint illnesses, and nonalcoholic steatohepatitis) as a second-line therapy prescribed after the failure of a multidisciplinary care programme carried out effectively over a period of six to 12 months [12]. The recommended surgical techniques include those based exclusively on gastric-restriction techniques: adjustable gastric band (AGB), sleeve gastrectomy (SG), and those that are combined with gastrointestinal malabsorption: gastric bypass (GBP) and biliopancreatic diversion surgery (BPD). Between 2005 and 2014, the number of bariatric surgery procedures conducted in France quadrupled, while AGB surgery has seen a significant decline in favour of SG, which is now the predominant technique followed by GBP and AGB [13, 14]. Of bariatric surgeries performed on 267,466 patients from 2005 until 2014, 86.4% were conducted on women with an average age of 40.3 years [13]. The growth of bariatric surgery among women of reproductive age is associated with an increase in the number of women becoming pregnant after this surgical procedure, raising issues for clinicians concerning the impact of bariatric surgery on pregnancy progress and screening procedures. Bariatric surgery lowers the risk of preeclampsia and gestational diabetes but increases the risk of maternal anaemia. Concerning neonatal complications, it could lower the risk of caesarean deliveries and large-for-gestational-age neonates but increase the risk of premature deliveries, small-for-gestational-age neonates (SGA), admission to neonatal intensive care units, and neonatal death [15–18]. Obesity is a risk factor for nutritional deficiencies that may be increased by both bariatric surgery and pregnancy-induced physiological changes [19, 20]. To our knowledge, no French study is reporting nutritional assessments in women after bariatric surgery during pregnancy.

The purpose of this study was to describe and compare the prevalence of maternal micronutrient deficiencies and obstetric and neonatal complications in pregnancy after bariatric surgery in terms of surgical technique, the time between surgery and conception, and BMI at the onset of pregnancy.

2. Methods

2.1. Background. Nutritional care of patients whose pregnancy was monitored at the Clermont-Ferrand Centre Hospitalier Universitaire (CHU) took the form of medical checkups in the CHU's Clinical Nutrition and Obstetrics Depts. The Clinical Nutrition Dept. was responsible for preoperative and postoperative assessments. Periconceptional and prenatal assessments were carried out jointly by the Clinical Nutrition and Obstetrics Depts. The *Association des Utilisateurs de Dossiers Informatisés en Pédiatrie, Obstetrique et*

Gynécologie (AUDIPOG) dossier is a common, electronic perinatal healthcare record intended for maternity units that collect all the data required for activities by healthcare professionals and patient monitoring systems. The individual, anonymised datasets were collected from two information sources: printed patient records at the Clinical Nutrition Dept. and the computer backup of AUDIPOG records at the Obstetrics Dept. (keywords: "sleeve gastrectomy", "by-pass", and "gastric band").

2.1.1. Design and Eligibility Criteria. A retrospective cohort study was carried out on adult women with a history of bariatric surgery who became pregnant between July 2011 and March 2016 and who were monitored in the Clinical Nutrition or Gynaecology-Obstetrics Depts. at Clermont-Ferrand University Hospital (CHU). Pregnancies that occurred after the removal of an AGB and those that were not monitored at the Clermont-Ferrand CHU were excluded.

2.1.2. Data Collected by the Researchers. Sociodemographic data included date of birth and professional activity.

Anthropometric data included height (metres) and weight (kg) before the operation, at the onset of pregnancy, and at each trimester of pregnancy. Body weight was measured at each checkup to the nearest 0.1 kg, with patients in their underwear and with their shoes off and the local scales calibrated. The patient's height and weight at the time of bariatric surgery were used to calculate their preoperative BMI (kg/m^2). Weight gain during pregnancy was defined as the weight on delivery less the weight at the onset of pregnancy.

Medical histories were collected at the time of the bariatric surgery. Anamnestic data included medical, obstetric, and surgical histories together with information on medical treatments. Data on the presence of cardiovascular risk factors such as high blood pressure (blood pressure greater than or equal to 140 and/or 90 mmHg, checked at least twice, WHO definition), type 2 diabetes (fasting blood glucose level greater than or equal to 1.26 g/L, taken twice), and age at the onset of weight gain were collected from the medical histories. Obstetric history included the number and outcome of pregnancies (miscarriages, therapeutic abortion, and births) and parity.

Surgical data included the date and type of surgical procedure. The types of surgical procedure included restrictive (AGB and SG) and mixed (GBP) techniques. The date of the operation was used to calculate the time that elapsed between surgery and conception. Data on surgical complications, compliance with nutritional supplementation, minimum postsurgery weight and the time taken to reach this weight, and monitoring frequency (number of medical consultations with nutritionist doctor per year) were collected during patient follow-up.

Nutritional status was determined using nutritional supplements, recording the start and finish dates of prescriptions and compliance with supplement intake. Fasting levels of haematological, biochemical, and micronutritional parameters in venous blood were recorded before and after surgery,

TABLE 1: Biological standards for haematological, biochemical, and micronutritional parameters in pregnant women.

	T1[a]	T2[b]	T3[c]
		min[d]–max[e]	
Haematology			
Haemoglobin (g/dL)	11.6–13.9	9.7–14.8	9.5–15
MCV[f] (fL)	81–96	82–97	81–99
Ferritin (μg/L)	6–130	2–230	0–116
Biochemistry			
Albumin (g/L)	31–51	26–45	23–42
Vitamins			
A (μmol/L)	1.12–1.64	1.22–1.54	1.01–1.47
B1 (nmol/L)	/[g]	/[g]	/[g]
B6 (nmol/L)	/[g]	/[g]	/[g]
B9 (nmol/L)	5.89–33.99	1.81–54.39	3.17–46.9
B12 (pmol/L)	87.08–323.24	95.94–484.13	73.06–388.2
C (μmol/L)	/[g]	/[g]	51.1–73.81
D (μg/L)	18–27	10–22	10–18
Minerals			
Magnesium (mmol/L)	0.66–0.90	0.62–0.90	0.45–0.90
Selenium (μmol/L)	1.47–1.85	0.95–1.85	0.90–1.69
Zinc (μmol/L)	8.72–13.47	7.65–13.47	7.65–11.78

[a]First trimester. [b]Second trimester. [c]Third trimester. [d]Minimum. [e]Maximum. [f]Mean Corpuscular Volume. [g]There are no standards specific to pregnant women.

during the periconceptional period, and at each trimester of pregnancy. Standards specific to pregnant women were used to interpret biological parameter values (Table 1) [21]. Women's standards were used in the absence of any standard specifically designed for pregnant women: vitamins B1 and B6 during the three trimesters of pregnancy [first trimester (T1), second trimester (T2), third trimester (T3)] and vitamin C in T1 and T2.

Blood samples for nutritional dosages were analyzed in the laboratory of the Clermont-Ferrand CHU. Concerning nutritional supplements, systematic supplements contain vitamins (A, B1, B2, B6, B12, C, D3, E, B5, B8, B9, and PP), calcium, magnesium, phosphorus, iron, manganese, copper, and zinc and specific supplements are prescribed in case of deficiency.

Patient *pregnancy-related parameters* were collected at each trimester of pregnancy and included maternal weight gain, gestational age (based on the craniocaudal length recorded on the fetal ultrasound), blood pressure, proteinuria, and stage of pregnancy. Ultrasound data included craniocaudal length, biparietal diameter, abdominal circumference, estimated fetal weight, the growth percentile estimated using Hadlock's formula, and the estimated abdominal perimeter percentile. Anomalies were interpreted based on AUDIPOG criteria. All data on comorbid conditions or complications that appeared during pregnancy and postpartum were collected. The pregnancy-induced hypertension diagnosis was defined by a systolic blood pressure greater than or equal to 140 mmHg and/or diastolic blood pressure greater than or equal to 90 mmHg, isolated, and appearing after 20 weeks of pregnancy based on the recommendations

of the International Society for the Study of Hypertension in Pregnancy. Preeclampsia was defined by the presence of chronic or pregnancy-related hypertension and proteinuria greater than or equal to 300 mg per day. Gestational diabetes was defined by the presence of two pathological values identified after oral hyperglycemia detected by an O'Sullivan screening test or by a blood glucose level greater than or equal to 2 g/L during the O'Sullivan test. An intrauterine growth restriction (below the 10th percentile) and its severe form (below the 3rd percentile) were recorded. The outcome of the pregnancy was recorded (miscarriage, birth, and medical termination of pregnancy). According to the AUDIPOG formula, hypotrophy was defined by a small weight for gestational age (SGA) below the 10th percentile and severe hypotrophy by a SGA below the 3rd percentile. Concerning birth and delivery, data on the manner of onset of labour (spontaneous or induced by prostaglandins and/or oxytocics), the methods of delivery (vaginal delivery, forceps delivery, and caesarean), and maternal complications such as postpartum bleeding (blood loss greater than or equal to 500 mL within 24 hours of delivery) were recorded. Lifestyle was assessed based on alcohol and tobacco consumption at the onset of pregnancy.

Neonatal data included sex, weight and size at birth, blood pH, the Apgar score at 5 minutes, neonatal complications such as shoulder difficulty or dystocia, the use of special procedures such as admission to a neonatal or intensive care unit, and gestational age expressed as weeks of amenorrhea (WA). Gestational age at birth was used to define the level of prematurity (below 37 WA), including severe prematurity (below 32 WA) and extreme prematurity (below

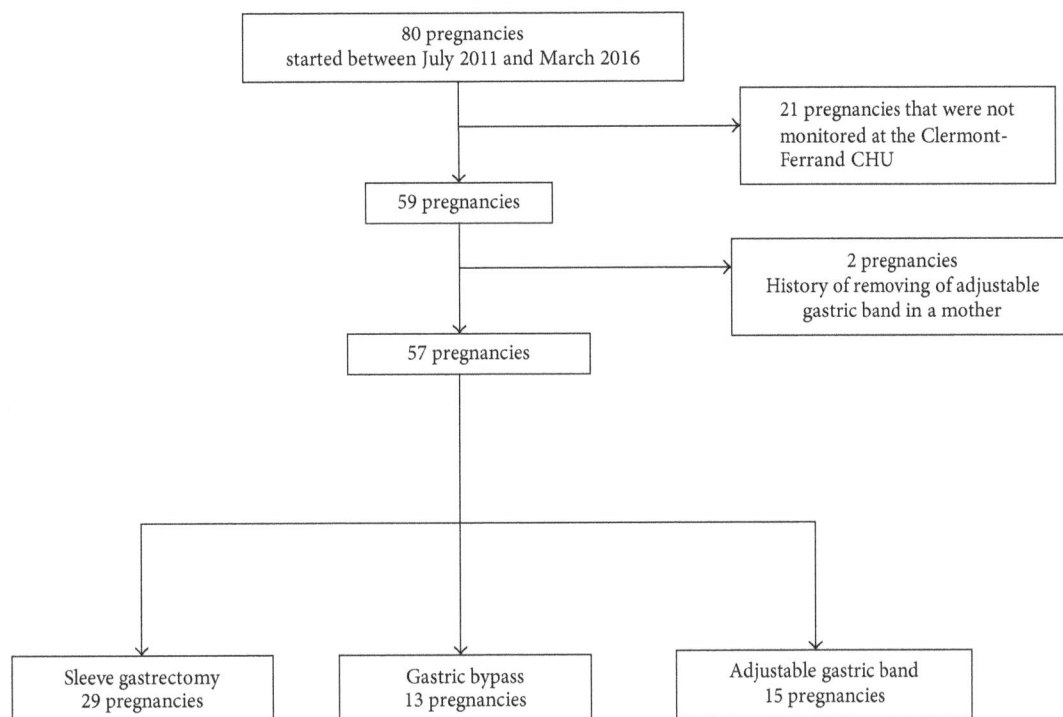

FIGURE 1: Flow chart.

28 WA). Birth weight and AUDIPOG data were used to distinguish between infants of normal weight (between the 10th and 90th percentile), small-for-gestational-age infants (below the 10th percentile), severe small-for-gestational-age infants (below the 3rd percentile), and large-for-gestational-age infants (above the 90th percentile). Apgar scores of less than 7 to 5 minutes of life and arterial blood pH below 7.20 were considered pathological. Therapeutic abortions (TA) administered due to fetal malformations and in utero fetal deaths were also recorded.

2.2. Statistical Analyses. In the descriptive analysis, qualitative variables were described by their numbers and percentages while quantitative variables were described by their means, standard deviations, and minimum and maximum values. The Chi-Squared Independence Test was used to compare ratios when theoretical numbers were greater than 5. In cases where this condition was not checked, Fisher's exact test was used. Comparisons of quantitative variable means were performed using the Student's test (2 groups) or by variance analysis based on ANOVA tests (more than 2 groups). All tests were bilateral and the acceptable risk of error was set at 5%. The statistical analyses were performed using Stata 12.0 software (STATACORP, Texas, USA).

3. Results

This study covered all adult obese women who had undergone bariatric surgery and become pregnant between July 2011 and March 2016 and who had been monitored in the Clinical Nutrition and Obstetrics Depts. at Clermont-Ferrand CHU.

Out of the 80 pregnancies involving patients with a history of bariatric surgery that began between March 2011 and July 2016, 59 were monitored in the Clinical Nutrition and Obstetrics Depts. at Clermont-Ferrand CHU. Two pregnancies in which the mother had had the AGB removed prior to becoming pregnant were excluded (Figure 1). In all, this study covered 57 singleton pregnancies in 48 patients. A total of nine women had two pregnancies within the study period. Tables 2 and 3 illustrate the maternal, neonatal, and pregnancy-related characteristics.

3.1. Maternal Characteristics. A total of 48 patients underwent bariatric surgery with an average preoperative BMI of $47.0 \pm 6.0\,kg/m^2$. There were a total of 57 singleton pregnancies in these 48 patients who had an average age of 31.0 ± 5.8 years and an average BMI of $30.5 \pm 7.4\,kg/m^2$ at the onset of pregnancy. A maternal history of AGB, SG, and GBP was recorded in 26.0%, 51.0%, and 23.0% of pregnancies, respectively (Table 2). Postoperative follow-up was conducted on a regular basis in 37.0% of patients, while 23.5% of patients declared having complied with their supplementation plan during the postoperative period. Maximum weight loss between surgery and pregnancy was generally around $52.0 \pm 15\,kg$.

3.2. Pregnancy-Related Characteristics. As regards nutritional status, 56.8% of pregnancies involved supplementation during the periconceptional period. Average weight gain during pregnancy was $11.5 \pm 5.5\,kg$. Gestational diabetes and pregnancy-induced hypertension were reported in 18.0% and 4.0% of pregnancies, respectively. Concerning pregnancy

TABLE 2: Maternal characteristics of 48 patients.

	$\%^a$ m^b ± sd^c [min–max^d]
Maternal characteristics (N = 48)	
Maternal age (years)	31.0 ± 5.8 [22–44]
Start of weight gain	
(i) Childhood	83.0
(ii) Adolescence	3.0
(iii) Adulthood	14.0
Antecedents	
(i) Type 2 diabetes	3.5
(ii) High blood pressure	15.5
(iii) Active smoking	35.0
Professional activities	
(i) Active or in training	60.5
(ii) Unemployed, at home, or on parental leave	39.5
Bariatric surgery	
(i) Preoperative weight (kg)	129 ± 18.0 [103.0–174.0]
(ii) Preoperative BMI^e (kg/m^2)	47.0 ± 6.0 [38.0–63.0]
(iii) AGB^f	25.0 (N = 12)
(iv) SG^g	47.9 (N = 23)
(v) GBP^h	27.1 (N = 13)
(vi) Postsurgery supplementations	23.5
(vii) Postsurgery monitoring^i (per year)	
(i) Regular ≥ 3	37.0
(ii) Irregular [1-2]	24.0
(iii) None, 0	39.0
(viii) Maximum weight loss	52.0 ± 15.0 [30.0–79.0]
Time between surgery and pregnancy (months)	40.7 ± 33.9 [5–130]
Gravidity	
(i) 1	36.8
(ii) 2	17.5
(iii) 3	22.8
(iv) >3	22.9
Parity	
(i) 0	42.1
(ii) 1	29.8
(iii) 2	10.5
(iv) >3	17.6

^{a}Percentage. ^{b}Mean. ^{c}Standard deviation. ^{d}Minimum–maximum. ^{e}Body Mass Index (kg/m^2). ^{f}Adjustable gastric band. ^{g}Sleeve gastrectomy. ^{h}Gastric bypass. ^{i}Medical consultation with nutritionist doctor.

outcome, 8.8% (i.e., 5) of outcomes involving three patients resulted in a TA due to malformation, including one case of spina bifida.

3.3. Neonatal Characteristics. Five cases of malformations with TA were counted in our study. Three out of five TA involved chromosomal rearrangements (trisomy 21) in the same patient. There was one case of polymalformative syndrome without detection of chromosomal rearrangements.

There was one case of spina bifida in a patient who had undergone SG and who presented with a folate deficiency.

No cases of malformation or neonatal death were reported among the 52 neonates. Concerning neonatal complications, 28.0% of newborns were premature, 36.0% were small-for-gestational-age, 4.0% were severely small-for-gestational-age, and 4.0% were large-for-gestational-age.

Concerning nutritional status, 77.8% of pregnancies involved supplementation during the periconceptional period

TABLE 3: Neonatal and pregnancy-related characteristics of 57 pregnancies in 48 patients.

	%[a] m[b] ± sd[c] [min–max[d]]
Pregnancy-related characteristics (N = 57)	
Nutritional supplementation in the periconceptional period	56.8
BMI[e] at the onset of pregnancy (kg/m^2)	30.5 ± 7.4
Maternal weight gain (kg)	11.5 ± 5.5
Pregnancy-induced hypertension	4.0
Gestational diabetes	18.0
Preeclampsia	0
IUGR[f]	3.0
Threat of premature delivery	11.1
Induction of labour	36.1
TA[g] for malformation	8.8 (N = 5)
Postpartum bleeding	3.0
Neonatal characteristics (N = 52)	
Gestational age at birth (WA[h])	38.0 ± 2.7 [27.0–41.0]
Birth weight (g)	3026.0 ± 553.0 [1065.0–3900.0]
Prematurity between 32 and 36 WA	11.0
(i) Severe prematurity < 32 WA	3.0
(ii) Extreme prematurity < 28 WA	14.0
AUDIPOG	
(i) Hypotrophy $P < 10$	32.0
(ii) Severe hypotrophy $P < 3$	4.0
(iii) Macrosomia $P > 90$	4.0
Shoulder difficulty	6.0
Shoulder dystocia	3.0
Apgar score < at 7 to 5 min.	12.5
Umbilical blood pH < 7.2	5.0
Transfer to the neonatal unit	12.0
Transfer to the intensive care unit	6.0

[a]Percentage. [b]Mean. [c]Standard deviation. [d]Minimum–maximum. [e]Body Mass Index. [f]Intrauterine growth restriction. [g]Therapeutic abortion. [h]Weeks of amenorrhea.

in T1, 96.3% in T2, and 100.0% in T3 (Table 4). The principal micronutrient deficiencies identified were vitamin A (T1: 36.4%, T2: 21.1%, and T3: 40.0%), D (T1: 33.3%, T2: 26.3%, and T3: 8.3%), C (T1: 66.7%, T2: 41.2%, and T3: 83.3%), B1 (T1: 45.5%, T2: 15.4%, and T3: 20.0%), B9 (T1: 14.3%, T2: 0%, and T3: 9.1%), and selenium (T1: 77.8%, T2: 22.2%, and T3: 50.0%). The mean of nutritional values showed no significant difference according trimesters of pregnancy. The rate of haemoglobin decreased significantly between T1 and the other trimesters of pregnancy, which is a physiological evolution due to expansion of plasma volume.

3.4. According to Surgical Technique. A few maternal, nutritional, and pregnancy-related parameters revealed significant differences depending on the surgical technique used (Table 5). Women who had undergone a SG had a higher BMI at the time of the surgery (49.0 ± 6.3 kg/m^2 versus 43.8 ± 4.1 kg/m^2 for AGB and 43.8 ± 4.4 kg/m^2 for GBP; p = 0.01) and a greater postoperative weight loss (57.6 ± 14.6 kg versus 42.6 ± 16.3 kg for AGB and 49.2 ± 9.4 kg for GBP; p = 0.03). The interval between surgery and conception and

BMI at the onset of pregnancy were greater in patients with a history of AGB. In T1, there were fewer patients with an AGB who took supplements (AGB: 25.0%, SG: 77.3%, and GBP: 100.0%; p = 0.01). The prevalence of neonatal complications and nutritional deficiencies showed no significant difference according to surgical technique.

3.5. According to the Time between Surgery and Conception. Among the women who became pregnant within 18 months of bariatric surgery, 47.1% were losing weight versus 7.7% for patients who waited for a period greater than or equal to 18 months (p = 0.008; Table 6). Other maternal characteristics and neonatal and pregnancy issues showed no significant difference according to the time between surgery and conception.

3.6. According to BMI at the Onset of Pregnancy. The time between bariatric surgery and minimum weight reached was shorter for obese women at the onset of pregnancy (13.4±7.2 months versus 21.6±9.4 months for nonobese patients at the onset of pregnancy; p = 0.02). A greater number of obese

TABLE 4: Mean values of parameters and prevalence of maternal nutritional deficiencies during pregnancy ($N = 57$).

	T1[a]	T2[b] $m^g \pm sd^h/\%^i$	T3[c]	p^d	p^e	p^f
Supplementation	77.8	96.3	100.0			
Haematology						
Haemoglobin (g/dL)	$12.9 \pm 1.6/5.0$	$11.9 \pm 1.2/7.1$	$11.6 \pm 1.0/0$	0.01	0.001	
Ferritin (ng/mL) μg/L	$43.9 \pm 42.3/5.9$	$28.2 \pm 34.0/0$	$35.7 \pm 57.8/0$			
Biochemistry						
Albumin (g/L)	$37.8 \pm 4.6/13.3$	$32.5 \pm 3.2/5.6$	$31.1 \pm 2.8/0$			
Vitamins						
A (μmol/L)	$1.2 \pm 0.19/36.4$	$1.3 \pm 0.25/21.1$	$1.2 \pm 0.5/40.0$			
B1 (nmol/L)	$125.1 \pm 43.8/45.6^j$	$138.0 \pm 34.5/15.4^j$	$134.7 \pm 41.8/20.0^j$			
B6 (nmol/L)	$85.8 \pm 27.0/0^j$	$110.6 \pm 80.4/0^j$	$77.4 \pm 20.1/0^j$			
B9 (nmol/L)	$21.8 \pm 9.8/14.3$	$22.5 \pm 20.0/0$	$24.0 \pm 19.0/9.1$			
B12 (pmol/L)	$215.0 \pm 73.0/0$	$204.0 \pm 78.0/4$	$184.0 \pm 51.0/0$			
C (μmol/L)	$23.0 \pm 18.0/66.7^j$	$34.0 \pm 21.0/41.2^j$	$32.0 \pm 19.0/83.3$			
D (μg/L)	$28.3 \pm 18.7/33.3$	$23.7 \pm 18/26.3$	$30.4 \pm 13/8.3$			
Minerals						
Magnesium (mmol/L)	$0.8 \pm 0.1/0$	$0.8 \pm 0.1/0$	$0.7 \pm 0.1/0$			
Selenium (μmol/L)	$0.9 \pm 0.2/77.8$	$0.9 \pm 0.2/22.2$	$0.8 \pm 0.1/50.0$			
Zinc (μmol/L)	$13.1 \pm 2.6/0$	$11.5 \pm 1.7/0$	$10.7 \pm 1.4/0$			

[a]First trimester. [b]Second trimester. [c]Third trimester. [d]Comparison T1-T2. [e]Comparison of T1-T3. [f]Comparison of T2-T3. [g]Mean. [h]Standard deviation. [i]Percentage of deficiency with specific standards for pregnant women. [j]Percentage of deficiency when no specific standards are used.

TABLE 5: Maternal, nutritional, and pregnancy-related characteristic according to surgical technique.

	AGB[a] ($N = 15$)	SG[b] ($N = 29$) $\%^d$ $m^e \pm sd^f$	GBP[c] ($N = 13$)	p
Maternal characteristics				
Weight at the time of surgery (kg)	118.0 ± 11.0	138.0 ± 18.0	118.0 ± 12.0	0.0002
BMI[g] at the time of surgery (kg/m^2)	43.8 ± 4.1	49.0 ± 6.3	43.8 ± 4.4	0.01
Maximum weight loss (kg)	42.6 ± 16.3	57.6 ± 14.6	49.2 ± 9.4	0.03
Pregnancy				
Time between surgery and pregnancy (months)	64.0 ± 40.0	33.0 ± 28.0	30.0 ± 25.0	0.006
Weight at the onset of pregnancy (kg)	90.0 ± 21.0	87.0 ± 20.0	71.0 ± 12.0	0.02
BMI at the onset of pregnancy (kg/m^2)	33.5 ± 7.9	31.0 ± 7.8	26.3 ± 4.2	0.03
Nutritional characteristics				
Supplementations at T1[h]	25.0	77.3	100.0	0.01

[a]Adjustable gastric band. [b]Sleeve gastrectomy. [c]Gastric bypass. [d]Percentage. [e]Mean. [f]Standard deviation. [g]Body Mass Index. [h]First trimester. All the maternal, neonatal, nutritional, and pregnancy-related characteristics presented in Tables 2 and 3 were compared according to the surgical technique used. The table only shows results that were statistically significant or were of borderline statistical significance.

TABLE 6: Maternal and pregnancy-related characteristics according to the time between bariatric surgery and pregnancy.

	Period < 18 months $N = 23$	Period $\geq$ 18 months $N = 34$ $\%^a$ $m^b \pm sd^c$	p
Time between surgery and pregnancy (months)	13 ± 4	57 ± 33.5	<0.0001
Minimum weight after surgery (kg)	81 ± 14	70 ± 9	0.01
Body weight dynamics at the onset of pregnancy			0.008
(i) Weight loss	47.1	7.7	
(ii) Weight stabilisation	53	84	
(iii) Weight gain	0	8.0	

[a]Percentage. [b]Mean. [c]Standard deviation. All the maternal, neonatal, nutritional, and pregnancy-related characteristics presented in Tables 2 and 3 were compared according to the time between bariatric surgery and pregnancy. The table only shows results that were statistically significant or were of borderline statistical significance.

TABLE 7: Maternal and pregnancy-related characteristics according to Body Mass Index at the onset of pregnancy.

	BMI[a] < 30 kg/m^2 (N = 27)	BMI ≥ 30 kg/m^2 (N = 30)	p
	%[b] m[c] ± sd[d]		
Weight at the time of surgery (kg)	122 ± 13	138 ± 20	0.001
Time between surgery and minimum weight (months)	21.6 ± 9.4	13.4 ± 7.2	0.02
Body weight dynamics at the onset of pregnancy			0.03
(i) Weight loss	13	37	
(ii) Weight stabilisation	87	53	
(iii) Weight gain	0	10	

[a]Body Mass Index. [b]Percentage. [c]Mean. [d]Standard deviation. All the maternal, neonatal, nutritional, and pregnancy-related characteristics presented in Tables 2 and 3 were compared according to BMI at the onset of pregnancy. The table only shows results that were statistically significant or were of borderline statistical significance.

women were losing weight at the onset of pregnancy (37.0% versus 13.0% of nonobese patients; $p = 0.03$, Table 7). Other maternal characteristics and neonatal and pregnancy issues showed no significant difference according to the maternal BMI at the onset of pregnancy.

4. Discussion

Our study demonstrates that women who were pregnant after bariatric surgery have a great risk of presenting with micronutritional deficiencies in vitamins A, B1, B9, B12, and D and selenium in each trimester of pregnancy. Maternal deficiencies in vitamins A, D, B1, B9, and B12 were also identified in the scientific literature [22, 23]. No study was found covering nutritional statuses for vitamin C, selenium, zinc, and magnesium in pregnant women with a history of bariatric surgery.

In accordance with the data in the scientific literature, our study did not reveal any significant association between micronutrient deficiencies and fetal malformations [22]. The prevalence of fetal malformations in our study was higher than in the literature, which can be explained by the fact that three out of five TA involved chromosomal rearrangements in the same patient [24]. One pregnancy was terminated following an antenatal diagnosis of spina bifida in a patient who had undergone SG and who presented with a folate deficiency. Pelizzo et al. described four cases of neural tube anomalies in patients deficient in folates, three of whom had a history of GBP and one had a history of BPD [25–27]. Given that neural tube anomalies are more frequent in overweight and obese women than in normal-weight women, it is impossible to deduce whether these malformations were caused by the folate deficiency [28].

We have demonstrated that all the surgical techniques investigated in the study, including restrictive procedures, showed a strong relationship with micronutritional deficiencies, with these findings supporting those found in the scientific literature [23]. It should be noted, however, that the prevalence of treatments using nutritional supplements in the first trimester of pregnancy in our study differed significantly depending on the techniques used. All the women with a history of GBP were actually taking supplements based on

the recommendations on good medical practice (professional agreement). French and international recommendations state that, in the event of pregnancy, and in particular after gastric bypass surgery, it is advisable for women to take supplements of iron, calcium, folates, vitamin B12, and vitamin D. In accordance with international recommendations, treatment with folate supplements should be set up as soon as a woman expresses the desire to become pregnant [12]. It is also advised that the multidisciplinary healthcare team should programme a nutritional monitoring plan during the pregnancy and postpartum period (professional agreement). The prevalence of the observed deficiencies illustrates the need for regular medical checkups after bariatric surgery coupled with a dietetic and nutritional, clinical, and biologic assessment during the periconceptional period or, failing this, at the onset of pregnancy [12]. In accordance with our findings, several studies have reported that approximately fifty percent of patients fail to take their vitamin supplements in the long term, a fact that could impact on the health of a pregnancy [29]. Patient compliance and ongoing information and support provided by caregivers are, therefore, important components of the efforts set up to prevent complications and deficiencies.

Regarding neonatal complications, the high prevalence of small-for-gestational-age neonates identified in our study mirrored the findings of the study by Johansson et al. that highlighted an increased risk of small-for-gestational-age neonates (defined by a birth weight below the 10th percentile) in patients with a history of bariatric surgery [17]. In the meta-analysis performed by Galazis et al., the incidence of small-for-gestational-age neonates in patients who had undergone bariatric surgery was higher with a level of risk that was approx. 80% greater than that for obese pregnant women (OR: 1.93 [1.52–2.44]; $p < 0.001$) [15]. These findings have been confirmed by other studies [30–34]. In our study, the prevalence of SGA and prematurity is greater than previous published data which could be explained by the heterogeneous definitions of these terms. Indeed, in the meta-analysis of Galazis et al., only seven studies out of eleven defined small neonates as having an SGA below the 10th percentile, similar to that reported in our study. In eight studies, prematurity was defined as birth before the 37th week of gestation, but in four studies no definition was provided. Moreover, in some previous published data, we do not know the nutritional status of these women at the beginning and during the pregnancy on one hand and their weight dynamics between the surgery and the conception on the other hand [15]. In clinical practice, a history of bariatric surgery should therefore be considered a risk factor for SGA. Maternal undernutrition and micronutrient deficiencies resulting from caloric restriction as part of bariatric surgery could be one of the mechanisms underlying SGA [35]. While nutritional status was not assessed, Johansson et al. suggested an association between the findings and pregnancy-related malnutrition concerning, in particular, deficiencies in iron, vitamins B12, and folates [17]. We put forward the hypothesis that special attention should be paid to assessing the protein-energy status in such patients. Protein deficiencies are frequently identified after bariatric surgery, especially after a GBP [36]. In keeping with the findings reported in the scientific literature, our study did not reveal any significant difference in the prevalence of small-for-gestational-age neonates in relation to surgical techniques [15]. Nevertheless, two studies reported that the prevalence of SGA was lower in pregnant women fitted with an AGB compared to obese women who had not undergone surgery [37, 38]. A case-control study reported a higher prevalence of SGA after GBP compared to restrictive surgical weight loss techniques (AGB and SG) [39]. These studies made no mention of preoperative BMI or of the time that elapsed between surgery and conception. This could indicate that the patients did not share similar weight dynamics in terms of the techniques used. Could restrictive surgical weight loss techniques really involve a lower risk of SGA or might it simply be that the weight dynamic of these patients is a decisive factor in assessing the risk of SGA? As the greatest weight loss occurs in the 12- to 18-month period after bariatric surgery, it is recommended that this time period prior to becoming pregnant should be respected so as to minimise the maternal, fetal, and neonatal complications associated with potential nutritional deficiencies and to optimise weight loss [40–43]. In line with the data found in the scientific literature, the prevalence of complications did not differ significantly according to time [44, 45]. This supports the hypothesis that the criteria for stabilisation of patient weight and correction of nutrient deficiencies would be of greater value when deciding on starting a pregnancy than the criteria for the time between surgery and conception. It should also be noted that rapid postoperative weight loss results in the distortion of body image. Weight gain during pregnancy may generate anxiety and decompensation of eating disorders, and restrictive behaviours in particular, due to the fear of regaining weight [41]. Waiting for the weight to stabilise prior to becoming pregnant could help to prevent such complications. The benefits of bariatric surgery in terms of reducing maternal metabolic and cardiovascular risks could be counteracted in the long term by the small-for-gestational-age adverse metabolic and cardiovascular effects [46]. Due to this potential risk of malnutrition and fetal growth restriction, more regular monitoring of fetal growth could be programmed for pregnant women with a history of bariatric surgery. Additional studies will be needed to establish recommendations on clinical-biological monitoring and supplementation treatments for women during both the periconceptional period and pregnancy after bariatric surgery. The prospective multicentric cohort study bAriatric sUrgery Registration in wOmen of Reproductive Age (AURORA) designed to monitor women of reproductive age prior to bariatric surgery and for up to 6 months after pregnancy will make it possible to assess the prevalence and incidence of maternal and neonatal nutritional deficiencies and fetal malformations and will support the establishment of recommendations on good clinical practice for pregnant women with a history of bariatric surgery [47].

Although this study did not include a control group and was of a fairly small cohort size, it is, nevertheless, the largest French study reporting on micronutrient assessments in each trimester of pregnancy. We also took into account the physiological variations in micronutrient rates during each trimester of pregnancy by referring to standardised micronutrient levels that are specific to pregnant women in order to avoid overestimating deficiency prevalence. Even if there is no other data, concerning standards given by Abbassi-Ghanavati et al., some normal intervals are large and population is different from the French pregnant women so that these values are perhaps not completely adequate for French pregnant women.

5. Conclusions

Deficiencies in vitamins A, D, C, B1, and B9 and selenium have been identified in women who become pregnant after bariatric surgery. The high prevalence of small-for-gestational-age neonates raises the issue of the protein-energy status of women who fall pregnant after bariatric surgery. These findings underscore the importance of regular monitoring and compliance with long-term nutritional supplement plans after bariatric surgery. These nutritional deficiencies and the high rate of small-for-gestational-age neonates justify the need for systematic screening and the development of specific protocols for pregnant women who have undergone bariatric surgery.

Conflicts of Interest

The authors declare that there are no conflicts of interest regarding the publication of this article.

References

[1] E. Eschwege, M. A. Charles, A. Basdevant, and C. Moisan, ObÉpi 2012. Enquête Épidémiologique Nationale sur le Surpoids et l'Obésité, Inserm/Kantar Health/Roch, Paris, France, 2012, http://www.roche.fr/innovation-recherche-medicale/decouverte-scientifique-medicale/cardio-metabolisme/enquete-nationale-obepi-2012.html.

[2] B. Blondel, N. Lelong, M. Kermarrec, and F. Goffinet, "Trends in perinatal health in france from 1995 to 2010. results from the french national perinatal surveys," Journal de Gynecologie Obstetrique et Biologie de la Reproduction, vol. 41, no. 4, pp. e1–e15, 2012.

[3] I. Guelinckx, R. Devlieger, K. Beckers, and G. Vansant, "Maternal obesity: pregnancy complications, gestational weight gain and nutrition," *Obesity Reviews*, vol. 9, no. 2, pp. 140–150, 2008.

[4] K. J. Stothard, P. W. G. Tennant, R. Bell, and J. Rankin, "Maternal overweight and obesity and the risk of congenital anomalies: a systematic review and meta-analysis," *Journal of the American Medical Association*, vol. 301, no. 6, pp. 636–650, 2009.

[5] L. Bellamy, J. P. Casas, A. D. Hingorani, and D. Williams, "Type 2 diabetes mellitus after gestational diabetes: a systematic review and meta-analysis," *The Lancet*, vol. 373, no. 9677, pp. 1773–1779, 2009.

[6] S. C. Bischoff, Y. Boirie, T. Cederholm et al., "Towards a multidisciplinary approach to understand and manage obesity and related diseases," *Clinical Nutrition*, vol. 36, no. 4, pp. 917–938, 2016.

[7] J. Cheng, J. Gao, X. Shuai, G. Wang, and K. Tao, "The comprehensive summary of surgical versus non-surgical treatment for obesity: a systematic review and meta-analysis of randomized controlled trials," *Oncotarget*, vol. 7, no. 26, pp. 39216–39230, 2016.

[8] T. Diamantis, K. G. Apostolou, A. Alexandrou, J. Griniatsos, E. Felekouras, and C. Tsigris, "Review of long-term weight loss results after laparoscopic sleeve gastrectomy," *Surgery for Obesity and Related Diseases*, vol. 10, no. 1, pp. 177–183, 2014.

[9] J. L. Colquitt, K. Pickett, E. Loveman, and G. K. Frampton, "Surgery for weight loss in adults," *The Cochrane Database of Systematic Reviews*, vol. 8, Article ID CD003641, 2014.

[10] D. E. Arterburn, M. K. Olsen, V. A. Smith et al., "Association between bariatric surgery and long-Term survival," *Journal of the American Medical Association*, vol. 313, no. 1, pp. 62–70, 2015.

[11] L. Sjöström, K. Narbro, C. D. Sjöström et al., "Effects of bariatric surgery on mortality in Swedish obese subjects," *The New England Journal of Medicine*, vol. 357, pp. 741–752, 2007.

[12] Obésité: prise en charge chirurgicale chez l'adulte - Recommandations pour la pratique clinique [Internet]. Haute Autorité de Santé; 2009 janv. Disponible sur: http://www.has-sante.fr/portail/jcms/c_765529/fr/obesite-prise-en-charge-chirurgicale-chez-l-adulte.

[13] T. Debs, N. Petrucciani, R. Kassir, A. Iannelli, I. B. Amor, and J. Gugenheim, "Trends of bariatric surgery in France during the last 10 years: analysis of 267,466 procedures from 2005–2014," *Surgery for Obesity and Related Diseases*, vol. 12, no. 8, pp. 1602–1609, 2016.

[14] K. Slim and Y. Boirie, "Superobesity and adjustable gastric banding.," *Journal of visceral surgery*, vol. 149, no. 2, pp. e83–85, 2012.

[15] N. Galazis, N. Docheva, C. Simillis, and K. H. Nicolaides, "Maternal and neonatal outcomes in women undergoing bariatric surgery: a systematic review and meta-analysis," *European Journal of Obstetrics Gynecology and Reproductive Biology*, vol. 181, pp. 45–53, 2014.

[16] N. Roos, M. Neovius, S. Cnattingius et al., "Perinatal outcomes after bariatric surgery: nationwide population based matched cohort study," *BMJ (Online)*, vol. 347, Article ID f6460, 2013.

[17] K. Johansson, S. Cnattingius, I. Näslund et al., "Outcomes of pregnancy after bariatric surgery," *The New England Journal of Medicine:*, vol. 372, no. 9, pp. 814–824, 2015.

[18] J. F. Berlac, C. W. Skovlund, and O. Lidegaard, "Obstetrical and neonatal outcomes in women following gastric bypass: A Danish national cohort study," *Acta Obstetricia et Gynecologica Scandinavica*, vol. 93, no. 5, pp. 447–453, 2014.

[19] C. Berti, T. Decsi, F. Dykes et al., "Critical issues in setting micronutrient recommendations for pregnant women: an insight," *Maternal and Child Nutrition*, vol. 6, no. 2, pp. 5–22, 2010.

[20] I. Guelinckx, R. Devlieger, and G. Vansant, "Reproductive outcome after bariatric surgery: a critical review," *Human Reproduction Update*, vol. 15, no. 2, pp. 189–201, 2009.

[21] M. Abbassi-Ghanavati, L. G. Greer, and F. G. Cunningham, "Pregnancy and laboratory studies: a reference table for clinicians," *Obstetrics and Gynecology*, vol. 114, no. 6, pp. 1326–1331, 2009.

[22] G. Jans, C. Matthys, A. Bogaerts et al., "Maternal micronutrient deficiencies and related adverse neonatal outcomes after bariatric surgery: a systematic review," *Advances in Nutrition*, vol. 6, no. 4, pp. 420–429, 2015.

[23] R. Devlieger, I. Guelinckx, G. Jans, W. Voets, C. Vanholsbeke, and G. Vansant, "Micronutrient levels and supplement intake in pregnancy after bariatric surgery: a prospective cohort study," *PLoS ONE*, vol. 9, no. 12, Article ID e114192, 2014.

[24] L. Fumery, M. Pigeyre, C. Fournier et al., "Impact of bariatric surgery on obstetric prognosis," *Gynecologie Obstetrique Fertilite*, vol. 41, no. 3, pp. 156–163, 2013.

[25] G. Pelizzo, V. Calcaterra, M. Fusillo et al., "Malnutrition in pregnancy following bariatric surgery: three clinical cases of fetal neural defects," *Nutrition Journal*, vol. 13, no. 1, article no. 59, 2014.

[26] L. Martin, G. Chavez, M. J. Adams Jr. et al., "GASTRIC bypass surgery as maternal risk factor for neural tube defects," *The Lancet*, vol. 331, no. 8586, pp. 640-641, 1988.

[27] J. Haddow, L. Hill, E. Kloza, and D. Thanhauser, "Neural tube defects after gastric bypass," *The Lancet*, vol. 1, no. 8493, p. 1330, 1986.

[28] S. V. Dean, Z. S. Lassi, A. M. Imam, and Z. A. Bhutta, "Preconception care: nutritional risks and interventions," *Reproductive Health*, vol. 11, article no. S3, 2014.

[29] C. B. Woodard, "Pregnancy following bariatric surgery," *The Journal of Perinatal & Neonatal Nursing*, vol. 18, no. 4, pp. 329–340, 2004.

[30] M. A. Maggard, I. Yermilov, Z. Li, M. Maglione et al., "Pregnancy and fertility following bariatric surgery: a systematic review," *Journal of the American Medical Association*, vol. 300, no. 19, pp. 2286–2296, 2008.

[31] M. M. Kjaer and L. Nilas, "Pregnancy after bariatric surgery - a review of benefits and risks," *Acta Obstetricia et Gynecologica Scandinavica*, vol. 92, no. 3, pp. 264–271, 2013.

[32] E. Sheiner, K. Willis, and Y. Yogev, "Bariatric surgery: impact on pregnancy outcomes," *Current Diabetes Reports*, vol. 13, no. 1, pp. 19–26, 2013.

[33] M. M. Kjær, J. Lauenborg, B. M. Breum, and L. Nilas, "The risk of adverse pregnancy outcome after bariatric surgery: a nationwide register-based matched cohort study," *American Journal of Obstetrics and Gynecology*, vol. 208, no. 6, pp. 464.e1–464.e5, 2013.

[34] A. Josefsson, M. Blomberg, M. Bladh, S. G. Frederiksen, and G. Sydsjö, "Bariatric surgery in a national cohort of women: Sociodemographics and obstetric outcomes," *American Journal of Obstetrics and Gynecology*, vol. 205, no. 3, pp. 206.e1–206.e8, 2011.

[35] C. Ciangura, J. Nizard, C. Poitou-Bernert, M. Dommergues, J. M. Oppert, and A. Basdevant, "Pregnancy and bariatric surgery: critical points," *Journal de Gynecologie Obstetrique et Biologie de la Reproduction*, vol. 44, no. 6, pp. 496–502, 2015.

[36] C. Poitou Bernert, C. Ciangura, M. Coupaye, S. Czernichow, J. L. Bouillot, and A. Basdevant, "Nutritional deficiency after gastric bypass: diagnosis, prevention and treatment," *Diabetes and Metabolism*, vol. 33, no. 1, pp. 13–24, 2007.

[37] L. Vrebosch, S. Bel, G. Vansant, I. Guelinckx, and R. Devlieger, "Maternal and neonatal outcome after laparoscopic adjustable gastric banding: a systematic review," *Obesity Surgery*, vol. 22, no. 10, pp. 1568–1579, 2012.

[38] G. Ducarme, A. Revaux, A. Rodrigues, F. Aissaoui, I. Pharisien, and M. Uzan, "Obstetric outcome following laparoscopic adjustable gastric banding," *International Journal of Gynecology and Obstetrics*, vol. 98, no. 3, pp. 244–247, 2007.

[39] A. Chevrot, G. Kayem, M. Coupaye, N. Lesage, S. Msika, and L. Mandelbrot, "Impact of bariatric surgery on fetal growth restriction: experience of a perinatal and bariatric surgery center," *American Journal of Obstetrics and Gynecology*, vol. 214, no. 5, pp. 655.e1–655.e7, 2016.

[40] American College of Obstetricians and Gynecologists, "ACOG Committee Opinion number 315, September 2005. Obesity in pregnancy," *Obstetrics & Gynecology*, vol. 106, no. 3, pp. 671–675, 2005.

[41] M. A. Kominiarek, "Preparing for and managing a pregnancy after bariatric surgery," *Seminars in Perinatology*, vol. 35, no. 6, pp. 356–361, 2011.

[42] American College of Obstetricians and Gynecologists, "ACOG practice bulletin no. 105: bariatric surgery and pregnancy," *Obstetrics & Gynecology*, vol. 113, no. 6, pp. 1405–1413, 2009.

[43] K. K. Mahawar, Y. Graham, and P. K. Small, "Optimum time for pregnancy after bariatric surgery," *Surgery for Obesity and Related Diseases*, vol. 12, no. 5, pp. 1126–1128, 2016.

[44] T. Dao, J. Kuhn, D. Ehmer, T. Fisher, and T. McCarty, "Pregnancy outcomes after gastric-bypass surgery," *American Journal of Surgery*, vol. 192, no. 6, pp. 762–766, 2006.

[45] G. Ducarme, V. Chesnoy, P. Lemarié, S. Koumaré, and D. Krawczykowski, "Pregnancy outcomes after laparoscopic sleeve gastrectomy among obese patients," *International Journal of Gynecology and Obstetrics*, vol. 130, no. 2, pp. 127–131, 2015.

[46] C. Levy-Marchal and D. Jaquet, "Long-term metabolic consequences of being born small for gestational age," *Pediatric Diabetes*, vol. 5, no. 3, pp. 147–153, 2004.

[47] G. Jans, C. Matthys, S. Bel et al., "AURORA: Bariatric surgery registration in women of reproductive age - a multicenter prospective cohort study," *BMC Pregnancy and Childbirth*, vol. 16, no. 1, article no. 195, 2016.

8

Danish Sonographers' Experiences of the Introduction of "Moderate Risk" in Prenatal Screening for Down Syndrome

Anne Møller (ID),[1,2] **Ida Vogel,**[2,3] **Olav Bjørn Petersen,**[2,4] **and Stina Lou**[2,5]

[1]*Department of Public Health, Aarhus University, Aarhus, Denmark*
[2]*Center for Fetal Diagnostics, Aarhus University Hospital, Aarhus, Denmark*
[3]*Department of Clinical Genetics, Aarhus University Hospital, Aarhus, Denmark*
[4]*Fetal Medicine Unit, Department of Obstetrics and Gynaecology, Aarhus University Hospital, Aarhus, Denmark*
[5]*DEFACTUM, Public Health & Health Services Research, Central Denmark Region, Aarhus, Denmark*

Correspondence should be addressed to Anne Møller; anmo@ph.au.dk

Academic Editor: Olav Lapaire

Objective. The aim of the study was to determine sonographers' experiences with the introduction of an offer of noninvasive prenatal testing (NIPT) to a new moderate-risk (MR) group at the combined first-trimester prenatal screening (cFTS). *Study Design.* A qualitative approach consisting of seven semistructured interviews with five sonographers (midwives and nurses). Data was analyzed using thematic analysis. *Main Outcome Measures.* Sonographers' perception of offering NIPT to women in MR. *Results.* The sonographers understood NIPT as a positive development in prenatal screening due to a safe procedure and high detection rates for trisomies 13, 18, and 21. Prior to the introduction of MR, the sonographers were concerned about inducing worry in pregnant women in this new risk group. However, the pregnant women responded very positively, which the sonographers attributed to several factors such as the women's overall reason for participating in prenatal screening, the simplicity of the NIPT procedure, and the communicative strategies used by the sonographers. The strategies included all sonographers using the same words and explanations, emphasizing that statistics were in the women's favor, initiating the presentation of MR with a positive message, and downplaying the MR category. *Conclusion.* Sonographers' communicative strategies succeeded in limiting worry in pregnant women in MR. As such, the findings are valuable for health professionals, who are responsible for communicating about prenatal screening results and diagnostic options.

1. Introduction

Over the past few decades, prenatal screening for chromosomal abnormalities in the fetus has been introduced in most Western countries. Prenatal screening technologies (such as combined first-trimester screening (cFTS)) allow for the identification of high-risk pregnancies. These women are subsequently offered a diagnostic test. Until recently, only invasive diagnostic tests involving a procedure-related risk of miscarriage were available (chorionic villus sampling (CVS) and amniocentesis). Recent studies have shown this risk of miscarriage to be as low as 0.1-0.2% [1]; however, it nevertheless remains a main concern amongst many high-risk pregnant women. Therefore, the noninvasive prenatal testing (NIPT) has potential to fundamentally change the

current framework of prenatal care and diagnosis. NIPT is performed on maternal blood and is thus noninvasive and risk-free. It is not a diagnostic test, and abnormal test results must be verified by invasive testing. NIPT has, however, high accuracy in detecting trisomies 13, 18, and 21 and is generally viewed as a positive advancement in prenatal screening by pregnant women and clinicians [2].

NIPT has been introduced differently in different countries. In the Netherlands, NIPT was recently introduced as an alternative to cFTS, and, in countries like Denmark and Sweden, NIPT is offered as an alternative to invasive testing in high-risk groups [3]. Moreover, in many countries, private providers now offer NIPT to pregnant women who were previously considered low risk. In Denmark, NIPT has been tested as an offer to pregnant women with a cFTS result just below the high-risk cut-off (>1:300). Hence, a new category of risk was created: moderate risk (MR) (cFTS result between 1:300 and 1:699), and the number of pregnancies categorized as "at risk" was consequently increased. The offer of NIPT to MR was introduced in an attempt to improve detection rates but also derived consequences for both pregnant women and the health professionals caring for them.

Several studies show that a high-risk prenatal screening result generates a significant increase in anxiety for pregnant women [4]. Studies suggest that it is falling into the high-risk category itself (more than the exact risk figure) that generates worry and anxiety in pregnant women [5–7]. Based on this, one could hypothesize that a MR screening result could generate similar increased anxiety in pregnant women, as the health of the baby is questioned and additional tests are offered. Additionally, studies have shown that prenatal screening is often considered a routine part of prenatal care and, consequently, pregnant women are often not prepared for abnormal results [6]. This situation places a great demand on the health professionals responsible for communicating the screening results, and previous studies indicate that this communication is of great importance for the subsequent coping methods of the patients [8, 9].

With the introduction of a new MR group, the importance of clinical risk communication is further highlighted. Although considerable research has been devoted to pregnant women's experiences with participating in prenatal screening, rather less attention has been paid to the health professionals, who perform the scans and inform pregnant women about the results and options available. Thus, the introduction of a new MR group serves as an interesting case to investigate the management of communication of risk. The aim of this study was to investigate how clinicians experience and manage the introduction of an offer of NIPT to a new MR group.

2. Methods

Qualitative interviews were conducted in order to explore sonographers' experiences with the introduction of an offer of NIPT to a new MR group [10, 11].

2.1. Setting. The research was conducted at a fetal medicine unit at Aarhus University Hospital in Denmark. Denmark has a comprehensive and free-for-all screening program including cFTS and second-trimester scans [12, 13]. All routine scans are performed by sonographers, who also handle routine pre- and posttest information and counselling, including the reporting of high-risk and MR screening results. The sonographers are nurses/midwives specially trained in fetal medicine and are all certified in ultrasound from the Fetal Medicine Foundation, London.

The offer of NIPT to MR was implemented in Central Denmark Region in September 2015 as an addition to the cFTS. In this setting, MR was defined as a cFTS result of 1:300-1:699. In January 2017, the offer of MR NIPT, as well as the MR category as such, was discontinued following new guidelines from the Danish Health Authority [14].

TABLE 1: Participant characteristics.

Name	Age	Education	Years of work experience
Isabel	50	Nurse	11
Emily	50	Midwife	12
Laura	46	Nurse	12
Tina	44	Nurse	12
Naomi	32	Nurse	2

2.2. Data Collection. Semistructured interviews were conducted by AM during February and March 2017. The interviews lasted approximately 30 minutes and were digitally recorded, anonymized, and transcribed verbatim. Recruitment was characterized by a convenience sample of five sonographers, of which two were interviewed twice (for participant characteristics, see Table 1). The main themes of the interview guide were the moderate-risk group, risk communication, consequences for the pregnant women, and the discontinuation (for examples of the interview questions, see Table 2). After interviews with four sonographers, the interviews were transcribed and initial findings were discussed among the authors. As there was a high degree of consensus among the interviewees, the interview guide was revised and probing questions were added. Subsequently, an additional sonographer was interviewed and two sonographers were interviewed again. However, these interviews added very limited new information to the material and researchers consequently estimated that data saturation was met [15, 16].

2.3. Data Analysis. Data was coded using NVivo 11.4 software (QSR International, Doncaster, Australia) and analyzed using thematic analysis, which is a theoretically flexible tool for analyzing qualitative data [17]. Data analysis was comprised of different steps. First, data familiarization was obtained by repeated reading of the transcripts. Second, the transcripts were coded into five main codes each with two to three subcodes. Third, the codes were clustered into themes by use of a thematic map to visualize the process. Fourth, reliability was ensured by reading through the coded data, which were compared to the themes. Finally, the themes were reviewed and named. Following this process, four themes were defined (see Figure 1).

2.4. Ethical Considerations. In Denmark, qualitative research does not require ethical approval from the National Committee on Health Research Ethics. Prior to the interviews, all sonographers at the fetal medicine unit received oral information about the study and informed consent was obtained. In the presentation of results, all participants have been carefully anonymized through the use of pseudonyms.

3. Results

The analysis resulted in the identification of four themes (see Figure 1) in the sonographers' experience with offering NIPT to MR: (1) Providing information is the objective.

TABLE 2: Topic guide.

Topic	Examples of questions
Implementation of NIPT	(i) Do you think implementing NIPT was a good idea? (Why/why not?)
	(ii) How was the pregnant women's reaction to NIPT?
The moderate-risk group	(i) Do you think there were any problems connected to the fact that pregnant women could be identified as in moderate risk? (Any benefits?)
	(ii) Did you think differently about the risk of the pregnant women that were in a moderate risk group compared to earlier times? (Why/why not?)
Risk communication	(i) Do you think about the word risk when you talk to the pregnant women?
	(ii) How exactly did you tell pregnant women that they were in a moderate risk group?
Consequences for the pregnant women	(i) How did the women react being identified as in moderate risk? (Examples?)
	(ii) Did you have a feeling of causing the women unnecessary anxiety?
The discontinuation	(i) How do you feel about that the moderate risk group no longer exists?
	(ii) What thoughts do you have about that pregnant women, who earlier would be in a moderate risk group and offered NIPT, today not are offered any additional tests?

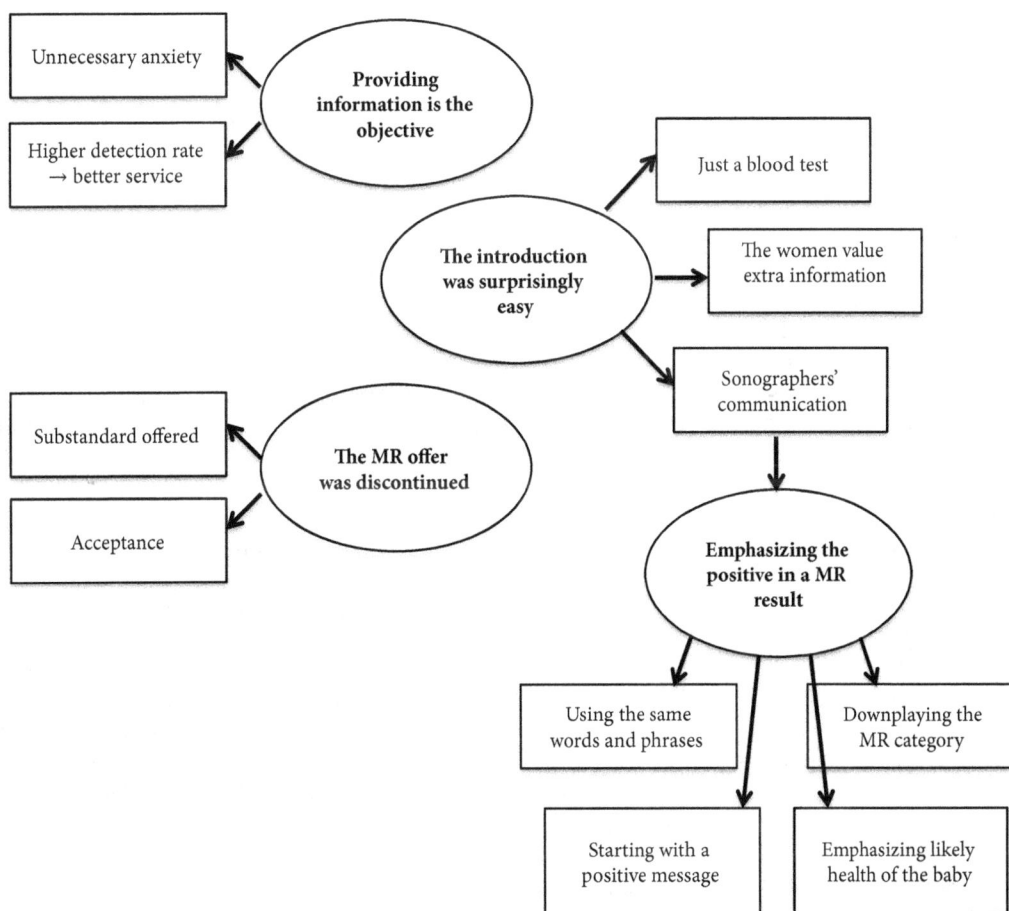

FIGURE 1: Thematic map.

(2) Introduction was surprisingly easy. (3) Emphasizing the positive in a MR result. (4) The MR offer was discontinued.

3.1. Providing Information Is the Objective. Prior to the introduction of NIPT for MR, the sonographers were predominantly positive. NIPT was perceived as a positive technology that would allow for detection of more cases of Down syndrome:

> *I think that when you are in this [field] you want to offer the pregnant women as many answers as you can and as big a security as possible that the*

baby is healthy. In that way I think it is a good offer for them. (Emily)

This quote reflects what the interviewed sonographers perceived their professional objective to be: to provide as detailed and accurate information about the fetus as possible. Their aim was to provide sufficient information for the prospective parents either to feel reassured of the fetus's normal development or, in case of detecting something, to provide reliable information about potential risks and/or malformations and diagnostic options. According to the sonographers, NIPT was a tool for improving this provision of detailed and accurate information.

The sonographers expressed initial concerns towards the MR category:

There is a risk that we "medicalize" them. You know, to suddenly go from being normal to being "maybe-normal". I had concerns about that. (Isabel)

The sonographers were cautious that the MR—also spoken of as a gray-zone result—would generate (in most cases unnecessary) increased anxiety in a larger group of women. The interviews reflected an effort among the sonographers to simultaneously *"tell it like it is."* These concerns influenced the communicative strategies that the sonographers employed when the MR category was introduced.

In sum, the sonographers were positive towards implementing NIPT for MR. They were not concerned with whether the pregnant women chose NIPT or not but valued the possibility to provide them a choice and as much information as possible. However, the sonographers had initial concerns on the women's behalf seeing that it could cause unnecessary worry.

3.2. The Introduction Was Surprisingly Easy. The sonographers described the pregnant women's reactions to MR as "untroubled" and "surprisingly easy."

They just accepted it and thought "well okay, then we have this [NIPT] offered". But they did not get concerned or surprised or shocked. Not at all. (Tina)

In the sonographers' experience, the MR women perceived the offer of NIPT as an extra test and reassurance of the baby's health. Interestingly, none of the sonographers had experienced conflicts or negative reactions and offered the following explanations: First of all, the sonographers all accepted that pregnant women attended the cFTS in order to see their unborn child and share the experience with their partner. However, it was also the sonographers' experience that pregnant women were well aware of the medical purpose of the scan and came to the cFTS to gain information about their babies' health, and they all reported that many women preferred as much information as possible from them. The offer of NIPT fitted well with this purpose. Secondly, the noninvasiveness of NIPT meant that it did not put the pregnancy at risk. Compared to the invasive procedures, NIPT was simply a blood test:

[With the CVS] there is a risk - even though it is very, very low, it is different. And the other [NIPT] is just a blood test. I think, they [the pregnant women] often think; "it is probably not as serious". (Naomi)

The sonographers argued that since most women have had a blood test taken, NIPT was an easier task for them to deal with. In comparison, an invasive test was more demanding for pregnant women, in terms of not only the risk of miscarriage, but also the discomfort of the invasive procedure, practical arrangements of getting extra days off, etc.

In sum, the pregnant women reacted surprisingly positively to MR and NIPT. The sonographers attributed this to the fact that the women were interested in information about their babies' health and the noninvasive, no-risk nature of NIPT. However, the sonographers assigned their own communication practice as the most important reason. This will be further described below.

3.3. Emphasizing the Positive in a MR Result. The sonographers were all attentive to the importance of appropriate clinical communication. Prior to the implementation of the MR, the sonographers had collectively discussed and agreed upon how to properly communicate the offer of NIPT to the MR group. One strategy was to ensure the collective use of approximately the same type of words and explanations in MR situations. This meant that the sonographers used collectively agreed on phrasing, examples, and figures of speech when communicating the MR result. This gave the sonographer a sense of security and speaking on behalf of her profession, not just her own experience and convictions. Another strategy was to emphasize that the fetus most likely was healthy. As one sonographer put it, this claim was fairly safe seeing that the risk was 1:300-1:699 and was earlier identified as low risk. Consequently, the sonographers felt confident enough using this strategy to not make the women feel unnecessarily worried. A third strategy was to avoid using the words *moderate risk* in the initial presentation of the screening result. The sonographers explained that, in their experience, the word *risk* had the power to trigger concern and worry in most pregnant women. Hence, they first underscored that the woman was *not* high risk, and the MR result was downplayed by referring to the offer of NIPT as something "extra" or "supplementary":

I used this phrase for a couple of months: "if you had come in 2 months ago [...] you would not have been offered anything, then you would just have been told that everything was fine and normal and no more tests, but now there is this, which is a good offer with a relatively little intervention." (Tina)

Thus, the sonographers emphasized NIPT as something the MR group were fortunate to be offered compared to earlier times.

In sum, with the introduction of NIPT for MR, the sonographers made use of the following communicative strategies: collectively using words and explanations, emphasizing the probability of a normal result, initiating the conversations with a positive message, and downplaying the MR category.

3.4. The MR Offer Was Discontinued. Shortly before the interviews were conducted, the offer of NIPT to women in MR was unexpectedly discontinued. The sonographers expressed some concern with not being able to offer NIPT to this group of pregnant women:

> *[Phasing out NIPT] is as if you all of a sudden had to stop measure their heads or something like that. (Naomi)*

This sonographer expressed a concern with delivering high-quality prenatal screening when no longer able to identify a MR group and offer NIPT. In her view, the discontinuation of MR increased the uncertainty for both the pregnant women and the sonographer herself. In principle, this made it more likely for the sonographers to overlook cases of Down syndrome. One sonographer explained her reaction when calculating a risk of 1:300-1:699 after the discontinuation:

> *Then I think "oh", which was not a problem before. But it is because we want to take good care of them [the pregnant women]. (Laura)*

The awareness of the former MR group made sonographers even more observant of risk results just above the high-risk cut-off. When asked if a woman's risk of giving birth to a Down syndrome baby was bigger after the discontinuation, one sonographer stated:

> *I have to say that I have not. If I start to go down that road I cannot be in this. So I have to be confident that this is normal. [. . .] I have to cope with scanning for many years to come and be able to stand being in it mentally and not lie awake at night [wondering] if I did it well enough. (Isabel)*

The sonographers expressed an intentional decision to accept the MR discontinuation as the right decision and they had collectively convinced themselves that they could still offer the same level of information (and reliability) in their scans. These decisions were reported to be necessary in order to be able to perform their daily work with confidence and satisfaction. Also, they did not want to contaminate the pregnant women with their own hesitance towards the discontinuation. One way to cope with this was to emphasize that they were not accountable for the decision to discontinue the MR group. They accepted it and perceived the argumentation to be fair. They agreed that it was vital for the number of cases detected to be in accordance with the financial expenses of the test.

In sum, the sonographers accepted the discontinuation of the MR group, despite it not being consistent with their wish to provide pregnant women with as much information about their babies' health as possible.

4. Discussion

Based on qualitative methods, this study aimed to investigate how sonographers experienced and managed the introduction of an offer of NIPT to a new MR group. The results show that in the sonographers' experience the pregnant women did not become particularly worried following a MR screening result. This untroubled response was largely attributed to the sonographers' communicative strategies: collectively using specific words and explanations, emphasizing that statistics were in the women's favor, initiating conversations with a positive message, and toning down the risk category. The sonographers were positive towards offering the new MR group NIPT, since it was consistent with their professional objective of providing detailed and high-quality information about the fetus to the pregnant women. Some sonographers found the discontinuation of the MR difficult, but they accepted the new guideline. The findings add new perspectives regarding how sonographers manage their daily work and regarding the significance of sonographers' communication within prenatal screening.

The results show that women with MR did not question the new risk category. This resonates with theories of modern society as a "risk society" where many health-related risks are invisible threats, whose presence is calculated through statistics and epidemiology [18]. Contrary to bodily symptoms, such as bleedings or pain, pregnant women cannot feel or observe symptoms of carrying a fetus with Down syndrome. Instead, the risk is calculated by computers and communicated by sonographers. Pregnant women rely on expert knowledge in order to identify and manage a number of invisible threats to the pregnancy and the fetus [19], and this context may help explain the ready acceptance of the MR category by the women in the study. Moreover, MR must be understood in the context of the Danish prenatal screening program that has a very consistent and high uptake (>90%) [20]. Studies have shown that Danish women are generally knowledgeable about and positive towards prenatal screening [21, 22], which means that the sonographers were communicating the MR to a—generally—proscreening and prochoice population, which may be another explanation why the MR result was so readily accepted. Moreover, the sonographers in this study were responsible for all risk communication without summoning a fetal medicine specialist, which may have downplayed and normalized MR women's experience of the situation.

The results show how the potentially worrisome and "invisible threat" to the baby's health—MR—was downplayed by the sonographers to "just" being a blood test and a current extra offer. A central premise in prenatal screening is neutral information and autonomous choice [23], and, consequently, one concern could be the potential undermining of pregnant women's autonomous choices by such communicative practices. Are pregnant women making informed choices, when the sonographers present NIPT as "just" a blood test? Health professionals play an important part in pregnant women's decision-making process [24]. However, studies have shown that, in order for women to make meaningful choices, more than neutral information about cut-off values and detection rates is needed [25]. Pregnant women also request experiential knowledge [26], alternative interpretations [7], and empathetic and collaborative communication [27]. Accepting these elements as central to good clinical communication, one must also take into account the specific situation that Danish pregnant women in MR are in: they have made an informed consent about participating in screening, they are NOT in high risk, and the test offered is risk-free. Thus, the context also supports a choice of NIPT. However, clinicians must always be careful and attentive to potential bias in their communication with patients, particularly to allow the less-likely choices to be made [21].

Ultimately, the discontinuation of MR put the sonographers in a position where they considered themselves unable to provide the same level of quality in their work. However, from the results, we can see how chosen standards (cut-offs, guidelines, and specific markers) are accepted and executed in order for clinical practice to function. Just like pregnant women trust the experts, the sonographers must trust the current guideline or protocol (MR or not) and act in accordance with it. This trust helps sonographers to navigate through gray zones (e.g., a "MR" result after the discontinuation) and to secure equal treatment for all patients. Thus, responsibility is delegated to the current cut-off, as the authoritative designator of high risk and low risk, around which the sonographers arrange their work and communication.

Consequently, the results point to two central motivations that underpin the sonographers' daily clinical work and communication with pregnant women: First, sonographers expressed a personal concern and responsibility for examining the fetus thoroughly and detecting as many cases of Down syndrome (and other abnormalities) as possible. Importantly, the sonographers were not concerned with whether the women chose NIPT or not, but with providing information and the possibility of choice. Secondly, the sonographers organized their work and their communication to ensure that pregnant women did not become unnecessarily worried by the information provided by ultrasound, including information about MR. Based on this study, it must be concluded that the sonographers—in their understanding—succeeded in balancing these paradigms in the implementation of NIPT to pregnant women with MR.

4.1. Limitations. The results are based on a small sample of sonographers recruited from an ultrasound clinic in Denmark, which limits generalizability of results. First, Danish sonographers are educated nurses and midwives and thus have expertise in clinical communication. Additionally, the sample of sonographers is small and relatively experienced, which may influence the results. Furthermore, there is a high uptake in cFTSs among Danish women, which may reflect a rather positive attitude towards screening compared to other countries. Finally, this study has focused on the sonographers' experiences and their impression of pregnant women's response to MR. Future research should include an investigation of pregnant women's own experiences.

5. Conclusion

This study is a step towards understanding how sonographers manage the introduction of a new technology (NIPT) and a new risk category (MR). The sonographers used different collective strategies to communicate a MR risk result. Overall, the sonographers experienced the pregnant women responding positively to the MR NIPT offer and they did not detect an increase in worry among the MR group. However, further research is needed to explore pregnant women's experiences of being categorized as MR, their assessment of the clinical communication, and their reasons for choosing/declining NIPT.

Conflicts of Interest

The authors declare that there are no conflicts of interest regarding the publication of this paper.

Acknowledgments

The work was supported by the Center for Fetal Diagnostics, Aarhus University Hospital, Denmark. Thanks are due to the head midwife at the fetal medicine unit, Marianne Raundal, for enabling and coordinating interviews. Also, thanks are due to the sonographers for a positive and collaborative approach and for sharing thoughts and experiences in the interviews.

References

[1] C. B. Wulff, T. A. Gerds, L. Rode, C. K. Ekelund, O. B. Petersen, and A. Tabor, "Risk of fetal loss associated with invasive testing following combined first-trimester screening for Down syndrome: a cohort of 147 987 singleton pregnancies : Procedure-related risk of fetal loss," *Ultrasound in Obstetrics & Gynecology*, vol. 47, no. 1, pp. 38–44, 2016.

[2] J. Bennett, L. Chitty, and C. Lewis, "Non-invasive Prenatal Diagnosis for BRCA Mutations – a Qualitative Pilot Study of Health Professionals' Views," *Journal of Genetic Counseling*, vol. 25, no. 1, pp. 198–207, 2016.

[3] T. J. Musci, G. Fairbrother, A. Batey, J. Bruursema, C. Struble, and K. Song, "Non-invasive prenatal testing with cell-free DNA: US physician attitudes toward implementation in clinical practice," *Prenatal Diagnosis*, vol. 33, no. 5, pp. 424–428, 2013.

[4] S. Lou, L. Mikkelsen, L. Hvidman, O. B. Petersen, and C. P. Nielsen, "Does screening for Down's syndrome cause anxiety in pregnant women? A systematic review," *Acta Obstetricia et Gynecologica Scandinavica*, vol. 94, no. 1, pp. 15–27, 2015.

[5] B. Heyman, G. Hundt, J. Sandall et al., "On being at higher risk: A qualitative study of prenatal screening for chromosomal

anomalies," *Social Science & Medicine*, vol. 62, no. 10, pp. 2360–2372, 2006.

[6] C. Baillie, J. Smith, J. Hewison, and G. Mason, "Ultrasound screening for chromosomal abnormality: Women's reactions to false positive results," *British Journal of Health Psychology*, vol. 5, no. 4, pp. 377–394, 2000.

[7] N. Schwennesen and L. Koch, "Representing and intervening: 'Doing' good care in first trimester prenatal knowledge production and decision-making," *Sociology of Health & Illness*, vol. 34, no. 2, pp. 283–298, 2012.

[8] A. Pilnick and O. Zayts, ""it's just a likelihood": Uncertainty as topic and resource in conveying "positive" results in an antenatal screening clinic," *Symbolic Interaction*, vol. 37, no. 2, pp. 187–208, 2014.

[9] K. O'Doherty and G. K. Suthers, "Risky communication: Pitfalls in counseling about risk, and how to avoid them," *Journal of Genetic Counseling*, vol. 16, no. 4, pp. 409–417, 2007.

[10] T. Tjørnhøj-Thomsen and S. R. Whyte, "Fieldwork and participant observation," in *Research methods in public health*, L. Koch and S. Vallgårda, Eds., pp. 90–118, Munksgaard, Copenhagen, 4 edition, 2011.

[11] N. E. Riley, "Book Review: STEINAR KVALE and SVEND BRINKMANN, Interviews: Learning the Craft of Qualitative Research Interviewing (2nd Edition). Thousand Oaks, CA: Sage, 2009. 354 pp. (including index). ISBN 9780761925422," *Qualitative Research*, vol. 10, no. 3, pp. 390–392, 2010.

[12] C. K. Ekelund, F. S. Jørgensen, O. B. Petersen et al., "Impact of a new national screening policy for Down's syndrome in Denmark: Population based cohort study," *BMJ*, vol. 338, no. 7692, pp. 449–452, 2009.

[13] O. B. Petersen, I. Vogel, C. Ekelund, J. Hyett, and A. Tabor, "Potential diagnostic consequences of applying non-invasive prenatal testing: Population-based study from a country with existing first-trimester screening," *Ultrasound in Obstetrics & Gynecology*, vol. 43, no. 3, pp. 265–271, 2014.

[14] Danish Health Authority. Retningslinjer for fosterdiagnostik : prænatal information, risikovurdering, rådgivning og diagnostik [Guidelines on fetal diagnostic]. 2nd ed. Copenhagen: Danish Health Authority; 2017.

[15] K. Malterud, V. D. Siersma, and A. D. Guassora, "Sample Size in Qualitative Interview Studies: Guided by Information Power," *Qualitative Health Research*, vol. 26, no. 13, pp. 1753–1760, 2016.

[16] J. M. Morse, "The significance of saturation," *Qualitative Health Research*, vol. 5, no. 2, pp. 147–149, 1995.

[17] V. Braun and V. Clarke, "Using thematic analysis in psychology," *Qualitative Research in Psychology*, vol. 3, no. 2, pp. 77–101, 2006.

[18] B. Smart, "Reviews : Ulrich Beck, Risk Society: Towards a New Modernity (London and New York, Sage, 1992)," *Thesis Eleven*, vol. 37, no. 1, pp. 160–165, 2016.

[19] A. Giddens, *The consequences of modernity*, Polity Press, Cambridge, 1993.

[20] National Database of Fetal Medicine. National Årsrapport 2014 [Annual Report 2014]. 2014; Available at: http://www.dfms.dk/images/foetodatabase/Arsrapport_FOTO_2014_final_anonymiseret.pdf. Accessed 5/5, 2017.

[21] L. Bangsgaard and A. Tabor, "Do pregnant women and their partners make an informed choice about first trimester risk assessment for Down syndrome, and are they satisfied with the choice?" *Prenatal Diagnosis*, vol. 33, no. 2, pp. 146–152, 2013.

[22] S. Lou, M. Frumer, M. M. Schlütter, O. B. Petersen, I. Vogel, and C. P. Nielsen, "Experiences and expectations in the first trimester of pregnancy: a qualitative study," *Health Expectations*, vol. 20, no. 6, pp. 1320–1329, 2017.

[23] E. García, D. R. M. Timmermans, and E. Van Leeuwen, "Rethinking autonomy in the context of prenatal screening decision-making," *Prenatal Diagnosis*, vol. 28, no. 2, pp. 115–120, 2008.

[24] S. G. Hertig, S. Cavalli, C. Burton-Jeangros, and B. S. Elger, "'Doctor, what would you do in my position?' Health professionals and the decision-making process in pregnancy monitoring," *Journal of Medical Ethics*, vol. 40, no. 5, pp. 310–314, 2014.

[25] A. Werner-Lin, J. L. M. McCoyd, and B. A. Bernhardt, "Balancing Genetics (Science) and Counseling (Art) in Prenatal Chromosomal Microarray Testing," *Journal of Genetic Counseling*, vol. 25, no. 5, pp. 855–867, 2016.

[26] F. E. Carroll, A. Owen-Smith, A. Shaw, and A. A. Montgomery, "A qualitative investigation of the decision-making process of couples considering prenatal screening for Down syndrome," *Prenatal Diagnosis*, vol. 32, no. 1, pp. 57–63, 2012.

[27] S. Lou, C. P. Nielsen, L. Hvidman, O. B. Petersen, and M. B. Risør, "Coping with worry while waiting for diagnostic results: A qualitative study of the experiences of pregnant couples following a high-risk prenatal screening result," *BMC Pregnancy and Childbirth*, vol. 16, no. 1, article no. 321, 2016.

9

Use of Over-the-Counter Medication among Pregnant Women in Sharjah, United Arab Emirates

Abduelmula R. Abduelkarem[1] **and Hafsa Mustafa**[2]

[1]*College of Pharmacy, University of Sharjah, Sharjah, UAE*
[2]*AME Global FZE, Sharjah, UAE*

Correspondence should be addressed to Abduelmula R. Abduelkarem; aabdelkarim@sharjah.ac.ae

Academic Editor: Fabio Facchinetti

Background. Over-the-counter medications are widely available in pharmacies Their safety profile, however, does not extend to pregnant women. Accordingly, there should be educational programs developed for pregnant women to protect them from the harms of the side effects. *Aim.* This study was planned and designed with the aim of exploring the awareness and assessing the usage of OTC medications among pregnant women in Sharjah, UAE. *Method.* A cross-sectional survey using a self-administered questionnaire. *Results.* More than three-quarters (75.7%) reported that they are familiar with the term "over-the-counter drugs." Interestingly, 40% of the respondents reported that they took OTC drugs during pregnancy, and the majority (94.2%) agreed with the survey statement "not all OTC medications are safe to be taken during pregnancy." Constipation was the most frequent side effect that most of the participants reported during the study period. Folic acid (36%), calcium (28.6%), and iron (35.1%) were the most common supplements used by the pregnant women responding. *Conclusion.* The reported 40% usage of OTC medications among pregnant women in this study is worrisome and calls for the need to educate, counsel, and increase awareness among pregnant women regarding the dangers of OTC drugs usage while pregnant in Sharjah, UAE.

1. Introduction

Self-medication is the treatment of common health problems with medicines designed and labeled for use without professional supervision and approved as safe and effective for such use, as defined by the World Self-Medication Industry. Over-the-counter (OTC) drugs have been widely used in self-medication, for many years, in the treatment of common pregnancy related health problems. Pregnancy is a dynamic process in which anatomic and physiological changes occur from fertilization to parturition. Any given over-the-counter agent has vastly different effects depending on the stage of embryo and fetal development [1]. Accordingly, when a pregnant female uses OTC products for self-medication, she is exposing herself and/or her baby to different toxicological effects brought about by these drugs. At any point in the gestation period, over 90% of pregnant women take a prescription or OTC medication [2]. The common symptoms of pregnancy such as nausea, vomiting, heartburn, backache, constipation, or even migraine, pains, and cough require medications that should be selected carefully to avoid side effects on the fetus and mother [3]. It is probably due to these symptoms that pregnant females are reaching out to OTC medications. Also, it has been demonstrated that the most common types of OTC medications used by pregnant women are allergy medications, analgesics, respiratory medications, gastrointestinal medications, and skin condition products [4–6].

The United Arab Emirates (UAE) is a federation of seven gulf emirates with an estimated population of 9 million people in 2016, with 80% of the population comprised of expatriates from different countries [7]. Despite being with an estimated GDP of $370 billion in 2016 and a rapidly increasing population, there is a paucity of published research regarding people living below the poverty level [8, 9]. This rapidly increasing population necessitates that pharmacists and other members of the healthcare teams have access to adequate and up-to-date information on OTC products and are able to provide advice on the benefits and risks of using such medications to consumers, including pregnant women. Currently, there is a scarcity of data about the practice and impact of OTC medication usage among pregnant women in UAE. Accordingly, this study was planned and designed with the aim of exploring the awareness and assessing the usage of OTC medications among pregnant women in Sharjah, UAE.

2. Method

2.1. Ethical Consideration. The study was conducted after the approval of the University of Sharjah Ethics Committee, Sharjah, UAE (reference number: REC-16-10-03-01-S).

2.2. Study Design. A cross-sectional survey was conducted to assess the level of awareness and knowledge of pregnant women concerning OTC drugs. The study took place in the Emirate of Sharjah, UAE, over a period of three months (October to December 2016).

2.3. Study Population. Sharjah is the third largest of the seven emirates that make up the UAE and is the only one to have land on both the Arabian Gulf Coast and the Gulf of Oman. Residents of Sharjah represent around 19% of the UAE's population (4.76 million) (Ministry of Economy, 2008) [10]. Within the UAE, it has been reported that the crude birth rate or birth rate per 1,000 population was 15.54 during the year of 2014. The reported birth rate declined to 10.59 in 2015 according to the World Bank collection of development indicators [11, 12].

This study was conducted at four different clinics/hospitals within Sharjah: Al Qassimi Hospital, Dr. Oras Medical Centre, Bait Al Seha Clinic, and Dr. Rabha Habib Al Sayegh Clinic. A total of 140 questionnaires were distributed among these locations as 140 pregnant patients (of varying trimesters) visited the clinic during the study period. All the women who visited the clinics during this period were invited to take part in the study; the response rate was 100%. If a woman was pregnant (at any trimester), she was eligible to participate in the study. The only other inclusion criterion for this study was the patient's ability to understand either English or Arabic. Every woman who agreed to participate in the study was informed that her name and her responses to the survey questions, as well as any statements, would be treated as confidential and would not be used for any other purpose, apart from the study and that only aggregated data would be published. As the women filled out the survey questions, the researchers were available to clarify any misinterpretation or answer questions the participants may have.

2.4. Questionnaire Development. A 19-item questionnaire (Appendix) was developed in both English and Arabic versions, using items from surveys from previous studies [13–15]. The Arabic questionnaire was read and modified by Arabic language experts in order to validate the accuracy from its English translation. The survey was modified and amended to fit the UAE society, and any outdated or unnecessary questions were eliminated. It should be emphasized that the development of the questionnaire in Arabic involved considerably more effort than just mere translation. Sometimes it was not possible to find an equivalent term in Arabic that expresses a medical term in English. Moreover, a direct translation of an English phrase might be meaningless in Arabic or, even worse, lead to misunderstandings, unless the phrase was elaborated on or further qualified. For this reason, the Arabic questionnaire was reviewed and modified by Arabic language experts to accurately reflect the meaning from the English version. Furthermore, the survey was not produced in other languages such as Urdu or Hindi, because, as mentioned in the study design and population description, pregnant women who were unable to speak/read English or Arabic were excluded from the study.

The survey was divided into six sections (a copy of the questionnaire is available from the authors). Section 1 comprised personal information (Q1–Q6). The aim of Section 1 was to assess the demographic data of the participants such as nationality, age, marital status, education level, employment situation, and parity. Level of knowledge (Q7–Q10) was assessed in Section 2. The purpose was to assess the attitude of the participants towards over-the-counter medication and herbal safety and the level of knowledge. Past and current medication use (Q11–Q12) was captured in Section 3. The aim of this section was to determine whether the participants were using any OTC medication or vitamins and whether they had suffered side effects. Current health status of the pregnant women (Q13-Q14) was solicited in Section 4. This was done to establish whether the participants had any chronic diseases that would encourage them to seek medications or smoking that may alter or interfere with, if any, over-the-counter medications they would be using. Section 5 consisted of information on previous children (Q15) born. This section established whether previous children were born with special needs or not. Assessment of over-the-counter drug use (Q16–Q19) was part of Section 6. The aim of this section was to determine the overall knowledge of participants of over-the-counter drugs and whether they intended to increase their knowledge of the OTC drugs they used by reading the accompanying leaflet.

At the completion of the study and as a special service, 31 participants who consented and agreed were provided with information about OTC drugs in the form of short paragraphs via the mobile application WhatsApp. This information was available in both English and Arabic and was provided to the consenting patients in accordance with their preferred language.

2.5. Validity and Reliability Testing. Face validity of the questionnaire was determined using the following approach. Despite the fact that the survey questions were taken from a validated study [15], it was sent to two faculty members and one physician to assess the face validity; this is because the original validity questionnaire was subjected to some modifications. Additionally, the survey was provided to four nonparticipants and they were asked to provide feedback.

To assess test-retest reliability, the questionnaire was sent on two separate occasions to ten participants randomly selected from the clinics and hospital. The second follow-up response was obtained two weeks later. Test-retest reliability was calculated using Spearman's correlation coefficient (r). The rho value was found to be 0.87, which implies an acceptable level of test-retest reliability.

2.6. Data Analysis. The participants' responses were encoded and the data were analyzed using Statistical Package for the Social Sciences (IBM SPSS Statistics for Windows, version 20.0, IBM Corp., Armonk, NY, USA). Descriptive analysis was used to calculate the response proportion of each group of respondents for each item in the questionnaire. Public responses options to the survey questions related to education level, use of over-the-counter drugs, medical history, and over-the-counter drug and vitamin use were reduced to three categories: yes, no, and sometimes. This enabled more reader comprehensible confidence intervals for the relative proportions to be calculated. The level $P < 0.05$ was considered as the cut-off value for statistical significance.

3. Results

A total of 140 questionnaires were distributed over the study period of 3 months (October 2016 to December 2016). All of them were returned fully complete, giving a response rate of 100%.

3.1. Demographics. Among the 140 pregnant females who participated in this study, the majority were married (137; 97.1%), Arab (nonlocal) (80; 57.1%), and between 21 and 35 years of age (115; 82.1%). Eighty-nine (65.7%) of the participants held a university degree and only 12 (8.6%) reported that they work as healthcare personnel. Details about participants' personal information are presented in Table 1.

3.2. Education Level, Use of Over-the-Counter Medication, and Medical History. When the participants were asked if they knew the term "over-the-counter medications," more than three-quarters (106; 75.7%) of the participants reported "yes" while 34 (24.3%) reported that they had no idea about the meaning of the term. They were then asked based on the previous question about their level of knowledge towards over-the-counter medications (low to medium to advanced); 36 (25.7%) of the participants believe that their knowledge about OTC drug use and safety was low. 81 (57.9%) and 23 (16.4%) of the participants reported their knowledge as medium and advanced levels, respectively. However, the majority (132; 94.3%) of the participants agreed with the survey statement that OTC drugs were not safe to be used during pregnancy. Even though pregnant women included in this study were not happy to use over-the-counter medication during pregnancy, 60 (42.9%) believed in the safety of herbal products during pregnancy.

Of the 140 women included in the study, 137 (97%) reported that they are nonsmokers, 3 (2.1%) were diabetics, 4 (2.9%) were hypertensive patients, and half of them (70;

TABLE 1: Demographic characteristics of the participants.

Characteristic	Frequency (%)
Nationality	
Local	42 (30%)
Arab (nonlocal)	80 (57.1%)
Non-Arab (nonlocal)	18 (12.9%)
Age (years)	
15–20	3 (2.1%)
21–25	35 (25%)
26–30	51 (36.4%)
31–35	29 (20.7%)
36–40	14 (10%)
41–55	8 (5.7%)
Marital status	
Married	137 (97.1%)
Divorced	2 (1.4%)
Widowed	0
Separated	1 (0.7%)
Educational level	
Primary/secondary school	10 (7.1%)
High school	35 (25%)
University or college	89 (63.6%)
Other	6 (4.3%)
Do you have previous children?	
None	40 (28.6%)
One	43 (30.7%)
Two	24 (17.1%)
More than two	33 (23.6%)
Occupation	
Student	9 (6.4%)
Housewife	92 (65.7%)
Healthcare personnel (physician, nurse, or pharmacist)	12 (8.6%)
Employed in the non-healthcare sector	23 (16.4%)
Other	4 (2.9%)
Do you smoke?	
Yes	3 (2.1%)
No	137 (97.9%)

50%) used at least one over-the-counter medication before their conception day. Participants were divided further; 40 (28.6%) participants reported "yes" to the survey question "Have you ever used an over-the-counter drug or vitamin in your current pregnancy?" Even though majority (129; 92.1%) of the sample pool did not experience any side effects from the drugs they used during their pregnancy, 11 (7.8%) reported some side effects. Constipation (6; 4.3%) and headache (5; 3.6%) were the most common side effects reported by the participants. The response from participants about the use and reading of the medication leaflet was positive and promising. Ninety-eight (70%) of the pregnant females under

TABLE 2: Public responses to the survey questions related to education level, use of over-the-counter drugs, and medical history.

Survey items	Yes n (%)	No n (%)	Sometimes n (%)	95% CI for single proportion for "yes"
Do you know what is meant by over-the-counter drugs?	106 (75.7%)	34 (24.3%)	0	68.6–82.8
Do you think that all over-the-counter drugs are safe to be taken during pregnancy?	8 (5.7%)	132 (94.3%)	0	1.9–9.5
Do you think that all herbal medications are safe to be taken during pregnancy?	60 (42.9%)	80 (57.1%)	0	34.7–51.1
Have you ever used an over-the-counter drug before pregnancy?	70 (50%)	70 (50%)	0	41.7–58.2
Do you read/check the accompanying leaflet?	98 (70%)	11 (7.9%)	31 (22.1)	62.5–77.5
Have you ever used an over-the-counter drug or vitamin in your current pregnancy?	40 (28.6%)	99 (70.7%)	0	21.1–36.1
Did you experience any side effects from the over-the-counter drugs?	11 (7.8%)	129 (92.1%)	0	3.4–12.3
Headache	5 (3.6%)	135 (96.4%)		
Constipation	6 (4.3%)	134 (95/7%)		
Do you have any chronic diseases (hypertension, diabetes, or asthma)?	9 (6.4%)	131 (93.6%)	0	2.4–10.5
Diabetes	3 (2.1%)	137 (97.9%)		
Disc and migraine	1 (0.7%)	139 (99.3%)		
Hypertension	4 (2.9%)	136 (97.1%)		
Do you have a child with special needs? Hereditary disease	1 (0.7%)	139 (99.3%)	0	1.0–2.1

investigation reported "yes" to the survey question "Do you read/check the accompanying leaflet?" Table 2 summarizes the education level towards over-the-counter drugs, their use, and medical history.

3.3. Over-the-Counter Medication Use and Vitamin Use by Pregnant Women. The participants' answers were analyzed and a variety of responses were recorded for the questions concerning the vitamins that the pregnant women took during their pregnancy. They were encouraged to select more than one answer. Folic acid was used by 100 (36.2%) participants, calcium by 79 (28.6%), and iron by 97 (35.1%). The participants were then asked to write down any other vitamins that they were taking. The following question asked them to choose any of the mentioned over-the-counter drugs used during their pregnancy; Panadol was used by more than half of the participants (43; 55.1%) followed by Panadol All in One, (Cold and Flu) (15; 19.2%), Prospan (ivy leaf extract) (11; 14.1%), and ibuprofen (8; 10.3%). Table 3 summarizes the vitamins and over-the-counter drugs used by the pregnant women.

Responses were recorded for the survey question "Do you know the critical time for the use of over-the-counter drugs during pregnancy?" More than half (73; 55.7%) indicated the first trimester, while 46 (32.9%) believed it depended on the drug. The rest decided on the second trimester (6; 4.3%) and third trimester (10; 7.1%).

4. Discussion

In UAE, healthcare, like many other gulf countries, is provided to all residents through primary healthcare centers. Patients gain access to secondary or tertiary care through referral from primary healthcare centers. Both local and insured patients can seek medical services and collect their prescription medications from a wide range of hospital pharmacies free of charge. However, outside the secondary care sector, a major portion of noninsured and expatriate patients obtain their medication from the growing number of private community pharmacies.

It has been reported that, in UAE, like the rest of the world, people tend to go for self-medication for many reasons, which include the high cost of medical consultations, lack of time, long hours of waiting at the physician's clinic, and lack of trust in the physicians' medical knowledge. Furthermore, previous experience with a medical condition and its drug management and the lack or the unavailability of nearby health facilities were identified as reasons for seeking OTC medications [5]. OTC medications are beneficial for the treatment of minor ailments only if there is sufficient knowledge about the correct use of the medicines. There are at least five pieces of information required for appropriate OTC medications use: information about the active ingredient, indication, dosage and administration, side effects, and contraindications. Even though the majority (94.3%) of

TABLE 3: Public responses on the survey questions related to over-the-counter drug and vitamin use.

Survey items (multiple responses)	Yes n (%)	No n (%)	95% CI for single proportion for "yes" answer option (%)
Vitamins used by pregnant women			
Folic acid	100 (36.2%)	0	63.9–78.8
Calcium	79 (28.6%)	0	48.3–64.6
Iron	97 (35.1%)	0	61.7–76.9
Others	12 (8.4)	0	3.9–13.2
Magnesium	2 (1.4%)	0	
Multivitamins	3 (2.1%)	0	
Medications used by pregnant women			
Panadol	43 (55.1%)		23.1–38.3
Ibuprofen	8 (10.3%)		1.9–9.5
Panadol All in One (Cold and Flu)	15 (19.2%)		10.5–27.9
Prospan or any cough syrup	11 (14.1%)		6.4–21.8

respondents of this study believed that not all OTC drugs are safe to be used during pregnancy, more than one-quarter (28.6%) of pregnant women respondents reported that OTC medications and other herbal supplements were used during their pregnancy.

This trend is similar to the use reported in Texas (23.0%) and Pakistan (37.9%) [13, 15] and is far less than the usage among women in USA [16]. More than three-quarters (82.0%) of women in USA reported that they have used OTC drugs in the previous six months [16, 17]. This is important if one considers that the level of knowledge that mothers had about medicine was considered to be inadequate to support safe and effective self-medication reported elsewhere [18]. In this study, more than half (57.1%) of the participants disagreed and 42.9% agreed on the survey statement "herbal products are safe in pregnancy." Such finding is similar to those studies that reported high usage of herbal products among pregnant women [14, 16, 19]. An interesting aspect to consider in this question is the cultural background of the patients answering the question. Even though cultural backgrounds were not asked in this survey, many pregnant women originating from countries like Pakistan or the Indian subcontinent utilized traditional medicines as part of their cultural heritage [20]. The ingredients of these traditional medicines are mostly uncontrolled and used as per traditional practices.

Drug use during pregnancy is common [21]. Commonly used OTC medications are analgesics, antipyretics, cough syrups, antiemetics, herbal products, and nutritional supplements. The incidence of prescribed drugs ranges from 40% to 93% [22, 23] in economically developed countries; variation in this range is explained by exclusion, or respective inclusion of vitamins. Even though not all the drugs are associated with medical complications to the fetus and mother, some may lead to severe damage to both fetus and mother. High doses of acetylsalicylic acid result in increased perinatal mortality, neonatal hemorrhage, low birth weight, prolonged gestation/labor, and possible birth defects. On the other hand, the use of folic acid is essential in the first trimester of pregnancy to prevent neural tube defects [24]. In this

study, the most commonly used supplements were folic acid (36.2%), followed by iron (35.1%) and then calcium (28.6%). These drugs are commonly recommended by doctors and are recommended for use during pregnancy.

Our study findings were similar to the study findings of Inamdar et al. [25] and Hanafy et al. [26]; these authors found that 39% of pregnant women used iron and 26.6% used calcium. However, the use of folic acid was higher than that reported in our study. The use of folic acid was 69% in India [25] and 51% in Egypt [26]. Calcium has the benefits of reducing preeclampsia and hypertension and maintaining a healthy heart for both fetus and mother [27]. Iron is known to fight depression and build resistance to stress and disease in the mother as well as being an important part of the red blood cells as mothers have an increased maternal red blood mass [28]. Low iron levels are associated with premature delivery, low birth weight, and infant mortality [29, 30]. Hence, it may be advised for healthcare professionals to advise pregnant women on the proper usage of these medications. Encouraging pharmacists, who are able to counsel patients more commonly, to talk to pregnant women upon the purchase of these products may be a beneficial idea.

The first trimester is an important period of pregnancy; more care should be taken as it is the period of organogenesis, and drug intake during this period has a profound effect on the fetus. Even though more than half (55.7%) of the respondents are aware that the first trimester remains the most critical time for the pregnant women to take any medication as it interferes with the development of the fetus, still 4.3% and 7.1% of the respondents believe that the second and third trimesters are more important than the first trimester.

Analgesic drug use is high, with more than half (55.1%) of the pregnant women using paracetamol during the study period. This is consistent with the findings from Pakistan (43.6%) [13] and Ethiopia (37.5%) [31]. It is common knowledge that every drug incurs a side effect within the human body which is consistent with the finding that paracetamol might have an adverse effect on neurological development (psychomotor, behavioral, and temperamental outcomes for the child), irrelevant of the trimester exposure that took place [32].

Interestingly, 70% of the pregnant females under investigation reported "yes" to the survey statement "read the accompanying leaflet content before using the OTC drugs". One can presume that one of the reasons behind reading the OTC medication leaflet before taking the OTC was either a lack of knowledge on how to take the drug or fear of side effects of the medication.

Limitations of the Study. Even though study participants were asked about which trimester was critical for OTC drug use during pregnancy (trimester timeline), it was not taken into consideration when participants were invited to be a part of the study. This is hence a limitation of this study and it is recommended to consider this for future studies. Secondly, the study was conducted over a period of only three months and patients who were available at the clinics/hospitals were considered for inclusion. The limited sample size and relatively short study period may not allow generalizing the research outcomes. Lastly, patient records are not available to pharmacists in UAE, and pregnant women displayed unwillingness to share personal information with researchers due to cultural sensitivities. This is an important limitation that may be experienced by other researchers within the Arab world as well.

5. Conclusion

The reported 40% usage of OTC medications among pregnant women in this study is high and not healthy. The perception of the safety of herbal drugs among the pregnant women is worrisome. There is a need to educate, counsel, and increase awareness among pregnant women regarding safe OTC drug and herbal medicine use while pregnant in Sharjah, UAE.

Appendix

Awareness and Use of Over-the-Counter Drugs in Pregnant Women

Tick only one answer

Nationality:

☐ Local
☐ Nonlocal (Arab)
☐ Non-Arab

Age (years)

☐ 15–20
☐ 21–25
☐ 26–30
☐ 31–35
☐ 36–40

☐ 41–55

Marital status:

☐ Single
☐ Married
☐ Divorced
☐ Widowed
☐ Separated

Highest education completed

☐ Primary/secondary school (8-9 years of education)
☐ High school (11–13 years of education)
☐ University or college
☐ Other education; please specify: ....

Work situation at the start of pregnancy

☐ Student
☐ Housewife
☐ Healthcare personnel (physician, nurse, or pharmacist)
☐ Employed in the non-healthcare sector
☐ Unknown

Previous children

☐ None
☐ One
☐ Two
☐ More than two

Do you know what is meant by over-the-counter drugs?

☐ Yes
☐ No

What is your level of knowledge towards over-the-counter drugs?

☐ Low
☐ Medium
☐ Advanced

Do you think that all the OTC drugs are safe to be taken during pregnancy?

☐ Yes
☐ No

Do you think natural remedies are safe to be taken during pregnancy?

☐ Yes
☐ No

Have you ever used an over-the-counter Drug before pregnancy?

□ Yes

□ No

Have you ever used an OTC drug including vitamins in your current pregnancy?

□ Yes

□ No

If your answer is yes, please answer the following questions:

(i) Name the OTC drug or vitamin that you are using
....

(ii) Have you ever experienced any side effects from the OTC drugs?

□ Yes

□ No

(iii) If the answer is yes, answer the question below: after taking the OTC drug or vitamins, have you experienced any of these side effects?

□ Headache

□ Cough

□ Constipation

□ Common cold

Do you have any chronic diseases (hypertension, diabetes, asthma, etc.)?

□ Yes

□ No

If yes, please specify ....
Do you smoke?

□ Yes

□ No

Do you have a child with special needs?

□ Yes

□ No

If yes, is it

□ hereditary disease

□ for the first time in your family

□ due to a side effect of an OTC drug, name of the drug ....

Do you know the critical time for OTC drug use during pregnancy?

□ First trimester

□ Second trimester

□ Third trimester

□ It depends on the drug

Do you use any of these vitamins (you can choose more than one answer)?

□ Folic acid

□ Calcium

□ Iron

□ Other; please specify: ....

Do you use any of these medications (you can choose more than one answer)?

□ Paracetamol

□ Ibuprofen

□ Any pain killer

□ Panadol All in One (Cold and Flu)

□ Prospan or any cough syrup

Do you read/check the accompanying leaflet content?

□ Yes

□ No

□ Sometimes

Conflicts of Interest

The authors declare that they have no conflicts of interest.

References

[1] D. W. Matt and J. F. Borzelleca, Toxic effects on the female reproductive system during pregnancy, parturition, and lactation. Witorsch RJ, ed reproductive toxicology. 2nd ed. New York: Raven; 1995. p. 175-193.

[2] A. A. Mitchell, S. M. Gilboa, M. M. Werler et al., "Medication use during pregnancy, with particular focus on prescription drugs," *American Journal of Obstetrics and Gynecology*, vol. 205, no. 1, 51 pages, 1976.

[3] L. L. Brunton, B. A. Chabner, and B. C. Knollmann, *Goodman and Gillmans Pharmacological Basis of Therapeutics*, McGraw-Hill, China, 12th edition, 2011.

[4] M. C. Blehar, C. Spong, C. Grady, S. F. Goldkind, L. Sahin, and J. A. Clayton, "Enrolling pregnant women: issues in clinical research," *Women's Health Issues*, vol. 23, no. 1, pp. e39–e45, 2013.

[5] J. Servey and J. Chang, "Over-the-counter medications in pregnancy," *American Family Physician*, vol. 90, no. 8, pp. 548–555, 2014.

[6] CDC. Use of Medication in Pregnancy 2017. Available from: https://www.cdc.gov/pregnancy/meds/treatingfortwo/data.html.

[7] U.A.E. Population. United Arab Emirates Population 2017 2017. Available from: http://worldpopulationreview.com/countries/united-arab-emirates-population/.

[8] U. A. Emirates. Best Countries for Business: Forbes; 2017. Available from: https://www.forbes.com/places/united-arab-emirates/.

[9] F. A. Kamali and H. A. Bastaki, Any poor Emiratis out there?: TheNational; 2017. Available from: http://www.thenational.ae/lifestyle/any-poor-emiratis-out-there.

[10] Sharjahmedia. About Sharjah 2017. Available from: http://sharjahmedia.ae/en/about-sharjah/history.aspx.

[11] I. Mundi, United Arab Emirates-Birth rate-Historical Data Graphs per Year. 2017. Available from: http://www.indexmundi.com/g/g.aspx?c=tc&v=25.

[12] Tradingeconomics. United Arab Emirates - Birth rate, crude 2015. Available from: https://tradingeconomics.com/united-arab-emirates/birth-rate-crude-per-1-000-people-wb-data.html.

[13] R. Bohio, Z. P. Brohi, and F. Bohio, "Utilization of over the counter medication among pregnant women; a cross-sectional study conducted at Isra University Hospital, Hyderabad," Journal of the Pakistan Medical Association, vol. 66, no. 1, pp. 68–71, 2016.

[14] A. F. Sawalha, "Consumption of prescription and non-prescription medications by pregnant women: a cross sectional study in palestine," The Islamic University Journal, vol. 15, no. 2, pp. 41–57, 2007.

[15] Chpa.org. Statistics on OTC Use: Chpa.org.; 2016. Available from: http://www.chpa.org/marketstats.aspx.

[16] S. H. Hong, D. Spadaro, D. West, and S. H. Tak, "Patient valuation of pharmacist services for self care with OTC medications," Journal of Clinical Pharmacy and Therapeutics, vol. 30, no. 3, pp. 193–199, 2005.

[17] K. L. Kline and S. M. Westberg, "Over-the-counter medication use, perceived safety, and decision-making behaviors in pregnant women," Innovation in Pharmacy, vol. 2, no. 1, pp. 1–14, 2011.

[18] S. Suryawati, "CBIA: improving the quality of self-medication through mothers active learning," Essential Drugs Monitor, vol. 32, pp. 22-23, 2003.

[19] M. C. Staff, Herbal supplements: What to know before you buy: MAYOCLINIC; 2016. Available from: http://www.mayoclinic.org/healthy-lifestyle/nutrition-and-healthy-eating/in-depth/herbal-supplements/art-20046714.

[20] S. Hussain, F. Malik, N. Khalid et al., Alternative and Traditional Medicines Systems in Pakistan: History, Regulation, Trends, Usefulness, Challenges, Prospects and Limitations, 2010.

[21] J. G. C. van Hasselt, M. A. Andrew, M. F. Hebert, J. Tarning, P. Vicini, and D. R. Mattison, "The status of pharmacometrics in pregnancy: highlights from the 3rd American conference on pharmacometrics," British Journal of Clinical Pharmacology, vol. 74, no. 6, pp. 932–939, 2012.

[22] S. Donati, G. Baglio, A. Spinelli, and M. E. Grandolfo, "Drug use in pregnancy among Italian women," European Journal of Clinical Pharmacology, vol. 56, no. 4, pp. 323–328, 2000.

[23] H. Nordeng, G. Jacobsen, B. Nesheim, and A. Eskild, "Drug use in pregnancy among parous Scandinavian women," Norsk Epidemiologi, vol. 11, no. 1, 2009.

[24] B. M. A. Board, Buying pregnancy multivitamins: BabyCenter; 2016. Available from: https://www.babycentre.co.uk/a561818/buying-pregnancy-multivitamins.

[25] I. F. Inamdar, N. R. Aswa, V. K. Snokar et al., "Drug utilization pattern during pregnancy," Indian Medical Gazette, vol. 146, pp. 305–311, 2012.

[26] A. S. Hanafy, A. S. Sallam, F. I. Kharboush et al., "Drug utilization pattern during pregnalncy in Alexandria, Egypt," European Journal of Pharmaceutical and Medical Research, vol. 3, no. 2, pp. 19–29, 2016.

[27] WHO.int. WHO Guideline: Calcium supplementation in pregnant women: WHO.int.; 2013. Available from: http://apps.who.int/iris/bitstream/10665/85120/1/9789241505376_eng.pdf.

[28] Clevelandclinic.org. Cleveland clinic Clevelandclinic.org.; 2015. Available from: http://my.clevelandclinic.org/.

[29] C. s. F. Guide. Folic acid, iron and pregnancy: Government of Canada 2016. Available from: https://www.canada.ca/en/public-health/services/pregnancy/folic-acid-iron-pregnancy.html.

[30] Centrum.ca. Are You Getting Enough Iron?: WebMD; 2016. Available from: http://www.webmd.com/baby/are-you-getting-enough-iron.

[31] C. Kassaw and N. T. Wabe, "Pregnant women and non-steroidal anti-inflammatory drugs: Knowledge, perception and drug consumption pattern during pregnancy in Ethiopia," North American Journal of Medical Sciences, vol. 4, no. 2, pp. 72–76, 2012.

[32] R. E. Brandlistuen, E. Ystrom, I. Nulman, G. Koren, and H. Nordeng, "Prenatal paracetamol exposure and child neurodevelopment: A sibling-controlled cohort study," International Journal of Epidemiology, vol. 42, no. 6, Article ID dyt183, pp. 1702–1713, 2013.

10

Latency after Preterm Prelabor Rupture of the Membranes: Increased Risk for Periventricular Leukomalacia

Annick Denzler,[1] Tilo Burkhardt,[1] Giancarlo Natalucci,[2] and Roland Zimmermann[1]

[1] *Department of Obstetrics, Zurich University Hospital, Frauenklinikstraße 10, 8091 Zurich, Switzerland*
[2] *Department of Neonatology, Zurich University Hospital, Frauenklinikstraße 10, 8091 Zurich, Switzerland*

Correspondence should be addressed to Tilo Burkhardt; tilo.burkhardt@usz.ch

Academic Editor: Rosa Corcoy

Objective. To identify the risk factors for cystic periventricular leukomalacia (cPVL) and their implications for deciding between immediate delivery and conservative management of preterm prelabor rupture of the membranes (pPROM). *Methods.* The following risk factors were compared between cPVL infants and 6440 controls: chorioamnionitis, sex, gestational age (GA), birth weight, pPROM, and pPROM-delivery interval. Factor impact on cPVL risk and clinical decision-making was determined by multivariate logistic regression. *Results.* Overall cPVL prevalence ($n = 32$) was 0.99/1000 births. All cPVL infants but one were born <34 weeks of gestation and were <2500 g; 56% had histological chorioamnionitis versus 1.1% of controls (OR 35.9; 95%-CI 12.6–102.7). Because chorioamnionitis is a postnatal diagnosis, logistic regression was performed with prenatally available factors: pPROM-delivery interval >48 hours (OR 9.0; 95%-CI 4.1–20.0), male gender (OR 3.2; 95%-CI 1.4–7.3). GA was not a risk factor if birth weight was included. Risk decreased with increasing fetal weight despite a prolonged pPROM-delivery interval. *Conclusion.* pPROM-delivery interval is the single most important prenatally available risk factor for the development of cPVL. Immediate delivery favors babies with chorioamnionitis but disfavors those with non infectious pPROM. In the absence of clinical chorioamnionitis fetal weight gain may offset the inflammatory risk of cPVL caused by a prolonged pPROM-delivery interval.

1. Introduction

Cerebral palsy includes a group of nonprogressive movement disorders due to brain lesions or abnormalities in early development [1]. Its prevalence of 2 per 1000 newborns overall rises to 77 per 1000 preterms born at below 28 0/7 weeks of gestation [2, 3]. A major cause is cystic periventricular leukomalacia (cPVL) comprising necrosis and subsequent cyst formation of the periventricular white matter: 60–100% of children with cPVL develop cerebral palsy [4–6]. Although the etiology and pathogenesis of cPVL remain unelucidated, several perinatal risk factors appear involved [7]. Birth asphyxia is no longer assumed the principal culprit [8].

Chorioamnionitis is thought to provoke a fetal inflammatory response syndrome associated with increased fetal cytokines that may lead to neonatal brain injury. Several studies indicate that the cytokines can themselves damage white matter without bacteremia being required [8–15]. An important predictor of chorioamnionitis is preterm prelabor rupture of membranes (pPROM) [16]. One-third of women with pPROM have positive amniotic fluid cultures [17]. Chorioamnionitis is quite common and often subclinical: fever and inflammatory marker elevation are rare in the early stages, making diagnosis difficult. Against this background the optimal management of pPROM remains unknown. The risks of prematurity from immediate delivery have to be balanced against those of ascending intrauterine infection and its probable consequences. Moreover subclinical chorioamnionitis is believed to cause pPROM. At a gestational age below 34 0/7 weeks, half the gynecologists in Australia and New Zealand preferred to induce labor, while the other half chose conservative management [18]. Several studies recommend an active management after 30 weeks [19, 20]. A Cochrane review from 2010 found no evidence about which strategy is favorable [21]. Despite a lack of randomized studies [22] new British and German guidelines advise active management before 34 weeks and active management between 34 and 36 weeks. Zurich University Hospital has hitherto favored conservative management, delaying delivery until clinically mandatory, on the grounds that the higher mortality and morbidity of newborns at lower gestational age are proven whereas the effect of increasing cPVL risk by prolonging pregnancy remains unknown. Only a prospective randomized trial can provide a definite answer. The more limited objectives of the present study were to identify the risk factors for PVL in the conservative pPROM management setting and determine whether prolonging gestation outweighs the risk of cPVL due to chorioamnionitis.

2. Materials and Methods

The study population comprised all babies with cPVL born in Zurich University Hospital's obstetric department between 1993 and 2008. Cranial ultrasound was obtained in infants with gestational age below 32 0/7 weeks or birth weight below 1500 g at days 1, 3, and 7 of life and repeated weekly until hospital discharge. cPVL was defined according to de Vries et al. [23]. All 6440 infants born between 2005 and 2007 and not affected by PVL served as controls.

During the study period women with premature contractions received tocolytic drugs (hexoprenaline only until 2001, nifedipine or hexoprenaline from 2002 to 2008) for 48 hours to allow lung maturation with 24 mg of betamethasone. Urinary tract infection or bacterial vaginosis was treated with antibiotics (co-amoxiclav or clindamycin). Steroids were repeated every 10 days until 2002. Since then, all women with threatened preterm delivery have received a single course of steroids. Tocolysis was maintained thereafter if contractions recurred after stopping tocolysis. Management of pPROM pregnancy was largely consistent with British Greentop Guideline no. 44 [17]. After pPROM co-amoxiclav was used until 2001 when it was changed to erythromycin [24], chorioamnionitis was monitored using blood tests (including leukocytes and C-reactive protein (CRP) 12 hourly for the first 48 hours), maternal temperature, and fetal heart rate. Clinical chorioamnionitis ($\geq$ 3 of following markers: leukocytes > 20,000/μL, CRP > 40 mg/dL, maternal temperature > 38°C, maternal tachycardia > 100 bpm, and fetal tachycardia > 160 bpm) was treated with antibiotics (co-amoxiclav) and prompt delivery. If the diagnosis was uncertain, delivery was deferred until chorioamnionitis became clinically obvious or delivery could be delayed no longer for other reasons. Diagnosis was based on placental histology, positive amniotic fluid cultures sampled at cesarean section, or clinical parameters.

Babies born below 25 0/7 weeks were excluded in both groups because in most instances neonatal care was restricted to comfort care. Infants with cPVL were monitored for long-term follow-up. Neurodevelopmental disability was classified according to Palisano et al. [25]. The risk factors recorded in both groups were chorioamnionitis, pPROM-delivery interval, gestational age at delivery, birth weight, gender, race, and parity.

All statistical analyses were performed with STATA 10 Statistics/Data Analysis Software (Stata Corporation, College Station, TX) using Pearson's χ^2 test for comparisons of

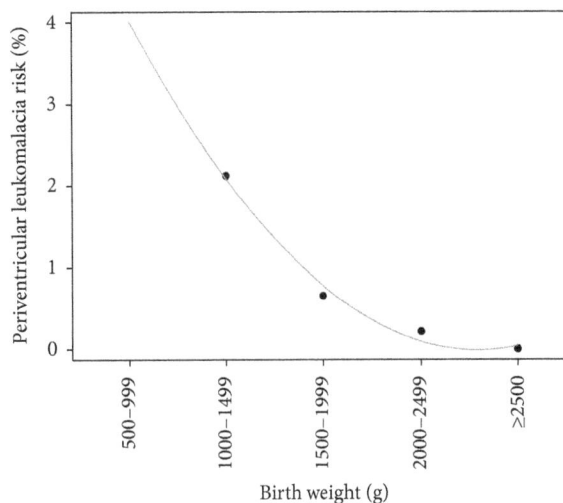

FIGURE 1: Exponential decrease in periventricular leukomalacia risk with increasing birth weight.

frequencies and Wilcoxon's rank-sum test for group comparisons. Odds ratios (OR) with 95% confidence intervals (CI) were calculated. Subsequent to univariate analysis, multivariate logistic regression was performed to test the impact of factors such as chorioamnionitis, gestational age, birth weight, gender, and pPROM-delivery interval on the incidence of cPVL. The results were used to calculate the risks of developing cPVL at different fetal weights and pPROM-delivery intervals.

Given that the analysis was of anonymized data, the study was exempt from local institutional review board approval. Follow-up data of study preterms below 32 0/7 weeks were extracted from the prospective national database of the Swiss Neonatal Network & Follow-up Group. According to the recommendations of our Research Ethics Committee the investigators were obliged to inform parents about the scientific use of anonymized data. Parents had the right to refuse participation of their child.

3. Results

Between 1993 and 2008, 32,276 infants were born at Zurich University Hospital, including 6027 (18.7%) preterms (below 37 0/7 weeks); over the same period 32 cases of cPVL were recorded, representing an overall prevalence of 0.99‰ (Tables 1 and 2).

cPVL prevalence among preterm infants was 5.3‰. All 32 infants with PVL were delivered preterm and all but one before 34 0/7 weeks. cPVL risk decreased exponentially with increasing birth weight (Figure 1) and increasing gestational age. Males were 3 times more affected than females (male : female ratio 24 : 8). All birth weights in newborns with cPVL were less than 2500 g (Table 1). The individual pPROM-delivery intervals of all PVL cases are shown in Figure 2.

Median infant age at cPVL diagnosis was 19 days (3–40 days). Of the 32 infants, five (16%) died within the first 6 weeks after birth. Of the 27 surviving infants, three (11%)

TABLE 1: Baseline cystic periventricular leukomalacia (cPVL) and control group characteristics.

Characteristic	cPVL ($n = 32$)	Controls ($n = 6,440$)	P
Gestational age (d)	207.5 (184–255)	273 (168–297)	<0.001
Below 34 gestational weeks (%)	97	9	<0.001
Multiparous (n [%])	12 (38)	3145 (49)	0.198
Birth weight (g, median [range])	1197.5 (740–2250)	3270 (300–5700)	<0.001
PROM (n [%])	18 (56)	714 (11)	<0.001
pPROM-delivery interval (h, median [range])	38 (0–960)	1.3 (0–2170)	0.004
Chorioamnionitis (n [%])	18 (56)	73 (1)	<0.001
Lung maturation administration (n [%])	27 (84)	281 (5)	<0.001
Infant sex (n [%])			
Female	8 (25)	3049 (47)	0.012
Male	24 (75)	3390 (53)	

PROM: premature rupture of the membranes; pPROM: preterm premature rupture of the membranes.

TABLE 2: Characteristics and management of the cystic periventricular leukomalacia (cPVL) group ($n = 32$) by study period.

Characteristic	Time period 1993–2001	Time period 2002–2008	Overall 1993–2008
Chorioamnionitis			
Yes	12 (60)	6 (50)	18 (56)
No	6 (30)	6 (50)	12 (38)
Unknown	2 (10)	0 (0)	2 (6)
Premature rupture of membranes			
Yes	11 (55)	7 (58)	18 (56)
No	9 (45)	5 (42)	14 (44)
Antenatal betamethasone			
Yes	15 (75)	12 (100)	27 (84)
No	5 (25)	0 (0)	5 (16)
Infant sex			
Male	15 (75)	9 (75)	24 (75)
Female	5 (25)	3 (25)	8 (25)
Total	20 (1.3‰)	12 (0.7‰)	32 (0.95‰)

Data are n (%).

were lost to follow-up (parental refusal), while 24 (89%) were neurodevelopmentally assessed at a median (range) age of 3.8 years (2.0–10.2 years): one (4%) was normal, nine (38%) were moderately disabled, defined as cerebral palsy grade <3 according to the Gross Motor Function Classification System (GMFCS), or cognitive impairment with developmental quotient 55–69, or moderate visual or hearing impairment, and 14/24 (54%) were severely disabled, defined as disabling cerebral palsy (grade 3–5 GMFCS), or severe cognitive disability with developmental quotient <55, or major visual or hearing impairment.

Histologically confirmed chorioamnionitis was present in 16 cPVL infants (50%). A further two infants, for whom placental histology was missing, had ≥3 markers of clinical chorioamnionitis: leukocytes > 20,000/μL, CRP > 40 mg/dL, maternal temperature > 38°C, maternal tachycardia > 100 bpm, and fetal tachycardia > 160 bpm. Thus, 18/32 cases (56%) were classified as having been complicated by chorioamnionitis. Two cases were assigned

to the nonchorioamnionitis group despite the absence of placental histology and a number of clinical parameters.

The control group included 134 cases of suspected chorioamnionitis. Review of the placental histology and clinical parameters reduced these to 71 cases of histological chorioamnionitis and two cases of clinical chorioamnionitis in the absence of placental histology. Chorioamnionitis thus complicated 73/6440 (1.1%) of control deliveries.

Preliminary logistic regression revealed significant associations between cPVL and chorioamnionitis, male sex, and birth weight. Chorioamnionitis had the highest impact on cPVL risk (OR 35.9, 95% CI 12.6–102.7). However, because a prenatal diagnosis of chorioamnionitis is often not possible, logistic regression was performed, replacing chorioamnionitis by the pPROM-delivery interval. This revealed significant impacts on cPVL by sex ($P = 0.008$), pPROM-delivery interval > 48 hours ($P < 0.001$), and fetal weight ($P < 0.001$; Table 3).

TABLE 3: Multivariate logistic regression analysis of the influence of fetal sex, preterm premature rupture of the membranes- (pPROM-) delivery interval, and birth weight on cystic periventricular leukomalacia (cPVL) prevalence.

Covariate	cPVL	P
Sex		
Female*	1	
Male	3.1 (1.3–7.1)	0.008
pPROM-delivery interval		
≤48 h*	1	
>48 h	8.2 (3.8–17.5)	<0.001
Per 100 g higher fetal weight	0.85 (0.81–0.89)	<0.001

Data are adjusted odds ratios (95% confidence intervals).
*Baseline category.

TABLE 4: Regression analysis of the impact of different birth weights and preterm premature rupture of membranes- (pPROM-) delivery intervals on periventricular leukomalacia risk, assuming fetal weight gains of 0 g in 24 h and 48 h, 200 g in 1 week, and 400 g in 2 weeks [26]. Data are estimated incidence of periventricular leukomalacia.

(a) Male infants

	Birth weight				
	500 g	1000 g	1500 g	2000 g	2500 g
pPROM-delivery interval					
0 h	0.268	0.096	0.035	0.012	0.004
24 h	0.279	0.100	0.036	0.013	0.005
48 h	0.291	0.105	0.038	0.014	0.005
1 week	0.240	0.086	0.031	0.012	0.004
2 weeks	0.214	0.077	0.028	0.010	0.004

(b) Female infants

	Birth weight				
	500 g	1000 g	1500 g	2000 g	2500 g
pPROM-delivery interval					
0 h	0.081	0.029	0.010	0.004	0.001
24 h	0.085	0.030	0.011	0.004	0.001
48 h	0.088	0.032	0.011	0.004	0.001
1 week	0.073	0.026	0.009	0.003	0.001
2 weeks	0.065	0.023	0.008	0.003	0.001

Further multiple logistic regression analyses revealed significant associations between chorioamnionitis and pPROM-delivery interval > 24 hours ($P = 0.002$) and gestational age ($P < 0.001$). No significant influence of ethnicity ($P = 0.49$), fetal weight ($P = 0.37$), or parity ($P = 0.79$) was observed.

According to logistic regression analyses tabulation of estimated cPVL incidence at varying pPROM-delivery intervals and birth weights for boys and girls (Table 4), assuming fetal weight gain of 200 g/week [26], revealed a slight rise in the first 48 hours, followed by a significantly lower risk after the first and second week of prolongation of pregnancy. Increasing fetal weight during pPROM latency had a far stronger protective effect despite a prolonged pPROM-delivery interval being a risk factor for cPVL.

4. Discussion

Zurich University Hospital's obstetrics department is a tertiary referral center. This accounts for the high prevalence of preterm deliveries compared to the national average (19% versus 9%) [27]. The prevalence of cPVL in our study group (0.99‰) appears lower than the few reports in the literature. Hamrick et al. reported an incidence of 1.8% at UC San Francisco in 1992, falling to 0.2% in 2002; the incidence of cPVL in children weighing <1500 g decreased from 2.9% to 0.5% over the same period [28].

The difference may be partly due to Zurich's conservative management of newborns below 25 0/7 weeks of gestation (restriction to comfort care in the majority of cases) [29]. We may also have missed some cases of late cPVL diagnosis in children born after 32 0/7 weeks (there were no instances of late diagnosis of brain lesions in preterms included in long-term follow-up). Given our small sample size, we could only extrapolate cPVL incidence for birth weights <1000 g (Figure 1). The Vermont Oxford Network reported approximately 3% cPVL at birth weights 751–1500 g; risk was highest (6%) at birth weights <751 g [30]. Our data confirm the reported exponential decrease in cPVL incidence with increasing birth weight [28, 30]. They also confirm a similar exponential decrease with advancing gestational age independently of birth weight [30]. Again, our data at below 26 0/7 weeks are not comparable to other centers due to our conservative management of newborns around 25 0/7 weeks.

Our data support the dependency of cPVL risk on the pPROM-delivery interval [8, 31], but not on either low parity or PROM [8, 10, 31]. The finding of a 4 : 1 male/female ratio confirms previous reports [8, 15, 31] but remains unelucidated.

We also confirmed the several reports of a significant association between cPVL and chorioamnionitis [8, 9, 11, 14, 15]. The fact that only one cPVL baby had a positive blood culture within 3 days of birth supports the hypothesis that fetal inflammatory response syndrome is perfectly capable of causing brain damage even in the absence of bacteremia [32–34]. Apart from being a risk factor for cPVL, chorioamnionitis is well-recognized as correlating with neonatal morbidity and mortality [32–34].

Unfortunately, these risk factors cannot resolve our strategic dilemma of immediate versus delayed delivery for lowering short-term mortality and long-term sequelae. Chorioamnionitis is a major complication of pPROM but probably even more often the cause of pPROM.

The increase in cPVL risk during the first 48 hours after pPROM and the substantial decrease thereafter at varying birth weights and pPROM-delivery intervals (Table 4) can be interpreted in several ways. For example, the initial increase may relate to the use of antenatal steroids to induce lung maturation. Steroids could facilitate the spread of bacterial infection; they could also modulate the fetal inflammatory cytokines thought to cause brain damage [14]. Corroborative evidence is that the incidence of cPVL in our group decreased from 1.3‰ on repeated steroid courses to 0.7‰ on single-course steroids (although we must admit to having concomitantly switched to erythromycin and introduced nifedipine

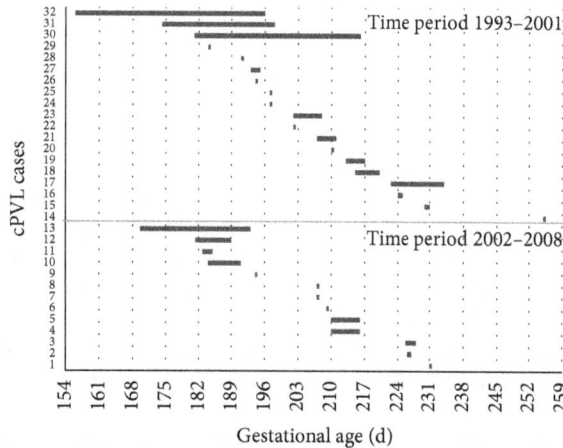

FIGURE 2: Data from 32 cPVL cases in two time periods. Each bar represents a pregnancy with pPROM-delivery interval beginning with gestational age of pPROM.

tocolysis). This study could not add any information about the impact of the different changed interventions to the lower cPVL incidence 2002–2008.

Another explanation is that the inverted U-shaped risk for cPVL with respect to the pPROM-delivery interval results from superposing two distinct groups of women: one with pPROM due to chorioamnionitis and the other with pPROM from a noninfectious cause. Most chorioamniotic pregnancies will deliver within a few days after pPROM. Thus, women still pregnant after one week of pPROM are more likely to have a noninfectious cause of fluid leakage. As a consequence, delaying delivery in these cases would lower cPVL risk by allowing birth weight to increase. At the same time, by increasing gestational age and birth weight, this strategy would substantially decrease all other complications of prematurity such as cerebral hemorrhage or lung pathology [35]. Conversely, a conservative strategy would increase cPVL risk in the infectious group. An increased risk for neurodevelopmental impairment in the first 48 to 72 hours after pPROM was also observed in a large French cohort with 1884 infants born at 24–32 weeks of gestational age [36].

Given this strong association between cPVL and chorioamnionitis, it is absolutely essential to diagnose intrauterine infection as early as possible. This points once again to the urgent need for a tool that reliably diagnoses chorioamnionitis.

In the absence of such a tool, either strategy carries a considerable risk of Pyrrhic victory. Because cPVL affects only a small proportion of newborns, with other problems of prematurity playing a much larger role, it seems not unreasonable to pursue a conservative strategy until prospective randomized trials provide a definitive answer or, at the least, until we have a reliable test for the early diagnosis of chorioamnionitis. Perinatal morbidity is strongly correlated with prematurity and latency does not appear to worsen outcome in pPROM [37].

The fact that chorioamnionitis and the pPROM-delivery interval seem to have a high impact on the risk of developing cPVL in our study could have important consequences for the future management of pPROM.

The strengths of this study are that all infants and mothers were monitored in the same department and that all preterms below 32 0/7 weeks received long-term follow-up, where possible (the actual follow-up rate was 89%). Only in midstudy were there any relevant changes in the management of pPROM (antibiotics, tocolytic, and steroid courses).

The study's limitations lie in its retrospective design and small cPVL sample size. We had particularly few birth weights below 1000 g, partly because the Swiss Society of Neonatology recommends restricting neonatal management to comfort care at gestational ages below 24 0/7 weeks. Between 24 0/7 and 25 6/7 weeks of gestation the decision to undertake intensive care is individual and influenced by prenatal factors such as birth weight, gender, antenatal steroid use, intrauterine growth restriction, chorioamnionitis, fetal malformation, multiple gestation, and clinical condition immediately after delivery (asphyxia, heart rate, activity, and response to initial resuscitation). Intervention continues in the neonatal intensive care unit with the primary goal of survival with an acceptable quality of life [29]. Our results are helpful for deliveries between 26 and 34 weeks of gestation only.

Other factors accounting for small sample size in any study of this kind include the fact that the true number of newborns with cPVL can be difficult to evaluate due to early postnatal death, especially when gestational age is very low. cPVL can often only be diagnosed weeks after birth because it takes time for the periventricular cysts to become visible on ultrasound. Failure of underreporting when making a late diagnosis of cPVL is another source.

Even if a prolonged pPROM-delivery interval may briefly increase the risk of cPVL, we believe that conservative management makes sense in the absence of clinical chorioamnionitis. Higher infant weight at delivery compensates for the impact of pPROM latency on neonatal outcome provided that the pregnancy can be prolonged by more than 48 hours.

Conflict of Interests

The authors declare that they have no financial or nonfinancial conflict of interests.

Authors' Contribution

Annick Denzler and Tilo Burkhardt have made substantial contributions to acquisition of obstetrical data and analysis and interpretation of all data. Giancarlo Natalucci has substantial contributions to acquisition of neonatal and outcome data. Roland Zimmermann conceived of the study and participated in coordination and helped to draft the paper. All authors read and approved the final paper. Annick Denzler and Tilo Burkhardt contributed equally to the study and paper.

References

[1] F. Stanley, E. Blair, and E. Alberman, "Pathways to cerebral palsy involving very preterm birth," in *Cerebral Palsies Epidemiology*

& Causal Pathways, F. Stanley, E. Blair, and E. Alberman, Eds., pp. 60–82, Mac Keith Press, London, UK, 2000.

[2] K. Himmelmann, G. Hagberg, E. Beckung, B. Hagberg, and P. Uvebrant, "The changing panorama of cerebral palsy in Sweden. IX. Prevalence and origin in the birth-year period 1995–1998," Acta Paediatrica, vol. 94, no. 3, pp. 287–294, 2005.

[3] S. Winter, A. Autry, C. Boyle, and M. Yeargin-Allsopp, "Trends in the prevalence of cerebral palsy in a population-based study," Pediatrics, vol. 110, no. 6, pp. 1220–1225, 2002.

[4] A. Leviton and N. Paneth, "White matter damage in preterm newborns: an epidemiologic perspective," Early Human Development, vol. 24, no. 1, pp. 1–22, 1990.

[5] J. J. Volpe and A. Zipurksy, "Neurobiology of periventricular leukomalacia in the premature infant," Pediatric Research, vol. 50, no. 5, pp. 553–562, 2001.

[6] Y. Murata, A. Itakura, K. Matsuzawa, A. Okumura, K. Wakai, and S. Mizutani, "Possible antenatal and perinatal related factors in development of cystic periventricular leukomalacia," Brain & Development, vol. 27, no. 1, pp. 17–21, 2005.

[7] I. Blumenthal, "Periventricular leucomalacia: a review," European Journal of Pediatrics, vol. 163, no. 8, pp. 435–442, 2004.

[8] M. M. Costantine, H. Y. How, K. Coppage, R. A. Maxwell, and B. M. Sibai, "Does peripartum infection increase the incidence of cerebral palsy in extremely low birthweight infants?" The American Journal of Obstetrics and Gynecology, vol. 196, no. 5, pp. e6–e8, 2007.

[9] R. Romero, J. Espinoza, L. F. Gonçalves, J. P. Kusanovic, L. Friel, and S. Hassan, "The role of inflammation and infection in preterm birth," Seminars in Reproductive Medicine, vol. 25, no. 1, pp. 21–39, 2007.

[10] Y. W. Wu, G. J. Escobar, J. K. Grether, L. A. Croen, J. D. Greene, and T. B. Newman, "Chorioamnionitis and cerebral palsy in term and near-term infants," Journal of the American Medical Association, vol. 290, no. 20, pp. 2677–2684, 2003.

[11] K. Tsukimori, H. Komatsu, T. Yoshimura et al., "Increased inflammatory markers are associated with early periventricular leukomalacia," Developmental Medicine and Child Neurology, vol. 49, no. 8, pp. 587–590, 2007.

[12] E. M. Graham, C. J. Holcroft, K. K. Rai, P. K. Donohue, and M. C. Allen, "Neonatal cerebral white matter injury in preterm infants is associated with culture positive infections and only rarely with metabolic acidosis," The American Journal of Obstetrics and Gynecology, vol. 191, no. 4, pp. 1305–1310, 2004.

[13] A. Bashiri, E. Burstein, and M. Mazor, "Cerebral palsy and fetal inflammatory response syndrome: a review," Journal of Perinatal Medicine, vol. 34, no. 1, pp. 5–12, 2006.

[14] G. Rocha, E. Proença, C. Quintas, T. Rodrigues, and H. Guimaríes, "Chorioamnionitis and brain damage in the preterm newborn," Journal of Maternal-Fetal and Neonatal Medicine, vol. 20, no. 10, pp. 745–749, 2007.

[15] E. Hatzidaki, E. Giahnakis, S. Maraka et al., "Risk factors for periventricular leukomalacia," Acta Obstetricia et Gynecologica Scandinavica, vol. 88, no. 1, pp. 110–115, 2009.

[16] B. M. Mercer, "Preterm premature rupture of the membranes," Obstetrics and Gynecology, vol. 101, no. 1, pp. 178–193, 2003.

[17] RCOG, "Guideline No. 44: Preterm prelabour rupture of membranes," November 2006.

[18] S. Buchanan, C. Crowther, and J. Morris, "Preterm prelabour rupture of the membranes: a survey of current practice," The Australian and New Zealand Journal of Obstetrics and Gynaecology, vol. 44, no. 5, pp. 400–403, 2004.

[19] L. Hartling, R. Chari, C. Friesen, B. Vandermeer, and T. Lacaze-Masmonteil, "A systematic review of intentional delivery in women with preterm prelabor rupture of membranes," Journal of Maternal-Fetal and Neonatal Medicine, vol. 19, no. 3, pp. 177–187, 2006.

[20] J. C. Pasquier, E. Bujold, M. Rabilloud et al., "Effect of latency period after premature rupture of membranes on 2 years infant mortality (DOMINOS study)," European Journal of Obstetrics Gynecology and Reproductive Biology, vol. 135, no. 1, pp. 21–27, 2007.

[21] S. L. Buchanan, C. A. Crowther, K. M. Levett, P. Middleton, and J. Morris, "Planned early birth versus expectant management for women with preterm prelabour rupture of membranes prior to 37 weeks' gestation for improving pregnancy outcome," The Cochrane Database of Systematic Reviews, no. 3, Article ID CD004735, 2010.

[22] AMWF-Leitlinien-Register: Empfehlungen zum Vorgehen bei vorzeitigem Blasensprung, http://www.awmf.org/.

[23] L. S. de Vries, P. Eken, and L. M. S. Dubowitz, "The spectrum of leukomalacia using cranial ultrasound," Behavioural Brain Research, vol. 49, no. 1, pp. 1–6, 1992.

[24] S. L. Kenyon, D. J. Taylor, and W. Tarnow-Mordi, "Broad-spectrum antibiotics for preterm, prelabour rupture of fetal membranes: the ORACLE I randomised trial," The Lancet, vol. 357, no. 9261, pp. 979–988, 2001.

[25] R. Palisano, P. Rosenbaum, S. Walter, D. Russell, E. Wood, and B. Galuppi, "Development and reliability of a system to classify gross motor function in children with cerebral palsy," Developmental Medicine & Child Neurology, vol. 39, no. 4, pp. 214–223, 1997.

[26] G. M. Beutler, J. Kurmanaviclus, M. Hoffmann, E. Welzl, R. Huch, and M. Bajka, "New nomogram for foetal weight estimation based on Hadlock's two-parameter formula," Ultraschall in der Medizin, vol. 25, no. 1, pp. 58–64, 2004.

[27] Bundesamt für Statistik (BFS), Neugeborene in Schweizer Spitälern 2004, Stat Santé, 2004.

[28] S. E. G. Hamrick, S. P. Miller, C. Leonard et al., "Trends in severe brain injury and neurodevelopmental outcome in premature newborn infants: the role of cystic periventricular leukomalacia," Journal of Pediatrics, vol. 145, no. 5, pp. 593–599, 2004.

[29] T. Berger, V. Büttiker, J. Fauchère et al., "ecommendations for the care of infants born at the limit of viability (gestational age 22-26 weeks)," in Swiss Society of Neonatology, 2002.

[30] Vermont Oxford Network, Vermont-Oxford Network Expanded Database Summary, Burlington, Burlington, Vt, USA, 2006.

[31] M. Bauer, C. Fast, J. Haas, B. Resch, U. Lang, and B. Pertl, "Cystic periventricular leukomalacia in preterm infants: an analysis of obstetric risk factors," Early Human Development, vol. 85, no. 3, pp. 163–169, 2009.

[32] J. M. Zhang, F. T. Kraus, and T. I. Aquino, "Chorioamnionitis: a comparative histologic, bacteriologic, and clinical study," International Journal of Gynecological Pathology, vol. 4, no. 1, pp. 1–10, 1985.

[33] J. V. Been, I. G. I. J. G. Rours, R. F. Kornelisse et al., "Histologic chorioamnionitis, fetal involvement, and antenatal steroids: effects on neonatal outcome in preterm infants," The American Journal of Obstetrics and Gynecology, vol. 201, no. 6, pp. 587.e1–587.e8, 2009.

[34] A. Wolfensberger, R. Zimmermann, and U. Von Mandach, "Neonatal mortality and morbidity after aggressive long-term

tocolysis for preterm premature rupture of the membranes," *Fetal Diagnosis and Therapy*, vol. 21, no. 4, pp. 366–373, 2006.

[35] T. P. Waters and B. M. Mercer, "The management of preterm premature rupture of the membranes near the limit of fetal viability," *The American Journal of Obstetrics and Gynecology*, vol. 201, no. 3, pp. 230–240, 2009.

[36] T. Mura, J.-C. Picaud, B. Larroque et al., "Cognitive impairment at age 5 years in very preterm infants born following premature rupture of membranes," *The Journal of Pediatrics*, vol. 163, no. 2, pp. 435.e2–440.e2, 2013.

[37] T. A. Manuck, C. C. Maclean, R. M. Silver, and M. W. Varner, "Preterm premature rupture of membranes: does the duration of latency influence perinatal outcomes?" *American Journal of Obstetrics & Gynecology*, vol. 201, no. 4, pp. 414.e1–414.e6, 2009.

11

The Relationship of Objectively Measured Physical Activity and Sedentary Behaviour with Gestational Weight Gain and Birth Weight

Anneloes E. Ruifrok,[1,2] Ellen Althuizen,[3] Nicolette Oostdam,[3] Willem van Mechelen,[3] Ben Willem Mol,[1] Christianne J. M. de Groot,[2] and Mireille N. M. van Poppel[3]

[1] Department of Obstetrics, Gynaecology and Fertility, Faculty of Medicine, University of Amsterdam (AMC-UvA), Meibergdreef 9, 1105 AZ Amsterdam, The Netherlands
[2] Department of Obstetrics and Gynaecology, Faculty of Medicine, VU University Medical Center, P.O. Box 7057, 1007 MB Amsterdam, The Netherlands
[3] Department of Public and Occupational Health, EMGO+ Institute for Health and Care Research, VU University Medical Center, Van der Boechorststraat 7, 1081 BT Amsterdam, The Netherlands

Correspondence should be addressed to Anneloes E. Ruifrok; anneloesruifrok@gmail.com

Academic Editor: Jeffrey Keelan

Objective. To evaluate the relationship of physical activity (PA) and sedentary behaviour with gestational weight gain (GWG) and birth weight. *Design.* Combined data from two prospective studies: (1) nulliparous pregnant women without BMI restrictions and (2) overweight and obese pregnant women at risk for gestational diabetes. *Methods.* Daily PA and sedentary behaviour were measured with an accelerometer around 15 and at 32–35 weeks of gestation. The association between time spent in moderate-to-vigorous PA (MVPA) and in sedentary activities with GWG and birth weight was determined. Main outcome measures were GWG between 15 and 32 weeks of gestation, average GWG per week, and birth weight. *Results.* We studied 111 women. Early in pregnancy, 32% of women spent ≥30 minutes/day in at least moderate PA versus 12% in late pregnancy. No significant associations were found between time spent in MVPA or sedentary behaviour with GWG or birth weight. *Conclusions.* We found no relation between MVPA and sedentary behaviour with GWG or birth weight. The small percentage of women meeting the recommended levels of PA indicates the need to inform and support pregnant women to maintain regular PA, as there seems to be no adverse effect on birth weight and maintaining PA increases overall health.

1. Introduction

Excessive weight gain during pregnancy is associated with an increased risk of obstetrical, maternal, and fetal complications [1–4] and postpartum weight retention [5]. It increases the risk of obesity in children [5–7]. This contributes to the prevalence of women who are overweight or obese and increases the long-term risk of body weight-associated diseases, which impose a great pressure on health care [5, 8–12].

The American Institute of Medicine (IOM) updated their evidence-based guidelines for weight development during pregnancy in 2009 [13]. However, 53% of all women gain more weight than advised by the IOM. This is even more pronounced in women with overweight or obesity, with 68.9% and 59.8%, respectively, exceeding the recommendations [14].

Many trials have been conducted evaluating the effect of different lifestyle interventions on gestational weight gain (GWG) and adverse pregnancy outcomes, which were recently reviewed and combined in a meta-analysis [15, 16]. Combining results of 15 interventions consisting of physical activity (PA) alone did not result in a statistically significant effect on GWG and showed a very small but statistically significant reduction in mean birth weight.

However, it must be noted that the compliance with the interventions was either not assessed or insufficient in some trials. Furthermore, the total number of PA of participants was often not measured. Therefore, a possible compensation of PA levels outside of the intervention sessions could not be taken into account. In most studies that did measure total PA, this was done with questionnaires, which might often not give a valid estimate of PA levels [17]. All in all, although the design of intervention studies in general allows for conclusions with regard to causality, the mentioned methodological shortcomings hamper causal inference of PA leading to lower GWG and birth weight.

The relationship between sedentary behaviour and weight (gain) has been found in women and adolescent girls outside of pregnancy [18, 19]. In pregnancy, US women spent more than half of the monitored day in sedentary behaviour [20]. However, whether the amount of time spent sedentary influences weight gain or birth weight is currently unknown.

The primary aim of this study was therefore to examine the relationship of objectively measured physical activity with sedentary behaviour at two time points in pregnancy with gestational weight gain and birth weight in a population with a wide range of BMI.

2. Methods

We performed a secondary analysis of data of the randomized controlled trials performed by Althuizen et al. [21] (ISRCTN85313483) and Oostdam et al. [22, 23] (NTR1139). The interventions evaluated in the two trials were not effective in reducing gestational weight gain in the total study population [23, 24]. Data from both trials were combined and analysed as a cohort, as the study design and procedures were similar for both trials. All participants were healthy pregnant women, only the BMI's were different (no BMI restrictions (Althuizen) and overweight or obese (Oostdam)). In both trials, the participants were followed from 15 weeks of gestation until delivery, with objective measurements of physical activity and sedentary behaviour and body weight at baseline (around 15 weeks of gestation) and at 32–35 weeks of gestation. Birth weight was reported in questionnaires. The Medical Ethics Committee of the VU University Medical Center had approved design, protocols, and informed consent procedures of both studies.

The first cohort consisted of nulliparous pregnant women without BMI restrictions. A complete description of the inclusion and exclusion criteria has been published in Althuizen et al. [21]. The second cohort consisted of pregnant women with a BMI of >25 kg/m^2 and at increased risk for GDM. Women were considered to be at an increased risk for GDM if they were obese (body mass index, BMI $\geq$ 30) or overweight (BMI $\geq$ 25) and had at least one of the three following characteristics: (1) history of macrosomia (offspring with a birth weight above the 97th percentile of gestational age), (2) history of GDM, or (3) first-grade relative with DM2. Exclusion criteria included recruitment after 20 weeks of gestation, age under 18 years, inadequate knowledge of the Dutch language, having been diagnosed with (gestational) diabetes mellitus before randomization, and severe chronic disease. A complete description of the inclusion and exclusion criteria has been published in Oostdam et al. [22]. For this paper, we excluded women with a twin pregnancy from the analyses.

The relationship of objectively measured physical activity (PA) and sedentary behaviour with gestational weight gain and birth weight was evaluated. The first measurements were at baseline (around 15 weeks of gestation), and the last measurements at 35 weeks of gestation in cohort 1 and at 32 weeks of gestation in cohort 2.

Maternal body weight was measured using calibrated electronic scales, with participants wearing only indoor clothing and no shoes. Prepregnancy weight was self-reported. On the first measurement, maternal body height was measured with bare feet and a (wall mounted) height scale. The measured height and weight were used to calculate BMI (kg/m^2). For the purpose of this paper, gestational weight gain (GWG) was defined as the weight gained between the first and the last measurements (kg). The neonatal outcome was birth weight, reported by the women in a questionnaire six weeks postpartum.

Daily physical activity (PA) was measured objectively using an accelerometer (ActiTrainer accelerometer; Acti-Graph, Pensacola, FL, USA). This accelerometer is a compact, lightweight, and uniaxial device that measures and records time-varying acceleration. Days with at least 8-hour registration time were used. Total counts per minute were converted into light, moderate, and vigorous PA (100 to 2019 counts/min for light PA, 2020 to 5998 counts/min for moderate PA and $\geq$5999 counts/min for vigorous PA) [25]. Sedentary behaviour was defined as <100 counts/min. In subsequent analysis, time spent by the participants was measured as a percentage of total registration time. These subsequent analysis were time spent in any physical activity (total PA), in moderate-to-vigorous physical activity (MVPA) and sedentary time.

Ethnicity was derived from the country of birth of the participant's parents. An individual was considered to be white European if both parents were born in Europe (with the exception of Turkey and Morocco; two groups with a higher risk for GDM) or North America. Furthermore, level of education was assessed as the highest level an individual reported to have achieved, which was then divided into lower, middle, or higher educational levels. Moreover, participants were asked to report on their status of employment (yes or no). Gestational age at delivery was self-reported.

The maternal characteristics of the study are presented as means and standard deviations for continuous variables and as percentages for ordinal variables. For the outcomes gestational weight gain and birth weight, standard linear regression analysis was used to test the association between the percentage of time spent sedentary or in physical activity at baseline and between the change in MVPA and sedentary time from 15 weeks to 32–35 weeks of gestation and the outcome. Regression models were controlled for allocation to intervention or control group, the difference in gestational age between the two measurements (weight gain and weight gain/week) or gestational age at birth (birth weight), BMI at first measurement during pregnancy, and parity and age.

The analyses were checked for effect modification by age and BMI. It was concluded that effect modification was present in case the P value of the interaction term was significant ($P < 0.10$). All analyses were performed using SPSS 20.0 (Statistical Package for the Social Sciences, SPSS Inc., Chicago, IL, USA) for windows, and the level of significance was set to <0.05.

3. Results

A total of 390 women were included in the two trials: 269 in cohort 1 and 121 women in cohort 2. Of these women, 139 completed both baseline and late pregnancy data collection. Due to lack of compliance of the participants, data on objectively measured PA and sedentary behaviour were available for 111 (80%) women with a singleton pregnancy. They comprised the study sample for the analyses. The baseline characteristics of the study population and the outcome measures are presented in Table 1. The mean GWG was 10.3 (SD 4.3) kg, with an average of 0.55 (SD 0.22) kg per week and mean birth weight was 3545 (SD 441) g.

Total daily physical activity (PA) measured with accelerometers at baseline showed an average of 286 (SD 103) minutes per day (range 45 to 512 minutes per day). At 32–35 weeks of gestation the mean total PA was 273 (SD 103) minutes/day. At both times this accounted for 35% of registration time. Overall, the minutes spent per day performing moderate and vigorous PA (MVPA) reduced during the pregnancy. At baseline, the mean number of minutes of moderate and vigorous PA spent per week was 24 (SD 16) minutes/day. At 32–35 weeks of gestation the mean number of minutes of moderate and vigorous PA performed per week had decreased to 18 (SD 22) minutes/day. This was a drop from 3% to 2% of the total registration time. At baseline, 31% of the women spent ≥ 30 minutes/day in MVPA and therefore met the guidelines of the ACOG for sufficient PA [26]. At 32–35 weeks, this proportion dropped to 12% of the women.

Sedentary behaviour remained relatively stable during pregnancy, with women spending more than 500 minutes/day (65% of the registration time) sedentary at both time points.

No statistically significant association was found between MVPA or sedentary behaviour at 15 weeks with GWG or GWG/week (Table 2). Also no significant associations were found for changes in PA and sedentary behaviour from 15 to 32–35 weeks of gestation. With birth weight as outcome, also no significant associations were found with the percentage of time in MVPA or sedentary behaviour (Table 2). Gestational age was not related to any PA or sedentary behaviour parameter (data not shown). No effect modifications of age or BMI were found.

4. Discussion

In this study, the association between objectively measured moderate to vigorous PA and/or sedentary behaviour with gestational weight gain (GWG) and birth weight was examined. We found that neither PA nor sedentary behaviour had an association with GWG or birth weight.

This is in line with the findings of a meta-analysis of 15 trials, showing no significant reduction in GWG in trials evaluating PA interventions [15, 16]. In the same meta-analysis, the pooled result of 14 PA trials showed a small (−60 g) but significant reduction in birth weight [15, 16]. A different meta-analysis, by Streuling et al. [27], showed a reduction of 61 g (CI −1.17 to −1.06) in GWG in the group receiving a PA intervention. Our sample size was very likely insufficient to detect such a small reduction in birth weight. It was certainly insufficient to study the effect of PA on the number of babies born small or large for gestational age.

The relationship between objectively measured sedentary behaviour and GWG or birth weight has not been studied so far, to our knowledge. Although outside pregnancy, sedentary behaviour is related to weight status in girls and women [18, 19], we could not establish an association with GWG or birth weight. This would indicate that trying to reduce sedentary behaviour in pregnant women would not likely lead to reduced GWG or changes in birth weight.

The data used for this study were collected in two separate trials [21, 22], and the results presented here are from secondary analysis of the data. However, since the interventions neither had an effect on GWG nor on birth weight, the design and procedures were similar for both trials, and all participants were healthy pregnant women [21, 23], we felt justified in analysing the data as a cohort. By combining the two datasets, there was a wider variation in PA levels in the data, which is needed for assessing an association with outcomes. However, the participants did not include women who participated in regular vigorous exercise. Our results can thus not be extrapolated to women who continue to participate in competitive exercise or elite sports during pregnancy.

The data on birth weight were self-reported by the mothers about six weeks after birth. This might have led to some inaccuracy in our outcome measure. Other studies showed, however, that self-reports of birth weight are accurate [28, 29], with small, clinically nonrelevant differences between birth weight in medical records and self-reports [29].

The data on physical activity and sedentary behaviour were objectively measured, reducing the reporting bias and increasing the accuracy of the results. The accelerometer, used for monitoring the amount of PA and sedentary behaviour, is a uniaxial device that measures and records vertical acceleration. In the Netherlands, many women cycle and continue to do so during pregnancy. The accelerometer does not record such activity well due to its uniaxial nature. Therefore the amount of PA measured might be underestimated. Furthermore, it has been shown that accelerometers might be less valid in pregnancy, mostly because of slower walking speeds of the women [30]. However, objective measurement of PA is to be preferred over using self-reported PA since most questionnaires show poor validity in pregnancy [31]. In this study, nutritional intake was not taken into account, which might have confounded the results presented in this paper. Weight gain is a function of energy expenditure through

TABLE 1: Characteristics of the study sample.

	Total population ($n = 111$)	
Age, years, mean (SD)	29.6	(3.8)
Ethnicity, N (%)		
White European	95	86%
Non-White	16	14%
Nulliparous, N (%)	81	73%
BMI at 15 wks (kg/m^2), mean (SD)	27.0	(5.5)
BMI category at 15 weeks, N (%)		
Normal weight	54	49%
Overweight	25	22%
Obese	32	29%
Gestational age at birth, weeks, mean (SD)	40.2	(1.2)
Gestational weight gain, kg, mean (SD)	10.3	(4.2)
Gestational weight gain per week, kg, mean (SD)	0.55	(0.22)
Birth weight, g, mean (SD)	3541	(429)
Total PA at 15 wks, mins/day, mean (SD)	286	(103)
% of registration time		35%
Total PA at 32–35 wks, mins/day, mean (SD)	273	(103)
% of registration time		35%
MVPA at 15 wks, min/day, mean (SD)	24	(16)
% of registration time		3%
MVPA at 32–35 wks, min/day, mean (SD)	18	(22)
% of registration time		2%
Sedentary behaviour at 15 wks, min/day, mean (SD)	530	(170)
% of registration time		65%
Sedentary behaviour at 32–35 wks, min/day, mean (SD)	505	(173)
% of registration time		65%

MVPA: moderate to vigorous physical activity; PA: physical activity; SD: standard deviation.

TABLE 2: Associations between PA, sedentary behaviour, gestational weight gain, and birth weight.

	Gestational weight gain between 15 and 32–35 weeks		Gestational weight gain per week		Birth weight	
	Beta	95% CI	Beta	95% CI	Beta	95% CI
15 weeks of gestation[*]						
% MVPA	−0.07	−0.48; 0.34	−0.002	−0.02; 0.02	26.93	−14.79; 68.65
% Sedentary behaviour	−0.07	−0.15; 0.01	−0.004	−0.01; 0.001	2.45	−5.53; 10.42
Change from 15 to 32–35 weeks of gestation[*]						
% MVPA	−0.16	−0.47; 0.15	−0.01	−0.03; 0.01	8.10	−23.83; 68.44
% Sedentary behaviour	−0.02	−0.12; 0.07	−0.001	−0.01; 0.004	0.59	−8.91; 10.09

[*]Moderate to vigorous PA (MVPA) and sedentary behaviour were entered into the same model, controlled for intervention group, age, parity, BMI, and (change in) gestational age. The model with MVPA and sedentary behaviour at 32–35 weeks was also controlled for baseline values and therefore reflects the betas for the changes in MVPA and sedentary behaviour.
CI: confidence interval; MVPA: moderate to vigorous physical activity; PA: physical activity.

physical activity and metabolism, as well as energy intake from food and drink consumption. Physical activity levels and sedentary time reflect only one half of the equation. Physical activity may affect appetite and food intake during pregnancy; furthermore, women who are health oriented may be more physically active and eat more healthily. Future studies are needed in which both sides of the energy balance are taken into account in relation to GWG and birth weight.

And although we did not find an interaction with BMI, it might be useful to study the relationship between PA and sedentary behaviour in different BMI categories separately.

5. Conclusion

This study showed that PA is not associated with GWG or birth weight, and also sedentary behaviour did not seem to contribute to GWG or birth weight of the infant. The findings regarding sedentary behaviour are new and need to be confirmed with studies using a design better suitable for studying causal relationships, such as randomized trials. The findings with regard to PA are not in line with the results of recent meta-analyses, and also here more research is needed to assess the relationship of objectively measured PA with GWG and birth weight. Another important finding is that only a small proportion of our pregnant women met the ACOG guidelines for sufficient MVPA [26] in early pregnancy (31%) and even fewer at the end of pregnancy (13%). This is much lower than the 58% of women 20–40 years of age meeting similar guidelines in the general Dutch population in 2010 according to the Dutch Bureau of Statistics (http://statline.cbs.nl). This indicates that pregnant women need to be better informed and advised about maintaining PA levels throughout pregnancy.

In summary, we have conducted analysis estimating the relationship between PA and sedentary behaviour and GWG and birth weight. Key finding of this study was that neither behaviour, physical or sedentary, at any time during pregnancy was associated with gestational weight gain or birth weight of the newborn.

6. Practical Implications

(i) Physical activity or sedentary behaviour does not seem to contribute to GWG.

(ii) Physical activity or sedentary behaviour does not seem to affect the birth weight of the newborn.

(iii) A small proportion of pregnant women meet the ACOG guidelines for sufficient MVPA in pregnancy, and pregnant women need to be informed and advised about physical activity throughout pregnancy.

Ethical Approval

The Medical Ethics Committee of VU University Medical Centre has approved the study design, protocols, and informed consent procedure of both studies (registration number 2004/184, approved November 11, 2004, and registration number 2007/133, approved September 12 2007). ISRCTN Trial Registration: http://www.controlled-trials.com/ISRCTN85313483 and NTR1139; http://www.trialregister.nl/trialreg/admin/rctview.asp?TC=1139.

Conflict of Interests

None of the authors declare any conflict of interests.

Authors' Contribution

Anneloes E. Ruifrok performed the analyses and drafted the paper. Ellen Althuizen and Nicolette Oostdam performed the studies. Mireille N. M. van Poppel had a role in the conception and planning of the study and partially drafted the paper. Willem van Mechelen had a role in the conception of the original studies and revised the paper critically. Ben Willem Mol and Christianne J. M. de Groot critically revised the paper. All authors approved this version for publication.

Acknowledgments

The authors would like to thank all participants, midwives, research nurses, and gynaecologists who participated in the studies. The studies in which the data were gathered were financially supported by a grant from the Netherlands Organisation for Health Research and Development (ZonMw, Grants 40100.0017 and 62300043).

References

[1] M. I. Cedergren, "Optimal gestational weight gain for body mass index categories," *Obstetrics and Gynecology*, vol. 110, no. 4, pp. 759–764, 2007.

[2] M. M. Hedderson, E. P. Gunderson, and A. Ferrara, "Gestational weight gain and risk of gestational diabetes mellitus," *Obstetrics & Gynecology*, vol. 115, no. 3, pp. 597–604, 2010.

[3] I. Thorsdottir, J. E. Torfadottir, B. E. Birgisdottir, and R. T. Geirsson, "Weight gain in women of normal weight before pregnancy: complications in pregnancy or delivery and birth outcome," *Obstetrics and Gynecology*, vol. 99, no. 5, part 1, pp. 799–806, 2002.

[4] X. Zhang, A. Decker, R. W. Platt, and M. S. Kramer, "How big is too big? The perinatal consequences of fetal macrosomia," *The American Journal of Obstetrics and Gynecology*, vol. 198, no. 5, pp. 517.e1–517.e6, 2008.

[5] E. Oken, E. M. Taveras, K. P. Kleinman, J. W. Rich-Edwards, and M. W. Gillman, "Gestational weight gain and child adiposity at age 3 years," *The American Journal of Obstetrics and Gynecology*, vol. 196, no. 4, pp. 322.e1–322.e8, 2007.

[6] S. R. DeVader, H. L. Neeley, T. D. Myles, and T. L. Leet, "Evaluation of gestational weight gain guidelines for women with normal prepregnancy body mass index," *Obstetrics and Gynecology*, vol. 110, no. 4, pp. 745–751, 2007.

[7] NIDDK Weight Control Information Network, "Healthy eating and physical activity across your life span: fit for two: tips for pregnancy," Tech. Rep. 02-5130 2002, NIH, 2002.

[8] J. M. Dodd, C. A. Crowther, and J. S. Robinson, "Dietary and lifestyle interventions to limit weight gain during pregnancy for obese or overweight women: a systematic review," *Acta Obstetricia et Gynecologica Scandinavica*, vol. 87, no. 7, pp. 702–706, 2008.

[9] F. Galtier-Dereure, C. Boegner, and J. Bringer, "Obesity and pregnancy: complications and cost," *The American Journal of Clinical Nutrition*, vol. 71, no. 5, pp. 1242S–1248S, 2000.

[10] N. Heslehurst, J. Rankin, J. R. Wilkinson, and C. D. Summerbell, "A nationally representative study of maternal obesity in England, UK: trends in incidence and demographic inequalities in 619 323 births, 1989–2007," *International Journal of Obesity*, vol. 34, no. 3, pp. 420–428, 2010.

[11] Y. Linné, L. Dye, B. Barkeling, and S. Rössner, "Long-term weight development in women: a 15-year follow-up of the effects of pregnancy," *Obesity Research*, vol. 12, no. 7, pp. 1166–1178, 2004.

[12] B. L. Rooney and C. W. Schauberger, "Excess pregnancy weight gain and long-term obesity: One decade later," *Obstetrics and Gynecology*, vol. 100, no. 2, pp. 245–252, 2002.

[13] Institute of Medicine, *Weight Gain during Pregnancy: Reexamining the Guidelines*, Committee to Reexamine IOM Pregnancy Weight Guideline, Ed., National Research Council, Washington, DC, USA, 2009.

[14] T. A. M. Simas, X. Liao, A. Garrison, G. M. T. Sullivan, A. E. Howard, and J. R. Hardy, "Impact of updated institute of medicine guidelines on prepregnancy body mass index categorization, gestational weight gain recommendations, and needed counseling," *Journal of Women's Health*, vol. 20, no. 6, pp. 837–844, 2011.

[15] S. Thangaratinam, E. Rogozińska, K. Jolly et al., "Interventions to reduce or prevent obesity in pregnant women: a systematic review," *Health Technology Assessment*, vol. 16, no. 31, pp. 1–191, 2012.

[16] S. Thangaratinam, E. Rogozińska, K. Jolly et al., "Effects of interventions in pregnancy on maternal weight and obstetric outcomes: Meta-analysis of randomised evidence," *BMJ*, vol. 344, Article ID e2088, 2012.

[17] K. R. Evenson, L. Chasan-Taber, D. D. Symons, and E. E. Pearce, "Review of self-reported physical activity assessments for pregnancy: summary of the evidence for validity and reliability," *Paediatric and Perinatal Epidemiology*, vol. 26, no. 5, pp. 479–494, 2012.

[18] F. B. Hu, T. Y. Li, G. A. Colditz, W. C. Willett, and J. E. Manson, "Television watching and other sedentary behaviors in relation to risk of obesity and type 2 diabetes mellitus in women," *Journal of the American Medical Association*, vol. 289, no. 14, pp. 1785–1791, 2003.

[19] S. A. Costigan, L. Barnett, R. C. Plotnikoff, and D. R. Lubans, "The health indicators associated with screen-based sedentary behavior among adolescent girls: a systematic review," *Journal of Adolescent Health*, vol. 52, no. 4, pp. 382–392, 2013.

[20] K. R. Evenson and F. Wen, "Prevalence and correlates of objectively measured physical activity and sedentary behavior among US pregnant women," *Preventive Medicine*, vol. 53, no. 1-2, pp. 39–43, 2011.

[21] E. Althuizen, M. N. M. van Poppel, J. C. Seidell, C. van der Wijden, and W. van Mechelen, "Design of the new life(style) study: a randomised controlled trial to optimise maternal weight development during pregnancy. [ISRCTN85313483]," *BMC Public Health*, vol. 6, article 168, 2006.

[22] N. Oostdam, M. N. M. van Poppel, E. M. W. Eekhoff, M. G. A. J. Wouters, and W. van Mechelen, "Design of FitFor2 study: The effects of an exercise program on insulin sensitivity and plasma glucose levels in pregnant women at high risk for gestational diabetes," *BMC Pregnancy and Childbirth*, vol. 9, article no. 1, 2009.

[23] N. Oostdam, M. N. M. Van Poppel, M. G. A. J. Wouters et al., "No effect of the FitFor2 exercise programme on blood glucose, insulin sensitivity, and birthweight in pregnant women who were overweight and at risk for gestational diabetes: results of a randomised controlled trial," *An International Journal of Obstetrics and Gynaecology*, vol. 119, no. 9, pp. 1098–1107, 2012.

[24] E. Althuizen, C. L. Van Der Wijden, W. Van Mechelen, J. C. Seidell, and M. N. M. Van Poppel, "The effect of a counselling intervention on weight changes during and after pregnancy: a randomised trial," *BJOG*, vol. 120, no. 1, pp. 92–99, 2013.

[25] R. P. Troiano, D. Berrigan, K. W. Dodd, L. C. Mâsse, T. Tilert, and M. Mcdowell, "Physical activity in the United States measured by accelerometer," *Medicine and Science in Sports and Exercise*, vol. 40, no. 1, pp. 181–188, 2008.

[26] R. Artal and M. O'Toole, "Guidelines of the American College of Obstetricians and Gynecologists for exercise during pregnancy and the postpartum period," *British Journal of Sports Medicine*, vol. 37, no. 1, pp. 6–12, 2003.

[27] I. Streuling, A. Beyerlein, E. Rosenfeld, H. Hofmann, T. Schulz, and R. Von Kries, "Physical activity and gestational weight gain: A meta-analysis of intervention trials," *BJOG*, vol. 118, no. 3, pp. 278–284, 2011.

[28] D. S. Seidman, P. E. Slater, P. Ever-Hadani, and R. Gale, "Accuracy of mothers'recall of birthweight and gestational age," *British Journal of Obstetrics and Gynaecology*, vol. 94, no. 8, pp. 731–735, 1987.

[29] J. E. Olson, X. O. Shu, J. A. Ross, T. Pendergrass, and L. L. Robison, "Medical record validation of maternally reported birth characteristics and pregnancy-related events: a report from the Children's Cancer Group," *The American Journal of Epidemiology*, vol. 145, no. 1, pp. 58–67, 1997.

[30] C. P. Connolly, D. P. Coe, J. M. Kendrick, D. R. Bassett, and D. L. Thompson, "Accuracy of physical activity monitors in pregnant women," *Medicine and Science in Sports and Exercise*, vol. 43, no. 6, pp. 1100–1105, 2011.

[31] C. L. Harrison, R. G. Thompson, H. J. Teede et al., "Measuring physical activity during pregnancy," *International Journal of Behavioral Nutrition and Physical Activity*, vol. 8, article 19, 2011.

12

Maternal Opioid Drug Use during Pregnancy and its Impact on Perinatal Morbidity, Mortality, and the Costs of Medical Care in the United States

Valerie E. Whiteman,[1] Jason L. Salemi,[2] Mulubrhan F. Mogos,[3]
Mary Ashley Cain,[1] Muktar H. Aliyu,[4] and Hamisu M. Salihu[1,2]

[1] Division of Maternal-Fetal Medicine, Department of Obstetrics and Gynecology, College of Medicine, University of South Florida,
 2 Tampa General Circle, 6th Floor, Tampa, FL 33606, USA
[2] Maternal and Child Health Comparative Effectiveness Research Group, Department of Epidemiology and Biostatistics,
 College of Public Health, University of South Florida, 13201 Bruce B. Downs Boulevard MDC 56, Tampa, FL 33612, USA
[3] Department of Community and Health Systems, School of Nursing, University of Indiana, 1111 Middle Drive, Indianapolis,
 IN 46202, USA
[4] Department of Health Policy and Medicine, Vanderbilt University, 2525 West End Avenue, Suite 750, Nashville, TN 32703, USA

Correspondence should be addressed to Hamisu M. Salihu; hsalihu@health.usf.edu

Academic Editor: Deborah A. Wing

Objective. To identify factors associated with opioid use during pregnancy and to compare perinatal morbidity, mortality, and healthcare costs between opioid users and nonusers. *Methods*. We conducted a cross-sectional analysis of pregnancy-related discharges from 1998 to 2009 using the largest publicly available all-payer inpatient database in the United States. We scanned ICD-9-CM codes for opioid use and perinatal outcomes. Costs of care were estimated from hospital charges. Survey logistic regression was used to assess the association between maternal opioid use and each outcome; generalized linear modeling was used to compare hospitalization costs by opioid use status. *Results*. Women who used opioids during pregnancy experienced higher rates of depression, anxiety, and chronic medical conditions. After adjusting for confounders, opioid use was associated with increased odds of threatened preterm labor, early onset delivery, poor fetal growth, and stillbirth. Users were four times as likely to have a prolonged hospital stay and were almost four times more likely to die before discharge. The mean per-hospitalization cost of a woman who used opioids during pregnancy was $5,616 (95% CI: $5,166–$6,067), compared to $4,084 (95% CI: $4,002–$4,166) for nonusers. *Conclusion*. Opioid use during pregnancy is associated with adverse perinatal outcomes and increased healthcare costs.

1. Introduction

Opioid pain medications are among the most prescribed drugs in the United States (US) [1]. In the past few decades, recent trends in increases in narcotic abuse overshadow successes in improved awareness and management of pain. Clinicians, administrators, and policymakers now face the consequential task of preventing opioid drug misuse and addiction without compromising their effective and appropriate use in the treatment of pain.

Opioid dependence in pregnancy complicates the clinical management of an already vulnerable group of patients.

Dependence increases the risk of poor maternal and perinatal outcomes [2–11]. Women of reproductive age who use and abuse opioid drugs, both prescription and illegal, are more likely to have a lower socioeconomic status, family instability, receive inadequate prenatal care, and suffer from alcohol, tobacco, and illicit drug use [12, 13]. In addition to the risks associated with opioid dependence, these comorbid conditions further increase the risk of adverse perinatal outcomes [3, 14].

Increasing at an alarming rate, opioid use in pregnancy underwent an estimated 3-4-fold increase between 2000 and

2009 [15, 16]. The 2011 National Survey on Drug Use and Health reports of the United States found 5% of pregnant women 15 to 44 years of age report using illicit drugs [17]. These data suggest an urgent need to evaluate, on a national level, not only the negative health outcomes associated with maternal opioid use during pregnancy, but also the related economic cost burden on the US healthcare system. In this study, we leveraged a large, nationally representative hospital discharge database to identify factors that are associated with an increased likelihood of opioid use during pregnancy. We then compared selected maternal and fetal outcomes between opioid users. Finally, we computed the direct inpatient medical costs associated with maternal opioid use.

2. Materials and Methods

A cross-sectional analysis of all pregnancy-related hospital discharges from 1998 to 2009 was conducted using the National Inpatient Sample (NIS), the largest publicly available all-payer inpatient database in the US, made available by the Healthcare and Cost Utilization Project (HCUP) [18]. To create the dataset each year, HCUP stratifies all nonfederal community hospitals from participating states by five major hospital characteristics: rural/urban location, number of beds, geographic region, teaching status, and ownership. A random sample of 20% of hospitals from each stratum is then drawn using a systematic random sampling technique [18].

Hospital discharges for women who were pregnant or delivered were identified using the variable "NEOMAT" in the NIS dataset. This indicator was created by HCUP to identify maternal and/or neonatal diagnosis records on the basis of International Classification of Diseases, Ninth Revision, Clinical Modifications (ICD-9-CM) diagnosis and procedure codes for pregnancy and delivery [19]. After identifying the study population, we scanned ICD-9-CM codes (principal and secondary) in each woman's discharge record for an indication of opioid use during pregnancy, as well as for selected maternal/fetal clinical outcomes. The complete list of ICD-9-CM codes used to characterize each condition is presented in the appendix.

Individual-level sociodemographic factors were extracted from the NIS databases. Maternal age in years was classified into five categories: <20, 20–24, 25–29, 30–34, and ≥35. Self-reported maternal race-ethnicity was first based on ethnicity (Hispanic or non-Hispanic [NH]), and the NH group further subdivided by race (white, black, or other). Relative median household income (in quartiles) was estimated by HCUP using the patient's zip code and served as a proxy for each woman's socioeconomic status. We grouped the primary payer for hospital admission into three categories: government (Medicare/Medicaid), private (commercial carriers, private health maintenance organization [HMOs], and preferred provider organization [PPOs]), and other sources (e.g., self-pay and charity). We also considered several hospital characteristics including teaching status (teaching, or a ratio of full-time equivalent interns and residents to nonnursing home beds ≥0.25, versus nonteaching), location (urban versus rural), and US region (Northeast, Midwest, South, or West).

The NIS databases also contain discharge-level charges for all hospitalized patients. Reported charges, however, are not a good estimate of actual cost, since there is significant variation in markup from what it costs a hospital to provide medical care to what it charges for services rendered [20]. To adjust for variation in markup across hospitals and over time, we multiplied the total charge for a hospital stay by a time- and hospital-specific cost-to-charge ratio (CCR) available from HCUP [21]. However, even within the same facility, sizeable differences in markup exist across different departments (e.g., higher markup for operating room services compared to routine bed services). Therefore, we incorporated into the computation of cost an "adjustment factor" (AF) that attempts to account for this intradepartmental variation to yield a more accurate cost estimate for each discharge record [22, 23]. Consider

$$\text{cost} = (\text{reported charges} * \text{CCR} * \text{AF}). \quad (1)$$

2.1. Statistical Analysis. We calculated descriptive statistics including frequencies, percentages, and rates to describe prevalence of opioid use during pregnancy across maternal age, racial/ethnic, household income strata, primary payer, selected behavioral characteristics, and comorbidities. National rate estimates were computed by weighting the analyses with discharge-level weights provided in the NIS databases. We constructed simple and multivariable survey logistic regression models (SURVEYLOGISTIC procedure) to identify factors associated with an increased likelihood of maternal opioid use during pregnancy. Since use of the NIS databases confers a large sample size and a limited number of available covariates, the multivariable model included all factors considered in bivariate analyses. In addition to identifying predictors for maternal opioid use, we also calculated the rate of selected clinical comorbidities by maternal opioid use status. These comorbidities were selected based on a review of the literature and expert opinion and identified using ICD-9-CM codes in the discharge record. The comorbidities included anxiety, chronic renal disease, depression, HIV status, insomnia, obesity, osteopenia, and prepregnancy diabetes and hypertension.

We compared the rate of selected maternal/fetal pregnancy outcomes between opioid users versus nonusers. We used unconditional survey logistic regression to generate the odds ratios (ORs) and 95% confidence intervals (CIs) for outcomes associated with maternal opioid use. In addition to an unadjusted model, we constructed two multivariable models. In the first multivariable model, we adjusted for sociodemographic, perinatal, and hospital characteristics. In the second multivariable model, we also adjusted for tobacco, alcohol, and drug use, as well as existing medical conditions (obesity, chronic renal failure, prepregnancy diabetes, and prepregnancy hypertension) that may be related to both maternal opioid use and the selected pregnancy outcomes.

After computing the direct inpatient medical costs for each pregnancy-related discharge, we compared mean maternal direct hospitalization costs by opioid use status. Considering the strong positive skewness of the cost data, we used a multivariable generalized linear model with a gamma distribution and a natural log link to estimate the mean difference in cost, after adjusting for potential confounders.

All statistical analyses accounted for the complex sampling design of the NIS. To account for NIS sampling design changes, we used the NIS-Trends files, supplied by HCUP, so that trend weights and data elements would be consistently defined over time [24]. Statistical tests were two-sided with level of significance set at 5%. In addition, for cost analyses, we reweighted all discharges to account for missing cost data by multiplying the original discharge weight provided by HCUP by the ratio of the summed weights across all discharges to the summed weight of discharges with nonmissing cost information. Since hospital-level CCR data were only available beginning in 2001, we restricted cost analyses to discharges for the period 2001–09. Analyses were performed using SAS software, version 9.3 (SAS Institute, Inc., Cary, MC) and Stata statistical software, release 11 (Stata Corp LP, College Station, TX). The Institutional Review Board of the University of South Florida determined that this study using deidentified, publicly available data did not meet the definition of human subjects research and was thus exempt from IRB approval.

3. Results

Of the estimated 55,781,965 pregnancy-related hospitalizations, 138,224 were associated with opioid use, a prevalence of 2.5 cases per 1,000 discharges (95% CI: 2.2–2.8). The rate of opioid use during pregnancy initially decreased from 2.5 per 1,000 in 1998 to 1.6 per 1,000 in 2001. This decreasing trend was followed by a 12% annual increase to a peak rate of 4.0 per 1,000 in 2009.

The rate of opioid use during pregnancy varied considerably across maternal sociodemographic, perinatal, behavioral, and hospital characteristics (Table 1). The highest crude rates (per 1,000 discharges) were seen among women using/abusing alcohol (81.0), women using tobacco during pregnancy (21.6), women on Medicare/Medicaid (4.5) or "Other" insurance (4.8), women in the lowest quartile of household income (3.6), and black-NH women (3.2). Conversely, low rates of opioid use during pregnancy were observed among teenage mothers (0.9), women on private insurance (0.7), women of other-NH race/ethnicity (1.0), and women in the highest quartile of household income (1.4). After adjusting for other covariates, compared to women with private insurance, women without private insurance had 9 times the odds of opioid use (Medicare/Medicaid; OR = 8.9; 95% CI: 7.7–10.3; "Other" insurance; OR = 9.2; 95% CI: 8.2–10.4). Alcohol and tobacco users were approximately 7 times as likely to use/abuse opioids, relative to nonusers. The likelihood of opioid use during pregnancy increased with increasing maternal age and decreased with increasing household income (Table 1). Although black-NH women had the highest crude rates of opioid use, after adjustment for other sociodemographic and behavioral characteristics, black-NH women were significantly less likely than white-NH women to use opioids (OR = 0.6, 95% CI: 0.5–0.8). Similar findings were obtained in Hispanic

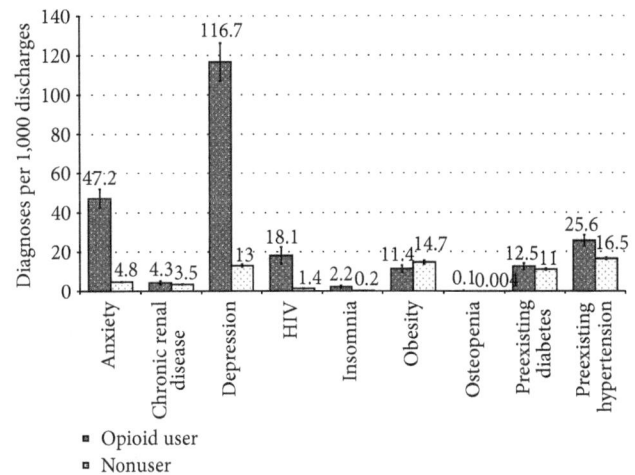

FIGURE 1: Rates (per 1,000 pregnancy-related discharges) of selected comorbidities, by opioid use status, among pregnancy-related discharges, NIS, 1998–2009. HIV = human immunodeficiency virus, NIS = Nationwide Inpatient Sample

and other-NH women when compared to their white-NH counterparts.

Figure 1 presents the rates of various comorbidities, by opioid use status. Compared to nonusers, women who used opioids during pregnancy had significantly higher rates of depression (per 1,000 discharges) (116.7 versus 13.0), anxiety (47.2 versus 4.8), HIV (18.1 versus 1.4), and insomnia (2.2 versus 0.2). Users were also more likely to have chronic medical conditions such as hypertension, diabetes, and renal disease but had a slightly lower rate of medically diagnosed obesity (11.4 versus 14.7).

Maternal opioid use during pregnancy was also associated with pregnancy-related maternal/fetal morbidity and mortality (Table 2). Even after adjusting for sociodemographic, behavioral, and chronic prepregnancy conditions, opioid use was associated with an increased odds of threatened preterm labor (OR = 1.3, 95% CI: 1.2–1.5), early onset delivery (OR = 1.7, 95% CI: 1.6–1.9), poor fetal growth (OR = 1.6, 95% CI: 1.5–1.8), and stillbirth (OR = 1.3, 95% CI: 1.2–1.5). Women who used/abused opioids during pregnancy were also 4 times as likely to have a prolonged hospital stay exceeding 5 days (95% CI: 3.4–4.7) and were almost 4 times as likely to die during their hospital stay (OR = 3.7, 95% CI: 2.3–5.9). These differences in morbidity and mortality also translated into differences in direct inpatient medical costs. The mean per-hospitalization cost of a woman who used opioids during pregnancy was $5,616 (95% CI: $5,166–$6,067), compared to $4,084 (95% CI: $4,002–$4,166) for nonusers. The estimated per-hospitalization difference in cost between opioid and non-opioid-related discharges was $2,602 (95% CI: $1,931–$3,272) after adjustment for potential confounders. With an estimated 138,224 pregnancy-related hospital discharges affected by opioid use nationally from 1998 to 2009, the excess direct inpatient medical cost associated with opioid use was estimated at $359 million, or approximately $30 million annually.

TABLE 1: Rates[a] of opioid use by maternal sociodemographic, perinatal, behavioral, and hospital characteristics, among pregnancy-related discharges, NIS, 1998–2009.

Characteristic	N^b	Rate[a] of opioid use (95% CI)	OR[c] (95% CI)	AOR[d] (95% CI)
Overall	55,781,965	2.48 (2.18–2.78)	n/a	n/a
Maternal age (years)				
13–19	6,198,796	0.93 (0.82–1.04)	0.35 (0.31–0.38)	0.23 (0.21–0.26)
20–24	13,822,023	2.47 (2.16–2.77)	0.91 (0.85–0.98)	0.62 (0.58–0.66)
25–29	15,001,057	2.70 (2.35–3.05)	Reference	Reference
30–34	12,797,406	2.76 (2.37–3.15)	1.02 (0.94–1.11)	1.36 (1.26–1.47)
≥35	7,921,464	2.84 (2.41–3.28)	1.05 (0.97–1.15)	1.37 (1.25–1.50)
Other/unknown	41,218	0.37 (<0.00–0.89)	0.14 (0.03–0.56)	0.15 (0.03–0.66)
Maternal race				
White, non-Hispanic	22,047,327	2.90 (2.52–3.28)	Reference	Reference
Black, non-Hispanic	6,025,913	3.24 (2.32–4.17)	1.12 (0.88–1.43)	0.61 (0.48–0.78)
Hispanic	9,444,177	1.33 (1.07–1.59)	0.46 (0.37–0.56)	0.31 (0.25–0.38)
Other, non-Hispanic	4,079,383	1.02 (0.80–1.24)	0.35 (0.28–0.44)	0.26 (0.21–0.34)
Missing/unknown	14,185,165	2.68 (2.02–3.35)	0.93 (0.70–1.22)	0.98 (0.78–1.23)
Tobacco use				
Yes	2,009,092	21.60 (18.71–24.50)	12.50 (11.41–13.70)	6.67 (6.07–7.33)
No	53,772,873	1.76 (1.56–1.97)	Reference	Reference
Alcohol use				
Yes	96,629	81.02 (71.00–91.04)	37.56 (33.98–41.52)	7.17 (6.42–7.99)
No	55,685,336	2.34 (2.06–2.62)	Reference	Reference
Hospital region				
Northeast	9,516,239	4.47 (3.66–5.28)	2.60 (1.88–3.60)	2.16 (1.60–2.92)
Midwest	12,032,900	2.35 (1.74–2.96)	1.37 (0.94–1.98)	0.88 (0.60–1.28)
South	20,796,015	2.13 (1.61–2.65)	1.24 (0.86–1.78)	0.87 (0.63–1.18)
West	13,436,811	1.72 (1.26–2.19)	Reference	Reference
Hospital location				
Rural	6,877,937	1.36 (1.15–1.58)	Reference	Reference
Urban	48,763,827	2.64 (2.30–2.98)	1.94 (1.58–2.38)	2.22 (1.80–2.74)
Hospital teaching status				
Nonteaching	29,501,465	1.63 (1.43–1.82)	Reference	Reference
Teaching	26,140,299	3.44 (2.85–4.04)	2.12 (1.72–2.62)	1.68 (1.33–2.12)
Hospital bed size				
Small	6,100,955	2.39 (1.84–2.94)	0.89 (0.63–1.28)	0.82 (0.59–1.13)
Medium	14,821,822	2.67 (1.94–3.39)	Reference	Reference
Large	34,718,987	2.42 (2.06–2.77)	0.91 (0.66–1.23)	0.95 (0.72–1.26)
Household income				
Lowest quartile	14,617,169	3.58 (3.06–4.10)	2.53 (2.19–2.93)	1.54 (1.36–1.82)
2nd quartile	14,070,584	2.50 (2.18–2.82)	1.76 (1.58–1.97)	1.20 (1.09–1.33)
3rd quartile	13,294,169	2.18 (1.89–2.47)	1.54 (1.41–1.67)	1.17 (1.08–1.26)
Highest quartile	12,830,659	1.42 (1.23–1.60)	Reference	Reference
Missing/unknown	969,383	3.63 (3.02–4.24)	2.56 (2.17–3.03)	1.43 (1.17–1.75)

TABLE 1: Continued.

Characteristic	N^b	Rate^a of opioid use (95% CI)	OR^c (95% CI)	AOR^d (95% CI)
Primary payer				
Medicare/medicaid	22,249,834	4.51 (3.89–5.14)	6.90 (6.07–7.84)	8.87 (7.66–10.27)
Private	29,701,613	0.66 (0.59–0.73)	Reference	Reference
Other	3,830,518	4.79 (4.18–5.41)	7.33 (6.54–8.22)	9.20 (8.16–10.38)

AOR = adjusted odds ratio, CI = confidence interval, NIS = Nationwide Inpatient Sample, OR = odds ratio.
^{a}Per 1,000 pregnancy-related discharges.
^{b}Weighted to estimate national frequency and may not add to total due to missing data.
^{c}Crude model comparing the odds of maternal opioid use across different levels of each characteristic, separately.
^{d}A single multivariable model includes all characteristics that appear in the table.

TABLE 2: Rates^a of selected clinical outcomes by opioid use status and odds ratios and 95% confidence intervals for the association between opioid use and each outcome among pregnancy-related discharges, NIS, 1998–2009.

Outcomes	Rate^a of outcome		OR (95% CI)		
	Opioid users	Nonopioid users	Model 1^b	Model 2^c	Model 3^d
Maternal					
Threatened preterm labor	30.1	22.3	1.36 (1.24–1.49)	1.34 (1.22–1.47)	1.32 (1.19–1.45)
Early onset delivery	124.0	65.2	2.03 (1.88–2.20)	1.92 (1.77–2.07)	1.72 (1.59–1.85)
PROM	38.5	35.4	1.10 (1.00–1.20)	1.12 (1.03–1.23)	1.06 (0.98–1.16)
Wound infection	7.0	5.0	1.41 (1.18–1.68)	1.19 (1.00–1.42)	1.17 (0.98–1.40)
Acute renal failure	2.1	0.5	4.10 (3.11–5.41)	2.78 (2.09–3.72)	2.84 (2.11–3.84)
Postpartum depression^f	24.7	2.1	12.04 (10.83–13.40)	2.09 (1.79–2.44)	1.75 (1.49–2.05)
Hospital stay >5 days^e	133.4	29.9	5.00 (4.16–6.02)	4.83 (4.10–5.69)	4.02 (3.41–4.74)
In-hospital maternal mortality	0.8	0.1	5.89 (3.74–9.28)	3.63 (2.32–5.68)	3.69 (2.32–5.87)
Fetal					
Poor fetal growth	35.9	15.9	2.31 (2.10–2.55)	2.21 (2.00–2.44)	1.61 (1.46–1.77)
Stillbirth	10.0	6.3	1.60 (1.39–1.83)	1.41 (1.23–1.62)	1.32 (1.15–1.51)

CI = confidence interval, NIS = Nationwide Inpatient Sample, OR = odds ratio, PROM = premature rupture of membranes.
^{a}Per 1,000 pregnancy-related discharges.
^{b}Crude model with maternal opioid use as the only independent variable.
^{c}Model 1 + adjustment for maternal age, household income, multiple birth, primary payer, and rural/urban status.
^{d}Model 2 + adjustment for tobacco, alcohol, maternal obesity, chronic renal failure, diabetes mellitus, and existing hypertension.
^{e}Model also adjusts for disposition at discharge.
^{f}Model also adjusts for history of depression.

4. Discussion

Consistent with previous studies, this multiyear population-based study found an increasing prevalence of opioids use/abuse among pregnant women in the US [1, 3–5, 7, 10, 17, 25, 26]. In our previous investigation of national trends of opioid use among pregnant mothers in the US, we discuss the alarming overall increase, as well as geographic, regional, and sociodemographic differences in both the rate and trends of opioid use over 12 years [16]. Due to concern for adverse effects on the mother and developing fetus, opioid abuse in pregnancy continues to be a major source of concern [1, 5–7, 13, 14]. As rates of opioid abuse in pregnancy are increasing the incidence of neonatal abstinence syndrome is rising [15]. This syndrome leads to prolonged neonatal hospitalizations, which in turn increase overall hospital costs among these mothers and their infants.

The current study builds on the existing literature by looking at the impact of opioid use and abuse during pregnancy on a wide range of maternal and infant birth outcomes. We found that pregnant women who used or abused opioids during pregnancy were more likely to have other comorbidities, including depression, anxiety, insomnia, diabetes, hypertension, renal diseases, and HIV infection. This finding was expected due to the association between these comorbid conditions and the development of chronic pain, poor response to pain medications, or experiencing the clinical condition during opioid withdrawal [26–28]. In our study, pregnant women who used or abused opioids were also more likely than nonusers to have a prolonged hospital stay; develop acute renal failure; and suffer mortality prior to hospital discharge. Their infants suffered from increased rates of growth restriction and stillbirth. Our findings were consistent with previous reports [29–31]. The source of worsening perinatal outcomes is likely multifactorial.

Opioid dependent women are more likely to have multiple comorbidities including mental health disorders such as depression and anxiety [32, 33]. Studies also associate

TABLE 3: List of International Classification of Diseases, Ninth Edition, Clinical Modification Codes used to identify selected perinatal conditions.

Condition	International Classification of Diseases, 9th Edition, Diagnosis Code
Exposure	
Opioid use	304.0x, 304.7, 305.5, 965.00, 965.01, E850.0, E935.0
Comorbidities	
Anxiety	300.0x, 309x, 293.84
Chronic renal disease	581x, 582x, 583x, 585x, 587x, 646.2x
Depression	296.2x, 296.3x, 298.0, 300.4, 301.12, 309.0, 309.1, 311
HIV	042, V08, 795.3
Insomnia	780.51, 780.52, 307.42, 327.0x, 327.15, 307.41
Obesity	278.00, 278.01, 278.03, 649.1x, V85.3x, V85.4x, V85.54, 793.91
Osteopenia	733.90
Prepregnancy diabetes	249x, 250x, 648.0x
Prepregnancy hypertension	401x, 402x, 403x, 404x, 405x, 642.0x, 642.1x, 642.2x, 642.7x
Perinatal outcomes	
Threatened preterm labor	644.0x
Early onset delivery	644.2x
Premature rupture of membranes	658.1x
Wound infection	674.1x, 674.3x, 998.3x, 998.5x
Acute renal failure	584x, 669.3x
Postpartum depression	648.40, 648.42, 648.44
Poor fetal growth	656.5x
Stillbirth	656.4x, V27.1, V27.3, V27.4, V27.6, V27.7

*The code suffix "x" represents all possible codes that follow the stated code prefix.
†Procedure codes, no diagnostic codes were used to define Cesarean section.

maternal anxiety during pregnancy with poor neurological development in the fetus [34]. In addition to mental health disorders, opioid dependent women are more often from socially disadvantaged backgrounds [35], lack healthy nutritional habits, have inadequate prenatal care, and engage in risky sexual practices [36]. These comorbid conditions may explain the adverse infant birth outcomes observed in our study. However, the association between opioid abuse during pregnancy and adverse maternal and infant birth outcomes persisted even after controlling for potential confounders. In addition to associated comorbidities, women with opioid abuse may have irregular menses leading to unintended pregnancy [37, 38]. Adverse perinatal outcomes occur at higher rates among unintended pregnancies alone [39]. Despite possible confounding due to associated comorbidities, the increase in hospital costs and adverse perinatal outcomes in the current study is likely due to neonatal abstinence syndrome and preterm deliveries as was seen in prior investigations [7, 15, 31, 40–42]. Due to a lack of sufficiently detailed data, this hypothesis could not be tested in our study.

This strength of the current study includes the large sample size and length of study. We used an extremely large multiyear hospital discharge database that enabled us to investigate a range of maternal/fetal outcomes. To our knowledge, this is the first study to report the impact of opioid dependence during pregnancy on maternal/fetal outcomes using over a decade of nationally representative data. We also looked at the distribution of comorbidities by maternal opioid dependence status to provide clinicians and other healthcare providers a broader understanding of the complexities surrounding opioid use/abuse during pregnancy.

Despite the noted strengths, our results need to be considered in light of the following limitations. First, the analyses were based on a database of inpatient hospitalizations and, therefore, cases of maternal opioid use not captured during pregnancy-related inpatient admissions were not included in this study. The missed cases are likely limited to home births which occurs in <1% of the US population [43]. Second, our operational definition of opioid use during pregnancy relied exclusively on ICD-9-CM codes documented in the NIS databases. These diagnostic codes lack the specificity to distinguish between use and abuse of prescription versus prescribed opioids. Thus, our analyses were not able to *directly* address the increasing concern for overprescription of opioids. Third, the deidentified nature of the publicly available NIS datasets do not permit linkage of maternal delivery and infant birth hospitalizations. Therefore, we were only able to investigate a small number of fetal outcomes and could not assess birth-related events available in the infant's birth record. Third, due to the lack of a unique patient identifier, we were unable to link hospitalizations for the same woman over time and may count the same woman more than once over time leading to an overestimation of opioid use in pregnancy. Finally, hospital discharge summaries have suboptimal sensitivity to capture all instances of maternal opioid use and may lead to underreporting. However, when compared to self-reports of substance abuse, discharge data contain greater objectivity [44]. Finally, our cost analyses were conducted from a third-party payer perspective and were only able to estimate direct medical care costs from the institutional portion of the hospital stay [45]. The NIS does not contain information on physician costs or indirect costs (e.g., lost wages).

In summary, we found increased rates of maternal comorbidities, prolonged hospital stays, in-hospital mortality, and poor fetal growth and survival among women who used or abused opioids during their pregnancy. These adverse pregnancy outcomes translated into significantly increased direct costs of inpatient care. The information provided in this study will be critical to the development and implementation of appropriate services for this high-risk group of women.

Appendix

See Table 3.

Conflict of Interests

The authors have no conflicts of interest to declare regarding the publication of this paper.

Acknowledgment

A preliminary version of the analyses used in this paper was presented at the 33rd annual meeting of Society of Maternal-Fetal Medicine, February 11–16, 2013 in San Francisco, CA.

References

[1] B. M. Kuehn, "Opioid prescriptions soar: increase in legitimate use as well as abuse," *The Journal of the American Medical Association*, vol. 297, no. 3, pp. 249–251, 2007.

[2] M. M. Benningfield, A. M. Arria, K. Kaltenbach et al., "Co-occurring psychiatric symptoms are associated with increased psychological, social, and medical impairment in opioid dependent pregnant women," *The American Journal on Addictions*, vol. 19, no. 5, pp. 416–421, 2010.

[3] K. Kaltenbach, V. Berghella, and L. Finnegan, "Opioid dependence during pregnancy: effects and management," *Obstetrics and Gynecology Clinics of North America*, vol. 25, no. 1, pp. 139–151, 1998.

[4] M. M. Benningfield, M. S. Dietrich, H. E. Jones et al., "Opioid dependence during pregnancy: relationships of anxiety and depression symptoms to treatment outcomes," *Addiction*, vol. 107, supplement 1, pp. 74–82, 2012.

[5] S. A. Shainker, K. Saia, and A. Lee-Parritz, "Opioid addiction in pregnancy," *Obstetrical and Gynecological Survey*, vol. 67, no. 12, pp. 817–825, 2012.

[6] W. M. Compton and N. D. Volkow, "Abuse of prescription drugs and the risk of addiction," *Drug and Alcohol Dependence*, vol. 83, supplement 1, pp. S4–S7, 2006.

[7] M. J. Hayes and M. S. Brown, "Epidemic of prescription opiate abuse and neonatal abstinence," *The Journal of the American Medical Association*, vol. 307, no. 18, pp. 1974–1975, 2012.

[8] A. S. Höflich, M. Langer, R. Jagsch et al., "Peripartum pain management in opioid dependent women," *European Journal of Pain*, vol. 16, no. 4, pp. 574–584, 2012.

[9] L. E. Kelly, M. J. Riede, K. Bridgman-Acker, A. Lauwers, P. Madadi, and G. Koren, "Are infants exposed to methadone in utero at an increased risk for mortality?" *Journal of Population Therapeutics and Clinical Pharmacology*, vol. 19, no. 2, pp. e160–e165, 2012.

[10] M. Meyer, A. Benvenuto, D. Howard et al., "Development of a substance abuse program for opioid-dependent nonurban pregnant women improves outcome," *Journal of Addiction Medicine*, vol. 6, no. 2, pp. 124–130, 2012.

[11] E. M. Park, S. Meltzer-Brody, and J. Suzuki, "Evaluation and management of opioid dependence in pregnancy," *Psychosomatics*, vol. 53, no. 5, pp. 424–432, 2012.

[12] B. Winklbaur, N. Kopf, N. Ebner, E. Jung, K. Thau, and G. Fischer, "Treating pregnant women dependent on opioids is not the same as treating pregnancy and opioid dependence: a knowledge synthesis for better treatment for women and neonates," *Addiction*, vol. 103, no. 9, pp. 1429–1440, 2008.

[13] A. Heberlein, L. Leggio, D. Stichtenoth, and T. Hillemacher, "The treatment of alcohol and opioid dependence in pregnant women," *Current Opinion in Psychiatry*, vol. 25, no. 6, pp. 559–564, 2012.

[14] K. A. Armstrong, M. G. Kennedy, A. Kline, and C. Tunstall, "Reproductive health needs: comparing women at high, drug-related risk of HIV with a national sample," *Journal of the American Medical Women's Association*, vol. 54, no. 2, pp. 65–78, 1999.

[15] S. W. Patrick, R. E. Schumacher, B. D. Benneyworth, E. E. Krans, J. M. McAllister, and M. M. Davis, "Neonatal abstinence syndrome and associated health care expenditures: United States, 2000–2009," *The Journal of the American Medical Association*, vol. 307, no. 18, pp. 1934–1940, 2012.

[16] H. M. Salihu, M. F. Mogos, A. A. Salinas-Miranda, J. L. Salemi, and V. E. Whiteman, "National trends in maternal use of opioid drugs among pregnancy-related hospitalizations in the United States, 1998 to 2009," *The American Journal of Perinatology*, 2014.

[17] "Results from the 2011 National Survey on Drug Use and Health: summary of national findings and detailed tables," in *NSDUH Series H-44, HHS, Publication No (SMA) 12-4713*, Substance Abuse and Mental Health Services Administration, Rockville, Md, USA, 2012.

[18] Health Care Cost and Utilization Project (HCUP), *Introduction to the NIS: 2009, HCUP NIS Related Reports*, Agency for Healthcare Research and Quality, Rockville, Md, USA, 2011.

[19] C. Merrill and P. L. Owens, "Reasons for being admitted to the hospital through the emergency department for children and adolescents, 2004," Statistical Brief 33, 2006.

[20] J. L. Salemi, M. M. Comins, K. Chandler, M. F. Mogos, and H. M. Salihu, "A practical approach for calculating reliable cost estimates from observational data: application to cost analyses in maternal and child health," *Applied Health Economics and Health Policy*, vol. 11, no. 4, pp. 343–357, 2013.

[21] "Cost-to-Charge Ratio Files," http://www.hcup-us.ahrq.gov/db/state/costtocharge.jsp#obtain.

[22] Y. Sun and B. Friedman, "Tools for more accurate inpatient cost estimates with HCUP databases, 2009. Errata added October 25, 2012," HCUP Methods Series Report 2011-04, U.S. Agency for Healthcare Research and Quality, 2012.

[23] X. Song and B. Friedman, "Calculate cost adjustment factors by APR-DRG and CCS using selected states with detailed

charges," HCUP Methods Series Report 2008-04, U.S. Agency for Healthcare Research and Quality, 2008.

[24] "Using the HCUP nationwide inpatient sample to estimate trends (updated for 1988–2004)," HCUP Methods Series Report #2006-05, 2006, http://www.hcup-us.ahrq.gov/reports/methods/2006_05_NISTrendsReport_1988-2004.pdf.

[25] B. M. Lester, L. Andreozzi, and L. Appiah, "Substance use during pregnancy: time for policy to catch up with research," *Harm Reduction Journal*, vol. 1, no. 1, article 5, 2004.

[26] H. Salihu, M. Mogos, A. Salinas-Miranda, J. Salemi, and V. Whiteman, "National trends in maternal use of opioid drugs among pregnancy-related hospitalizations in the United States, 1998–2009," *American Journal of Perinatology*, 2014.

[27] S. N. Davison, "Pain in hemodialysis patients: prevalence, cause, severity, and management," *The American Journal of Kidney Diseases*, vol. 42, no. 6, pp. 1239–1247, 2003.

[28] B. Doolittle and W. Becker, "A case series of buprenorphine/naloxone treatment in a primary care practice," *Substance Abuse*, vol. 32, no. 4, pp. 262–265, 2011.

[29] G. L. Bell and K. Lau, "Perinatal and neonatal issues of substance abuse," *Pediatric Clinics of North America*, vol. 42, no. 2, pp. 261–281, 1995.

[30] S. K. Lam, W. K. To, S. J. Duthie, and H. K. Ma, "Narcotic addiction in pregnancy with adverse maternal and perinatal outcome," *Australian and New Zealand Journal of Obstetrics and Gynaecology*, vol. 32, no. 3, pp. 216–221, 1992.

[31] U. A. Pritham, J. A. Paul, and M. J. Hayes, "Opioid dependency in pregnancy and length of stay for neonatal abstinence syndrome," *JOGNN—Journal of Obstetric, Gynecologic, and Neonatal Nursing*, vol. 41, no. 2, pp. 180–190, 2012.

[32] T. Field, M. Diego, M. Hernandez-Reif et al., "Depressed pregnant black women have a greater incidence of prematurity and low birthweight outcomes," *Infant Behavior and Development*, vol. 32, no. 1, pp. 10–16, 2009.

[33] J. R. W. Fisher, M. M. Morrow, N. T. N. Ngoc, and L. T. H. Anh, "Prevalence, nature, severity and correlates of postpartum depressive symptoms in Vietnam," *BJOG*, vol. 111, no. 12, pp. 1353–1360, 2004.

[34] J. Fisher, T. Tran, B. T. La, K. Kriitmaa, D. Rosenthal, and T. Tran, "Common perinatal mental disorders in northern Viet Nam: community prevalence and health care use," *Bulletin of the World Health Organization*, vol. 88, no. 10, pp. 737–745, 2010.

[35] B. C. Moore, C. J. Easton, and T. J. McMahon, "Drug abuse and intimate partner violence: a comparative study of opioid-dependent fathers," *American Journal of Orthopsychiatry*, vol. 81, no. 2, pp. 218–227, 2011.

[36] G. K. Hulse, E. Milne, D. R. English, and C. D. J. Holman, "Assessing the relationship between maternal opiate use and neonatal mortality," *Addiction*, vol. 93, no. 7, pp. 1033–1042, 1998.

[37] M. J. Kreek, J. Schluger, L. Borg, M. Gunduz, and A. Ho, "Dynorphin A1-13 causes elevation of serum levels of prolactin through an opioid receptor mechanism in humans: gender differences and implications for modulation of dopaminergic tone in the treatment of addictions," *Journal of Pharmacology and Experimental Therapeutics*, vol. 288, no. 1, pp. 260–269, 1999.

[38] S. H. Heil, H. E. Jones, A. Arria et al., "Unintended pregnancy in opioid-abusing women," *Journal of Substance Abuse Treatment*, vol. 40, no. 2, pp. 199–202, 2011.

[39] R. J. Mercier, J. Garrett, J. Thorp, and A. M. Siega-Riz, "Pregnancy intention and postpartum depression: secondary data analysis from a prospective cohort," *BJOG: An International Journal of Obstetrics and Gynaecology*, vol. 120, no. 9, pp. 1116–1122, 2013.

[40] N. Goel, D. Beasley, V. Rajkumar, and S. Banerjee, "Perinatal outcome of illicit substance use in pregnancy—comparative and contemporary socio-clinical profile in the UK," *European Journal of Pediatrics*, vol. 170, no. 2, pp. 199–205, 2011.

[41] M. A. Huestis and R. E. Choo, "Drug abuse's smallest victims: in utero drug exposure," *Forensic Science International*, vol. 128, no. 1-2, pp. 20–30, 2002.

[42] A. J. W. Liu, M. P. Jones, H. Murray, C. M. Cook, and R. Nanan, "Perinatal risk factors for the neonatal abstinence syndrome in infants born to women on methadone maintenance therapy," *Australian and New Zealand Journal of Obstetrics and Gynaecology*, vol. 50, no. 3, pp. 253–258, 2010.

[43] FETUS, "Newborn: planned home birth," *Pediatrics*, vol. 131, no. 5, pp. 1016–1020, 2013.

[44] J. Zhao, T. Stockwell, and S. Macdonald, "Non-response bias in alcohol and drug population surveys," *Drug and Alcohol Review*, vol. 28, no. 6, pp. 648–657, 2009.

[45] J. Rogowski, "Measuring the cost of neonatal and perinatal care," *Pediatrics*, vol. 103, no. 1, pp. 329–335, 1999.

13

Can Preterm Labour Be Predicted in Low Risk Pregnancies? Role of Clinical, Sonographic, and Biochemical Markers

Reva Tripathi,[1] Shakun Tyagi,[1] Nilanchali Singh,[1] Yedla Manikya Mala,[1] Chanchal Singh,[1] Preena Bhalla,[2] and Siddhartha Ramji[3]

[1] Department of Obstetrics and Gynaecology, Maulana Azad Medical College, New Delhi 110002, India
[2] Department of Microbiology, Maulana Azad Medical College, New Delhi, India
[3] Department of Paediatrics, Maulana Azad Medical College, New Delhi, India

Correspondence should be addressed to Nilanchali Singh; nilanchalisingh@gmail.com

Academic Editor: R. L. Deter

Background and Objectives. This is a prospective nested cohort study conducted over a period of 3 years. 2644 women were recruited, out of which final analysis was done for 1884 women. *Methods.* Cervicovaginal and blood samples were collected for all recruited women. Out of these, 137 women who delivered before 35 weeks were treated as cases and equal number of matched controls were chosen. Analysis of samples for serum G-CSF, AFP, ferritin, and cervicovaginal interleukin-6 and IGFBP-1 was done. *Results.* Poor orodental hygiene, which can be a social marker, was significantly more common in women who delivered preterm ($P = 0.008$). Serum alkaline phosphatase and serum ferritin were found to be significantly associated with preterm deliveries. The 90th percentile value of these parameters was considered as cut-off as there is no specific cut-off. *Conclusions.* Our study did not prove usefulness of any predictive marker. Serum ferritin and alkaline phosphatase were found to have correlation but their values are affected in many conditions and need to be elucidated with caution. Larger studies are needed for predicting preterm labour in asymptomatic women.

1. Introduction

Prematurity continues to be the major cause of neonatal morbidity and mortality across the world accounting for an enormous 70% of neonatal deaths in nonanomalous babies [1]. Despite decades of research, we are no closer to finding answers in terms of prediction and hence prevention of preterm labour. This is in sharp contrast to the increasing rates of preterm births across the world. This increase is in part attributable to increase in artificial reproductive techniques and multiple pregnancies. Efforts to predict preterm delivery have classically been based on history and examination findings only. But these risk assessment scores have poor predictive values [2, 3]. Some studies have found cervical length as measured by transvaginal ultrasound and cervicovaginal IGFBP-1 as most strongly and consistently associated with subsequent spontaneous preterm birth [4]. Increased level of cervicovaginal interleukin-6 (IL-6) at 24 weeks has also been associated with preterm delivery [5]. New biochemical markers like increased levels of serum ferritin, serum granulocyte colony-stimulating factor, serum alkaline phosphatase, and serum alpha-fetoprotein have also been associated with increased incidence of preterm delivery [6, 7]. Combining these markers with clinical findings and ultrasonography has also contributed significantly to increased predictive values [4]. We wanted to validate various screening tests for predicting preterm labour in low risk women as there is a known effective intervention (i.e., progesterone) for its prevention. This study was undertaken to evaluate the role of biomarkers and cervical length in prediction of preterm labour in asymptomatic low risk women in an Indian population.

2. Materials and Methods

This prospective study was conducted at a tertiary care teaching hospital over a period of 3 years. All low risk women with singleton pregnancy who visited the antenatal clinic of a single unit between 24 and 27 weeks and 6 days were consecutively recruited after counseling and an informed consent. Women either with certain last menstrual periods or having a first trimester ultrasound were recruited in study. The study was approved by the ethical committee of the hospital.

Considering the rate of preterm delivery at 35 weeks being approximately 5% at our centre, for a 95% confidence level and 80% power for majority of factors to be studied, 2600 pregnant women needed to be studied. Only low risk women were included in the study. Women with history suggestive of cervical incompetence, previous preterm delivery (defined as less than 37 weeks) or previous cervical surgery, preexisting medical disorders like chronic hypertension, diabetes mellitus, heart disease, and SLE, and so forth, were excluded from the study. Women with major degree placenta previa or gross congenital anomaly in the foetus were also excluded. All women underwent routine antenatal care with thorough history taking and obstetric examination.

A 10 mL venous blood sample was collected in a vacutainer from all the women recruited in study and transported within three hours to be stored at −70° Celsius for assessment of the following biomarkers: serum ALP, AFP, ferritin, G-CSF, and interleukin-6. Sterile speculum examination was done and cervical swab taken for smear examination after gram staining. Nugent score was calculated. pH of cervical secretion was determined using litmus paper and a pH value of more than 4.5 was taken as "abnormal." Cervicovaginal secretion was collected for assessment of insulin like growth factor binding protein (IGFBP-1) and interleukin-6.

For this study a nested cohort was used; that is, samples of all recruited patients were collected and stored. A smear was made on slide using swab and air-dried to fix it. Two dacron swabs were soaked in cervical secretions by placing them at the external os for 15 seconds to absorb cervical secretions and stored in a buffer solution containing sodium phosphate, sodium chloride, EDTA, Tween-20, bovine serum albumin, aprotinin, and proclin 300. These were then stored in deep freeze (−70° Celsius) to be tested later for IGFBP-1 and interleukin-6.

Those who delivered at less than 35 weeks gestation were treated as *cases*. An equal number of women matched with respect to parity and age amongst the remaining recruited women delivering at more than 37 weeks were treated as *controls*. Using efficient transport and storage of samples, only samples of cases and controls were analyzed, to reduce the financial burden of kits required for biochemical analysis. Analysis of the samples was done for patients who eventually delivered preterm and their matched controls. Analysis of samples for serum granulocyte colony-stimulating factor, serum alpha-fetoprotein, serum ferritin, and cervicovaginal interleukin-6 was done in microbiology department of the institution using ELISA kits for these parameters. For testing IGFBP-1, the swabs were placed into the specimen extraction solution provided with the kit (*Rapid Actim Partus test, Medix Biochemica, Kauniainen, Finland*) and swirled around vigorously for 10 seconds. The swab was then withdrawn and the dipstick provided in the kit was placed in the specimen extraction solution and held there till the liquid front reaches

the result area. The dipstick was then withdrawn and results were interpreted after 5 minutes. The appearance of two blue lines was taken as positive whereas only one blue line at the end of five minutes was taken as negative. Tests for cervicovaginal IGFBP-1 and IL-6 were standardized prior to analyses. Serum levels of iron and alkaline phosphatase were tested.

A transvaginal scan was done in the same sitting. All the scans were performed by the same sonographer using 5 MHz to 9 MHz transvaginal transducer of HD 11 Philips ultrasound machine and cervical length was measured as recommended. A cervical length of less than 25 mm was defined as "short" cervix. The treating obstetricians were blinded to the results of these tests. All women were followed till delivery and obstetric and neonatal outcomes noted. The primary outcome was preterm delivery defined as delivery before 37 weeks. Women who required iatrogenic preterm delivery were excluded from the final analysis. Serum AFP, ALP, IL-6, and GCSF and serum ferritin were measured in the stored samples of women who had spontaneous preterm delivery before 37 weeks and an equal number of matched controls. Since there are no defined cut-offs for these biomarkers, values of more than 90th percentile were taken as high. Serum ferritin less than the 25th percentile was taken as "low."

2.1. Statistical Analysis. SPSS Version 17 and Microsoft Excel 2007 have been used for statistical analyses. χ^2-test has been used for comparison of categorical variables and Student's t-test has been used for comparison of continuous variables. P values < 0.05 have been considered as significant. Odds ratios have been computed subsequently.

3. Results

A total of 2644 women were recruited for the study. 532 women required iatrogenic preterm delivery prior to 37 weeks and were excluded. One woman underwent cerclage at 24 weeks and was excluded from the analysis. There were 3 maternal mortalities which were excluded. 224 (8.4%) women were lost to follow-up. Thus the final analysis was done for 1884 women. Demographic data for the study population is summarized in Table 1. Most of the demographic characteristics were similar in both the groups except family type and orodental hygiene. Although mental stress was not studied separately; family type was studied in an attempt to analyse whether this could be a surrogate indicator of mental stress which in turn is associated with preterm deliveries. Extended family staying together with a young couple is a feature typical of Indian culture. In our study joint family setup was significantly associated with preterm delivery ($P = 0.042$). This might be explained by the increased physical and mental stress associated with larger extended families. Good orodental hygiene was significantly more common in case of women who delivered at term as compared to women who delivered preterm ($P = 0.008$). The association of poor orodental hygiene with preterm birth needs further elucidation in the Indian scenario.

TABLE 1: Population characteristics in both the groups.

Characteristics	Preterm $n = 137$ (%)	Term $n = 138$ (%)	P value
B.M.I (mean ± SD)	22.858 (±4.147)	23.483 (±3.908)	0.1992
Literacy			
Illiterate	33 (24.09)	22 (15.94)	
Primary	22 (16.06)	18 (13.04)	
Secondary	70 (51.09)	78 (56.52)	0.172
Graduate and above	12 (8.76)	20 (14.49)	
Family type			
Joint	82 (59.85)	99 (71.74)	0.042
Nuclear	55 (40.15)	39 (28.26)	
Tobacco use			
Present	1 (0.73)	1 (0.72)	1.000
Absent	136 (99.27)	137 (99.28)	
Profession			
Home maker	133 (97.08)	135 (97.83)	
Working	4 (2.92)	3 (2.17)	0.723
Type of work			
Heavy	2 (1.46)	0 (00)	
Moderate	135 (98.54)	138 (100)	0.247
Sedentary	00 (00)	00 (00)	
Domestic violence			
Present	3 (2.19)	1 (0.72)	
Absent	134 (97.81)	137 (99.28)	0.370
Parity			
0	56 (40.88%)	59 (42.75%)	
1	57 (41.61%)	55 (39.86%)	0.966
2	21 (15.33%)	22 (15.94%)	
3	3 (2.19%)	2 (1.45%)	
Abortions			
0	107 (78.10%)	102 (73.91%)	
1	24 (17.52%)	30 (21.74%)	0.875
2	4 (2.92%)	4 (2.90%)	
3	2 (1.46%)	2 (1.45%)	
Poor orodental hygiene	10 (7.30%)	14 (10.14%)	0.008

The various predictive markers in both the cases and control group are shown in Table 2. Only serum alkaline phosphatase and serum ferritin were found to be significantly associated with preterm deliveries. The serum alkaline phosphatase which was studied in this study was not placental-specific and hence could have been raised due to many other reasons. The serum ferritin could be raised in anaemia, which is so prevalent in Indian women; hence, serum iron was done in these women. Hence, before taking into account the interpretation of these markers, other possible pathologies should be ruled out. The difference in the level of serum iron in the preterm and control group was not statistically significantly.

The 90th percentile value of biochemical laboratory parameters was considered as cut-off when deciding relevance as there is no specific cut-off for these markers. The

distribution of the various biochemical laboratory parameters with respect to 90th percentile value in the cases and controls has therefore also been depicted in Table 3. Serum alkaline phosphatase (>90th percentile) was significantly more common in preterm group with high odds ratio of 3.0315. No significant association was seen in other markers. Table 4 shows sensitivity, specificity, and positive and negative likelihood ratios (LR) of some of the markers.

4. Discussion

Prematurity is a leading cause of neonatal and infant morbidity and mortality and many times it occurs unexpectedly in low risk women. Many biochemical and imaging predictors have been evaluated as screening test of preterm labour in low risk women. An ideal screening test should have a high sensitivity and specificity and should be widely available, easy to perform, reproducible, and accurate. More importantly, an effective intervention should be available to ameliorate the condition for which the screening test is positive. With a solid body of evidence establishing the role of vaginal progesterone in prevention of preterm labour, the search for predictors of spontaneous preterm labour has intensified [8, 9]. Though many biochemical markers have been evaluated, sonographic cervical length, IGFBP-1, and fetal fibronectin in cervicovaginal secretions are most widely used in preterm labour prediction [10]. We wanted to evaluate their success in predicting it in low risk women.

The pathogenesis of preterm labour is not well understood but multifactorial etiology has been postulated. A significant amount of evidence suggests that preterm labour is mediated via infection and inflammation [11]. From study of placentae of preterm deliveries it was found that histological chorioamnionitis was more common in preterm than term deliveries [12]. Therefore, if presence of subclinical infection can be detected between 24 and 28 weeks by various biochemical markers of infection, it would be a step forward towards predicting preterm delivery. This study was planned on this premise. Various clinical, ultrasonographic, and biochemical parameters were studied.

In this study, the cases and controls were matched with respect to age, parity, and socioeconomic status; hence, these parameters were not studied. However, previous studies have reported increased risk of preterm delivery if the maternal age is less than 18 years and more than 35 years [13]. Previous studies have shown association between history of second trimester abortions and preterm delivery; no such association was observed in our study [14, 15]. The association of poor orodental hygiene with preterm birth is a relatively new area of study and though proven to have some association with preterm delivery needs further elucidation in the Indian scenario.

Cervical length less than or equal to 22–25 mm and presence of funneling have been suggested as an important marker for prediction of preterm labour and delivery [16–18]. In a systematic review, it was found that shorter the cervical length, the higher the positive likelihood ratio for preterm delivery [19]. The most common cervical length cut-off used was <25 mm. Combination with other markers like IGFBP-1

TABLE 2: Various predictive markers in both the groups.

	Preterm (n = 137)	Term (n = 138)	P value
Nugent's score ≥8	15	13	0.725 (NS)
Sonographic			
Cervical length (cm)	3.424 (±0.6582)	3.535 (±0.627)	0.2120 (NS)
Funneling	3	1	
Length of funnel (cm)	1.475 (±0.459)	1.72 (±0)	
Diameter of os (cm)	0.25 (0.15–1.08)	0.71 (±0)	
S. interleukin-6 (pg/ml)	0 (0–100)	0 (0–100)	0.4205 (NS)
S. alpha-fetoprotein (ng/ml)	68 (0–208)	62 (0–280)	0.5462 (NS)
S. alkaline phosphatase (U/I)	212.511 (±98.538)	172.835 (±79.214)	**0.0003 (Sig)**
S. ferritin (ng/ml)	10 (2–90)	15 (1–98)	**0.0134 (sig)**
S. iron (μg/dl)	54.5 (17–211)	60 (16–424)	0.2741 (NS)
S. granulocyte colony-stimulating factor (pg/ml)	10 (0–360)	15 (0–560)	0.4728 (NS)
Insulin growth factor binding protein-1 (in cervicovaginal secretion)			
Negative	24 (88.89)	46 (88.46)	1.000 (NS)
Positive	3 (11.11)	6 (11.54)	
Interleukin-6 (pg/ml) (in cervicovaginal secretion)	0 (0–2)	0 (0–2)	0.312 (NS)

TABLE 3: Showing number of patients with more than 90th percentile of various predictive markers in both the groups.

	Preterm (n = 137)	Term (n = 138)	P value	Odds ratio (95% CI)
Serum IL-6 (>90th percentile)	14	16	0.42	0.662 (0.3053 to 1.4354)
Serum ferritin (>90th percentile)	10	20	0.05	0.464 (0.2089 to 1.0333)
Serum G-CSF (>90th percentile)	16	21	0.36	0.9205 (0.4505 to 1.8807)
Serum ALP (>90th percentile)	20	7	0.003	3.0315 (1.1812 to 7.7803)
Serum alpha-fetoprotein (>90th percentile)	13	14	0.546	0.7016 (0.316 to 1.5576)
Cervicovaginal IL-6 (>90th percentile)	17	12	0.312	1.487 (0.6818 to 3.2454)
Cervicovaginal IGFBP (positive)	3	6	1.0	1.2 (0.2624 to 5.4874)

improves the predictive value [20]. Various other studies have concluded that sonographic cervical assessment may be useful in the prediction of preterm delivery, but it should be considered in association with the previous history of preterm delivery rather than in isolation [20]. However in our study cervical length and funneling were not significantly associated with preterm delivery ($P = 0.212$) refuting their efficacy in low risk women.

Various studies show that asymptomatic patients with increased serum IL-6 values between 24 and 36 weeks of gestation are at high risk for preterm delivery [21, 22]. However in our study there was no statistical correlation between levels of IL-6 in serum and preterm delivery ($P = 0.4205$). Granulocyte colony-stimulating factor is elevated in the amniotic fluid and plasma of women with chorioamnionitis and active preterm labour. A study evaluated the association of plasma granulocyte colony-stimulating factor and subsequent spontaneous preterm birth in asymptomatic pregnant women [23]. It reported that compared to term controls, increased values of granulocyte colony-stimulating

factor tested at 24 weeks of gestation were found in women delivering before 28 weeks. In our study no such association was found ($P = 0.472$).

Alkaline phosphatase and alpha-fetoprotein have also been found to be significantly elevated in pregnancies associated with spontaneous preterm birth. In preterm prediction study, Moawad et al. reported association of alkaline phosphatase and alpha-fetoprotein levels with preterm birth. When alkaline phosphatase levels at 24 weeks were studied, the odds ratio for spontaneous preterm birth at <32 weeks was 6.8 (1.4–32.8) and at <35 weeks was 5.1 (1.7–15.6) [24]. In our study there was significant correlation between preterm birth and serum alkaline phosphatase levels at 24 to 28 weeks ($P = 0.009$). In the same study, increased serum alpha-fetoprotein levels at 24 weeks were associated with spontaneous preterm birth at <32 weeks (OR-8.3) and <35 weeks (OR-3.5). There was no statistically significant correlation between preterm birth and serum alpha-fetoprotein levels in our study.

Some prior studies have analysed association between serum ferritin and preterm delivery. One of them reported

TABLE 4: Showing sensitivity, specificity, and positive and negative likelihood ratios (LR) of some markers.

Marker	Biological sample	Sensitivity (%) (95% CI)	Specificity (%) (95% CI)	Positive LR	Negative LR
phIGFBP-1	Cervicovaginal fluid	2 (0.005–0.062)	97 (0.96–0.98)	90 (0.28–2.8)	100 (0.97–1.02)
ALP	Serum	14 (0.09–0.21)	99 (0.991–0998)	**35.18** (15.21–81.41)	86 (0.80–0.91)
AFP	Serum	8 (0.04–0.14)	90 (0.84–0.94)	93 (0.45–1.92)	100 (0.95–1.05)
GCSF	Serum	12 (0.08–0.19)	99 (0.984–0.994)	**13** (6.96–24.67)	88 (0.82–0.93)
IL6	Serum	8 (0.04–0.14)	99 (0.984–0.994)	**8.96** (4.44–18.10)	92 (0.87–0.96)
Cervical length	—	14 (0.09–0.21)	98 (0.97–0.99)	**9.85** (5.65–17.16)	80 (0.81–0.92)

that, after adjusting for various possible confounding factors, the odds ratio for extreme quartiles (>64.5 versus <26.0 ng/mL) of ferritin was 1.3 (95% CI 0.8, 2.1). Stratified analyses indicated that elevated maternal serum ferritin was associated with an increased risk of preterm premature rupture of membranes (OR = 2.1; 95% CI 1.1, 4.1), but not with spontaneous preterm labour (OR = 0.9; 95% CI 0.4, 1.7) or induced preterm delivery (OR = 1.1; 95% CI 0.6, 2.0) [25]. Considering 60% prevalence rate of anaemia during pregnancy in India, serum iron levels were also done to eliminate anaemia as the confounding factor. In our study both serum ferritin and serum iron levels were less in women who delivered preterm as compared to the women who delivered at term but the difference was not statistically significant ($P = 0.053$). This reflects that in developing countries like India the etiology of preterm birth might be more related to nutrition and specifically deficiency of micronutrients like iron. Further studies are indicated.

Insulin-like growth factor binding protein-1 (IGFBP-1) is mainly secreted from fetal and adult liver. It leaks into cervical secretions when fetal membranes detach from decidua. Studies have shown that a bedside rapid strip test (Actim Partus Test) for detection of IGFBP-1 in cervical secretions provides an additional diagnostic tool for the assessment of patients presenting with preterm labour [26, 27]. In another study in which cervicovaginal sample was collected at 22-23 weeks, IGFBP-1 > 6.4 μg/L had a likelihood ratio of +1.8 (95% CI 0.7–2.9) [10]. However in our study group comprised of only low risk women, IGFBP-1 levels did not significantly correlate with preterm delivery. This parameter is possibly more relevant in those patients who have already gone into preterm labour process. We also evaluated IL-6 levels in cervicovaginal secretions for predicting preterm birth; however, no significant correlation was observed. Another study evaluated cervical IL-6 levels in patients who delivered at less than 32 and 35 weeks and found it to be significantly higher in preterm deliveries as compared to their matched controls [28].

Some newer markers have been evaluated in various studies like vitamin D-binding protein, triggering receptor expressed on myeloid cells-1 (sTREM-1), matrix metalloproteinases- (MMP-) 9, MMP-3, tissue inhibitor of metalloproteinases- (TIMP-) 1, TIMP-2, TIMP-3, and TIMP-4, and a panel of various cytokines, chemokines, and growth factors. But they all are still in experimental phase [29, 30].

The lack of association between serum and cervicovaginal makers of inflammation with preterm labour in low risk women points towards some etiology other than inflammation or infection for the occurrence of preterm delivery. Considering 60% prevalence rate of anaemia during pregnancy in India, serum iron levels were also done to eliminate anaemia as the confounding factor. In our study both serum ferritin and serum iron levels were less in women who delivered preterm as compared to the women who delivered at term ($P = 0.053$) but the difference was not statistically significant. This reflects that in developing countries like India the etiology of preterm labour birth might be more related to nutrition and specifically deficiency of micronutrients like Iron.

The strengths of this study were its study design, strict inclusion criteria pertaining to low risk women with no prior history of preterm delivery, and blinding of results to treating physicians. On the other hand, the drawback was smaller samples of preterm cases and controls. Since preterm labour is multifactorial, several factors may have been unaccounted for and further studies are indicated in this important arena.

5. Conclusion

Our study did not prove usefulness of predictive markers like serum AFP, G-CSF, and interleukin-6 and cervicovaginal insulin like growth factor binding protein (IGFBP-1) and interleukin-6. Serum ferritin and alkaline phosphatase were found to have correlation but value of the former is affected in conditions like anaemia and the latter in many other conditions like hemolysis, liver disorders, and so forth. Hence, these markers cannot be relied upon in predicting preterm labour in asymptomatic women. Larger studies evaluating these biomarkers are needed for predicting preterm labour in asymptomatic women. Role of newer markers including genetic markers and micronutrient deficiency needs elucidation.

Conflict of Interests

The authors declare that there is no conflict of interests regarding the publication of this paper.

Acknowledgments

The authors acknowledge the Indian Council of Medical Research for providing grants for conducting this study. This study was planned in the Department of Obstetrics and Gynaecology, Lok Nayak Hospital and Maulana Azad Medical College, with grants from Indian Council of Medical Research. Funding was obtained from ICMR.

References

[1] S. W. Wen, G. Smith, Q. Yang, and M. Walker, "Epidemiology of preterm birth and neonatal outcome," *Seminars in Fetal and Neonatal Medicine*, vol. 9, no. 6, pp. 429–435, 2004.

[2] A. Lembet, D. Eroglu, T. Ergin et al., "New rapid bed-side test to predict preterm delivery: phosphorylated insulin-like growth factor binding protein-1 in cervical secretions," *Acta Obstetricia et Gynecologica Scandinavica*, vol. 81, no. 8, pp. 706–712, 2002.

[3] K. Kwek, C. Khi, H. S. Ting, and G. S. H. Yeo, "Evaluation of a bedside test for phosphorylated insulin-like growth factor binding protein-1 in preterm labour," *Annals of the Academy of Medicine Singapore*, vol. 33, no. 6, pp. 780–783, 2004.

[4] F. Akercan, M. Kazandi, F. Sendag et al., "Value of cervical phosphorylated insulinlike growth factor binding protein-1 in the prediction of preterm labor," *Journal of Reproductive Medicine for the Obstetrician and Gynecologist*, vol. 49, no. 5, pp. 368–372, 2004.

[5] S. E. Elizur, Y. Yinon, G. S. Epatein, D. S. Seidman, E. Schiff, and E. Sivan, "Insulin-like growth factor binding protein-1 detection in preterm labor: evaluation of a bedside test," *American Journal of Perinatology*, vol. 22, no. 6, pp. 305–309, 2005.

[6] P.-Y. Ancel, M.-J. Saurel-Cubizolles, G. C. Di Renzo, E. Papiernik, and G. Breart, "Very and moderate preterm births: are the risk factors different?" *The British Journal of Obstetrics and Gynaecology*, vol. 106, no. 11, pp. 1162–1170, 1999.

[7] N. B. Kyrldund-Blomberg and S. Cnattingius, "Preterm birth and maternal smoking: Risks related to gestational age and onset of delivery," *American Journal of Obstetrics and Gynecology*, vol. 179, no. 4, pp. 1051–1055, 1998.

[8] S. S. Hassan, R. Romero, D. Vidyadhari et al., "Vaginal progesterone reduces the rate of preterm birth in women with a sonographic short cervix: a multicenter, randomized, double-blind, placebo-controlled trial," *Ultrasound in Obstetrics & Gynecology*, vol. 38, no. 1, pp. 18–31, 2011.

[9] R. Romero, K. Nicolaides, A. Conde-Agudelo et al., "Vaginal progesterone in women with an asymptomatic sonographic short cervix in the midtrimester decreases preterm delivery and neonatal morbidity: a systematic review and metaanalysis of individual patient data," *The American Journal of Obstetrics & Gynecology*, vol. 206, pp. 124.e1–124.e19, 2012.

[10] M. Kurkinen-Räty, A. Ruokonen, S. Vuopala et al., "Combination of cervical interleukin-6 and -8, phosphorylated insulin-like growth factor-binding protein-1 and transvaginal cervical ultrasonography in assessment of the risk of preterm birth," *British Journal of Obstetrics and Gynaecology*, vol. 108, no. 8, pp. 875–881, 2001.

[11] J. Lumley, "The epidemiology of preterm birth," *Bailliere's Clinical Obstetrics and Gynaecology*, vol. 7, no. 3, pp. 477–498, 1993.

[12] D. S. Guzick and K. Winn, "The association of chorioamnionitis with preterm delivery," *Obstetrics and Gynecology*, vol. 65, no. 1, pp. 11–16, 1985.

[13] P.-Y. Ancel, M.-J. Saurel-Cubizolles, G. C. di Renzo, E. Papiernik, and G. Breart, "Very and moderate preterm births: are the risk factors different?" *British Journal of Obstetrics and Gynaecology*, vol. 106, no. 11, pp. 1162–1170, 1999.

[14] N. B. Kyrldund-Blomberg and S. Cnattingius, "Preterm birth and maternal smoking: risks related to gestational age and onset of delivery," *American Journal of Obstetrics and Gynecology*, vol. 179, no. 4, pp. 1051–1055, 1998.

[15] S. Cnattingius, F. Granath, G. Petersson, and B. L. Harlow, "The influence of gestational age and smoking habits on the risk of subsequent preterm deliveries," *The New England Journal of Medicine*, vol. 341, no. 13, pp. 943–948, 1999.

[16] J. Owen, N. Yost, V. Berghella et al., "Mid-trimester endovaginal sonography in women at high risk for spontaneous preterm birth," *Journal of the American Medical Association*, vol. 286, no. 11, pp. 1340–1348, 2001.

[17] W. W. Andrews, R. Copper, J. C. Hauth, R. L. Goldenberg, C. Neely, and M. Dubard, "Second-trimester cervical ultrasound: associations with increased risk for recurrent early spontaneous delivery," *Obstetrics and Gynecology*, vol. 95, no. 2, pp. 222–226, 2000.

[18] V. C. Heath, G. Daskalakis, A. Zagaliki, M. Carvalho, and K. H. Nicolaides, "Cervicovaginal fibronectin and cervical lenth at 23 weeks of gestation: relative risk of early preterm delivery," *British Journal of Obstetrics and Gynaecology*, vol. 107, no. 10, pp. 1276–1281, 2000.

[19] J. M. G. Crane and D. Hutchens, "Transvaginal sonographic measurement of cervical length to predict preterm birth in asymptomatic women at increased risk: a systematic review," *Ultrasound in Obstetrics and Gynecology*, vol. 31, no. 5, pp. 579–587, 2008.

[20] M. H. B. de Carvalho, R. E. Bittar, M. D. L. Brizot, C. Bicudo, and M. Zugaib, "Prediction of preterm delivery in the second trimester," *Obstetrics and Gynecology*, vol. 105, no. 3, pp. 532–536, 2005.

[21] M. A. G. Coleman, J. A. Keelan, L. M. E. McCowan, K. M. Townend, and M. D. Mitchell, "Predicting preterm delivery: comparison of cervicovaginal interleukin (IL)-1β, IL-6 and IL-8 with fetal fibronectin and cervical dilatation," *European Journal of Obstetrics Gynecology and Reproductive Biology*, vol. 95, no. 2, pp. 154–158, 2001.

[22] J. Dowd, N. Laham, G. Rice, S. Brennecke, and M. Permezel, "Elevated interleukin-8 concentrations in cervical secretions are associated with preterm labour," *Gynecologic and Obstetric Investigation*, vol. 51, no. 3, pp. 165–168, 2001.

[23] R. L. Goldenberg, W. W. Andrews, B. M. Mercer et al., "The preterm prediction study: granulocyte colony-stimulating factor and spontaneous preterm birth," *American Journal of Obstetrics & Gynecology*, vol. 182, no. 3, pp. 625–630, 2000.

[24] A. H. Moawad, R. L. Goldenberg, B. Mercer et al., "The Preterm Prediction Study: the value of serum alkaline phosphatase, α-fetoprotein, plasma corticotropin-releasing hormone, and other serum markers for the prediction of spontaneous preterm birth," *The American Journal of Obstetrics and Gynecology*, vol. 186, no. 5, pp. 990–996, 2002.

[25] R. Xiao, T. K. Sorensen, I. O. Frederick et al., "Maternal second-trimester serum ferritin concentrations and subsequent risk of preterm delivery," *Paediatric and Perinatal Epidemiology*, vol. 16, no. 4, pp. 297–304, 2002.

[26] H.-S. Ting, P.-S. Chin, G. S. Yeo, and K. Kwek, "Comparison of bedside test kits for prediction of preterm delivery: phosphorylated insulin-like growth factor binding protein-1 (pIGFBP-1) test and fetal fibronectin test," *Annals of the Academy of Medicine*, vol. 36, no. 6, pp. 399–402, 2007.

[27] A. Lembet, D. Eroglu, T. Ergin et al., "New rapid bed-side test to predict preterm delivery: phosphorylated insulin-like growth factor binding protein-1 in cervical secretions," *Acta Obstetricia et Gynecologica Scandinavica*, vol. 81, no. 8, pp. 706–712, 2002.

[28] P. S. Ramsey, T. Tamura, R. L. Goldenberg et al., "The preterm prediction study: elevated cervical ferritin levels at 22 to 24

weeks of gestation are associated with spontaneous preterm delivery in asymptomatic women," *The American Journal of Obstetrics and Gynecology*, vol. 186, no. 3, pp. 458–463, 2002.

[29] S. Liong, M. di Quinzio, G. Fleming, M. Permezel, G. Rice, and H. Georgiou, "New biomarkers for the spontaneous labour symptomatic pregnant women: a comparison with fetal fibronectin," *BJOG*, 2014.

[30] I. Tency, M. Temmerman, and M. Vaneechoutte, "Inflammatory response in maternal serum during preterm labour," *Facts, Views & Vision in Obgyn*, vol. 6, no. 1, pp. 19–30, 2014.

14

Male Partner's Involvement in HIV Counselling and Testing and Associated Factors among Partners of Pregnant Women in Gondar Town, Northwest Ethiopia

Alemu Zenebe,[1] Abebaw Gebeyehu,[2] Lemma Derseh,[3] and Kedir Y. Ahmed[4]

[1]*Department of Pediatric Operation Theatre, Black Lion teaching Hospital, Addis Ababa, Ethiopia*
[2]*Department of Reproductive Health, Institute of Public Health, College of Medicine and Health Science,*
 University of Gondar, P.O. Box 196, Gondar, Ethiopia
[3]*Department of Epidemiology and Biostatistics, Institute of Public Health, College of Medicine and Health Science,*
 University of Gondar, P.O. Box 196, Gondar, Ethiopia
[4]*Department of Public Health, College of Medicine and Health Science, Debre Markos University, P.O. Box 269, Debre Markos, Ethiopia*

Correspondence should be addressed to Kedir Y. Ahmed; kedirymam331@gmail.com

Academic Editor: Fabio Facchinetti

Background. Despite the existence of several programmes promoting male involvement in HIV counselling and testing during their wife's pregnancy as a part of PMTCT, few men have heeded the call. The aim of this study was to assess male partner's involvement in HCT and its associated factors. *Methods.* This study was based on institution based cross-sectional study design that used systematic random sampling technique. A total of 416 partners were interviewed in the data collection. Multivariable logistic regression model was fitted to identify the independent predictors. *Result.* In this study, the prevalence of male involvement in HCT was found to be 40.1% (95% CI: 35.3%–44.7%). The independent predictors of male involvement were partners who were younger, were cohabitant, were with multigravida wives, were knowledgeable on route of mother-to-child transmission, and discussed HCT. *Conclusion.* The prevalence of male involvement in HCT was found to be suboptimal compared to similar studies in Ethiopia. There is a need of interventions on partners who are older, separated, and with lower gravidity wife. Awareness creation campaign should also be created on the route of mother-to-child transmission of HIV and on the importance of discussion with wife.

1. Introduction

HIV pandemic created an enormous challenge to the survival of mankind worldwide [1]. Worldwide there are an estimated 33.3 million people infected with HIV; Sub-Saharan Africa bears the greater burden with an estimated 22.5 million people infected with HIV [2]. According to UNAIDS, women represent 52% of those infected with HIV worldwide and in Sub-Saharan Africa 60% of those infected with HIV are women [2]. With a national adult HIV prevalence of 1.5% (1.9% in women and 1.0% in men), Ethiopia is one of the country's most severely hit by the epidemic [3].

Mother-to-child transmission (MTCT) is an important source of HIV infection among Ethiopian children, which accounts for more than 90% of pediatric AIDS [1, 4].

Prevention of Mother-to-Child Transmission (PMTCT) programmes have been proven to be effective in reducing the risk of HIV transmission from infected mothers to their children [5]. Without intervention, the risk of MTCT of HIV ranges from 20% to 45%. With specific interventions in nonbreast-feeding populations, the risk of MTCT can be reduced to less than 2% and to 5% or less in breastfeeding populations [6]. Antenatal care (ANC) is a major entry point for PMTCT programmes especially in countries with a high prevalence of HIV. It creates an opportunity to capture pregnant mothers and their male partners to reverse the transmission of HIV during pregnancy, labour, and breastfeeding [7]. Male involvement is necessary for improving women's uptake of core PMTCT services; it is a key contributor to community acceptance and support of PMTCT [8].

However, actual involvement of male partners in PMTCT programmes in several counties of Sub-Saharan Africa is low and programmes report difficulties in attracting the involvement of male partners. Studies conducted in African countries showed that male involvement in PMTCT during pregnancy ranges from 11% to 58.3% [5, 9–11]. In Ethiopia, studies conducted in Arba Minch and Debre Markos town reported that 53.6% and 55.4% of partners accompanied their wives for HIV testing and counselling [12, 13].

Despite the existence of several programmes promoting male involvement in HIV counselling and testing during their wives' pregnancy as a part of PMTCT, few men have heeded the call. Numerous reasons for nonparticipation of male partners in HIV counselling and testing as PMTCT programmes have been gained from studies that primarily focused on women as respondents. This study primarily focused on men to gain understanding of factors that influence their involvement in these programmes. Thus, this study was aimed at assessing male involvement and associated factors in HCT among partners of pregnant women in Gondar town, Northwest Ethiopia.

2. Methods

2.1. Study Design and Study Setting. Institution based cross-sectional study was used to assess the prevalence and associated factors of male involvement in HCT among partners of pregnant women in Gondar administrative city from July to November 2014. Gondar is an ancient town located 727 Km North of Addis Ababa with an estimated population of 207,044 of which 50.8% were females and the rest are males. There are eight health centers that provide ANC service with HCT of both pregnant women and their husbands.

2.2. Source and Study Population. Partners of all pregnant women who did voluntary HCT in the current pregnancy were the study population. Those partners selected by systematic random sampling technique were included in this study. Partners who are unable to communicate for different reasons and those who are not living together were excluded from the study.

2.3. Sample Size Determination and Sampling Procedure. By using single population proportion formula, as there is no information about it, about 50% prevalence of male involvement was used. Considering 5% margin of error and 95% confidence interval with 10% nonresponse rate, the final minimum sample size was found to be 422. Based on the number of mothers who were on ANC follow-up, the samples were distributed to all eight health centers proportionate to their number. After the first participant was selected using lottery method, systematic random sampling technique was used to select eligible participants.

2.4. Data Collection. Data was collected by using pretested structured questionnaire. The tool was developed in English and translated to Amharic and then back to English to check for its consistency. Ten data collectors and three supervisors who can speak Amharic language were recruited. Partners

involved in HCT were interviewed at the facility level and those who did not involve in HCT were at the household level. To assure the quality of the data, three-day training was given to data collectors and supervisors, and on each data collection day some percent of the collected data were reviewed by principal investigator; any problems faced in the time of data collection were discussed and immediate solution was made.

2.5. Operational Definitions. Operational definitions are as follows:

(i) Male involvement: when husbands or partners of pregnant women attended both HIV counselling and testing (HCT) during ANC visit for the purpose of PMTCT service.

(ii) Knowledge about route of MTCT: when respondents know at least one route of transmission of MTCT of HIV from three questions.

(iii) Knowledge about PMTCT: when respondents know at least one way of PMTCT from three questions.

2.6. Data Processing and Analysis. The data were checked, coded, and entered to Epi-info software version 3.5.1 and cleaning was performed by using SPSS 20. Frequencies, proportions, and measures of central tendency and variation were used to describe the study participant. Binary logistic regression was used to examine association between dependent and each independent variable. All variables with $p < 0.2$ in bivariate analysis were entered into multiple logistic regression model to identify factors independently associated with male involvement in HCT during pregnancy. Backward stepwise likelihood ratio was used to select the final independent predictors. The significance of Odds Ratios (OR) was determined with 95% CI and $p < 0.05$.

2.7. Ethical Consideration. Ethical clearance was obtained from University of Gondar, and letter of permission was obtained from the respected health institutions. Informed consent from each study participant was being obtained after explaining the purpose of the study. Confidentiality of the information was assured by omitting names from the questionnaire and maximum effort was made to maintain privacy of the respondents during the interview. No question was asked about their serostatus. No incentives were provided to the respondents as a way of motivating them to participate in the study. All the identified potential participants agreed to participate in the study.

3. Result

3.1. Sociodemographic Characteristics of Partners. The nonresponse rate of this study was found to be 6 (1.42%). The mean (±SD) age of partners who participated in this study was 34.38 years (±6.0). The majority, 210 (50.5%) of them, reported the current pregnancy as wife's first pregnancy (Table 1).

Among respondents, 206 (49.5%) reported that the average distance of the living area from health institution used to perform HCT was less than five Km. Regarding the amount

TABLE 1: A sociodemographic characteristic of partners of pregnant women in Gondar town, Northwest Ethiopia, 2013.

Variables	Frequency	Percentage (%)
Age		
20–29	79	19
30–39	237	57
40+	100	24
Marital statues		
Married	403	96.9%
Unmarried	13	3.1%
Religion		
Orthodox christian	287	69
Muslim	97	23.3
Others (protestant or catholic)	32	7.7
Educational status		
No formal education	66	15.9
Primary education	97	23.3
Secondary and above	253	60.8
Occupation		
Private business	143	34.4
Government employee	88	21.2
NGO	74	17.8
Daily labor	62	14.9
Farmer and others	49	11.8
Wife's number of pregnancies		
1	166	39.9
2-3	210	50.5
4-5	34	8.2
6+	6	1.4
Time of living together		
Not living together	11	2.6
1–5 years	254	61.1
6–10 years	108	26
11–15 years	33	7.9
16+ years	10	2.4
Distance to nearby health facility		
Less than 5 km	206	49.5
5–10 km	128	30.8
More than 10 km	82	19.7
Money paid for transportation		
Did not pay	34	8.2
<5 Ethiopian birr	182	43.8
5–10 Ethiopian birr	165	39.6
>10 Ethiopian birr	35	8.4

TABLE 2: Knowledge and attitude towards PMTCT and risk perception of male partners of pregnant women in Gondar town, Northwest Ethiopia, 2013.

Variables	Frequency	Percentage (%)
Occurrence of MTCT ($n = 386$)		
During pregnancy	301	78
During childbirth	199	51.6
During breastfeeding	298	77.7
PMTCT methods ($n = 384$)		
ART	324	84.4
Caesarean section	13	3.4
Avoiding of breastfeeding	221	57.6
Presence of HCT during ANC visit		
Yes	375	90.1
No	16	3.9
I do not know	25	6
Necessity of partner testing		
Yes	396	95.2
No	20	4.8
Discordant test result		
Yes	356	85.6
No	60	14.4
Feeling when seen with pregnant women in clinic		
Feel nothing	214	51.4
Feel happiness	197	47.4
Feel ashamed	5	1.2
Risk perception		
Yes	98	23.6
No	318	76.4
Reasons of risk perception ($n = 98$)		
Used unsterile sharp object	57	58.2
Had multiple sexual partner	44	44.9
Had sexual contact without condom	39	39.8
Had sex with positive person	10	10.2

of money they paid for transports, 182 (43.8%) of the them paid less than five Ethiopian birr for the trip (Table 1).

3.2. *Knowledge and Attitude towards PMTCT.* About 386 (92.8%) of them knew at least one route of MTCT and 301 (78%), 298 (77.2%), and 199 (51.6%) of them reported MTCT of HIV during pregnancy, breastfeeding, and childbirth, respectively. The majority, 384 (92.3%) of respondents, knew

at least one method of PMTCT and 324 (84.4%) of them knew that provision of ARTs for the mother could help to reduce MTCT of HIV. On the other hand, 221 (57.6%) of them knew that avoiding breastfeeding is one of the alternatives for preventing HIV transmission from mother to child, but only 3.4% [12] of respondents were aware that risk of MTCT of HIV could be reduced by caesarean section. Among respondents, 375 (90.1%) of them knew the presence of HCT for pregnant women during their ANC visit. Three hundred ninety-six (95.2%) of them agreed on the necessity of partner testing. About 356 (85.6%) of partners knew that discordant result can be found among married partners (Table 2).

3.3. *Perceived Risk to Acquire the Virus.* Perceived risk of acquiring the virus was reported in about 98 (23.6%) of male

TABLE 3: Level of involvement of partners of pregnant women towards HCT in Gondar town, Northwest Ethiopia, 2013.

Variables	Frequency	Percentage (%)
Discussed about HCT with their wife		
Yes	278	66.8
No	138	33.2
Willingness to visit PMTCT clinic with his wife		
Yes	288	69.2
No	128	30.8
Visited PMTCT clinic with his wife		
Yes	212	51
No	204	49
Involved in counselling only		
Yes	174	41.8
No	242	58.2
Involved for both counselling and testing		
Yes	167	40.1
No	249	59.9
Reasons for partners involvement ($n = 167$)		
Feel responsibility	100	59.9
Initiated by provider	65	38.9
Initiated by wife	44	26.3
Reasons for partners noninvolvement ($n = 249$)		
Work overload	131	52.6
Fear of acquiring the virus	116	46.6
Confidentiality issue	47	18.9
Fear of inaccurate test result	12	4.8

partners. Of these, 57 (58.2%) used unsterile sharp object and 44 (44.9%) of them had multiple sexual partners (Table 2).

3.4. Level of Male Involvement in HCT. Among partners, 278 (66.8%) discussed HCT with their pregnant wives. And more than two-thirds (69.2%) of them had willingness to accompany PMTCT clinic with their pregnant wife together. Two hundred twelve (51%) of them visited PMTCT clinic with their wife. About 174 (41.8%) of respondents were involved in the counselling part only and 167 (40.1%) of them with 95% CI (35.2–44.2) participated in both counselling and testing, meaning the overall involvement in HCT (Table 3). Among those involved in HCT, 100 (59.9%) were involved because they felt responsibility. Work overload which was mentioned by 131 (52.6%) of them was the main reason for noninvolvement of partners (Table 3).

3.5. Factors Associated with Male Involvement in HCT. In multivariable analysis, being at younger age group, couples living together, wife's number of pregnancies, having knowledge on the timing of MTCT, and husbands discussing HCT

with their wives were positively and significantly associated with male involvement in HCT. The odds of male involvement in HCT was higher in 20–29-year (AOR = 4.94 95% CI: 1.97–12.39) and 30–39 years' (AOR = 2.82 95% CI: 1.37–5.81) age groups as compared to those who were 40 years of age and above.

Those partners who are living together with their wives were 5.5 (95% CI: 1.97–15.39) times more likely to be involved in HCT. Wife's gravidity of 2-3 (AOR = 5.34 95% CI: 1.38-20.69) and 4-5 (AOR = 8.10 95% CI: 1.52-43.32) was significantly associated with male involvement in HCT compared to those who had only one pregnancy. The likelihood of male involvement in HCT was found to be higher (AOR = 7.41 95% CI: 1.80–30.45) among those who knew the timing of mother-to-child transmission. Those partners who reported discussion about HCT with their wives had increased (AOR = 8.60 95% CI: 4.30–17.21) odds of involvement in HCT compared to their counterparts (Table 4).

4. Discussion

In this study, about 40.1% of the partners escorted their wives to ANC and received HIV counselling and testing together. This finding is relatively similar to study conducted in Addis Ababa and Tanzania community which was 44% and 46.3%, respectively [9, 14]. However, the finding is lower than that reported in Cameroon which was 58.3% [5], while it was higher than pooled estimate of studies conducted in India, Cameroon, Georgia, and the Dominican Republic which was 36.1% and another study conducted in Cape Town, South Africa, which was 32% [11, 15]. Thus, the finding of this study implies that there is already an encouraging platform for male involvement in the study area, and this could serve as a springboard to achieve full scale male involvement in HCT in the city of Gondar and other similar urban areas.

This study demonstrated that the level of male involvement in HCT was found to be higher among younger male partners. This finding is consistent with reviewed literatures which found that males involved in HCT were younger than those who received HCT alone in the same clinic [16]. This might be due to increased communication between couples and level of knowledge expected to be reduced with age. This is supported by study conducted in South Africa, 23.5% of individuals 50 years of age and above did not know the route of transmission of HIV from mother to child [17]. Moreover, an operational research conducted in Zimbabwe showed that as age increased majority of men fear going for HIV tests [18]. However, similar studies conducted in Cameroon and Western Uganda showed that the proportion of males accompanying their partner increased with age, for example, in rural western Uganda males older than 35 years were 2.89 times more likely to receive VCT than those of 35 years or younger [5, 19]. The difference with these studies could be explained by the existence of social support and difference in health service utilization in the later studies.

This result showed that male partners of pregnant women who were living with their wives were significantly more likely to be tested than those partners of pregnant women living in separated place. Absence of the male partner for

TABLE 4: Factors associated with male involvement in HCT in Gondar town, Northwest Ethiopia, 2013.

Variables	Male involvement		COR with 95% CI	AOR with 95% CI
	Yes	No		
Age				
20–29	36	43	2.51 (1.33, 4.73)	**4.94 (1.97, 12.39)**[**]
30–39	106	131	2.43 (1.44, 4.08)	**2.82 (1.37, 5.81)**[*]
40+	25	75	1	1
Living together				
Yes	161	199	6.74 (2.82, 16.12)	**5.50 (1.97, 15.39)**[**]
No	6	50	1	1
Wife's total pregnancy				
One	66	100	1	1
Two-three	87	123	1.07 (0.71, 1.62)	**5.34 (1.38, 20.69)**[*]
Four-five	13	21	0.94 (0.44, 2.0)	**8.10 (1.52, 43.32)**[*]
Six and above	1	5	0.30 (0.04, 2.65)	1.35 (0.09, 20.23)
Knew time of MTCT				
Yes	164	222	6.65 (1.98, 22.29)	**7.41 (1.80, 30.45)**[*]
No	3	27	1	1
Discussed HCT				
Yes	153	125	10.84 (5.94, 19.77)	**8.60 (4.30, 17.21)**[*]
No	14	124	1	**1**

[*] p value < 0.05, [**] p value <= 0.001, COR = crude odds ratio, and AOR = adjusted odds ratio.

discussion at home and decreased likelihood of accompanying his pregnant wife during ANC follow-up could be the possible explanation for the above finding. In this study, male involvement in HCT was significantly associated with wife's number of pregnancies. This could be explained by the fact that for each additional pregnancy there is increased frequency of contact of mothers with health care workers which increases their awareness and their chance of discussion with their husbands. Furthermore, these findings contradict with studies conducted in India and Kenya and showed that males who had fewer children were more likely to assist their partner in pregnancy and childbirth than males who had large number of children [20, 21].

Those partners who know at least one mode of transmission of HIV from MTC were 7.4 times more involved in HCT compared to their counterparts. This finding is similar to the study conducted in Zambia which showed that knowledge and the total score on level of involvement were positively and significantly associated [22]. This might be due to increased level of knowledge and awareness about HCT expected to have a positive influence on men's involvement in HCT. Having history of discussion about HIV testing with pregnant wife remained significantly associated with male attendance at the antenatal clinic for HCT. This finding was similar to another study conducted in Zambia [22]. Having discussion with their wives might help them to get what they heard from the health care workers during their wives' ANC visit which could be the possible explanation for increased uptake of partners.

The possibility of social desirability bias due to sensitiveness of issues and cross-sectional nature of the study which fails to show causal relationship were among the limitations of this study. Study was conducted both in health institution and in community level to address both involvers and noninvolvers which is the strength of this study.

5. Conclusion

Despite the existence of several programmes promoting male involvement in HIV counselling and testing during their wives' pregnancy as a part of PMTCT, still lower proportion of them accompany their wives for HCT. The prevalence of male involvement was found to be significantly higher among partners who are younger, living with their wives, are living with multigravida wives, are knowledgeable about mode of mother-to-child transmission of HIV, and discussed HCT with their wives. Therefore, there is a need of an intervention in the independent predictors.

Competing Interests

The authors declared that they have no conflict of interests.

Acknowledgments

The authors would like to forward their thanks to all supervisors and data collectors for their willingness and timely submission of questionnaires. Their thanks also go to University of Gondar for their library service and academic support. In addition, they thank Gondar health office and all health institutions for facilitation of data collection.

References

[1] Federal HIV/AIDS Prevention and Control Office, *Federal Ministry of Health: Guidelines for Prevention of Mother-to-Child Transmission of HIV in Ethiopia*, Federal HIV/AIDS Prevention and Control Office, Addis Ababa, Ethiopia, July 2007.

[2] WHO, *Global Report on the Global AIDS Epidemic. Joint United Nations Programme on HIV/AIDS (UNAIDS)*, WHO, Geneva, Switzerland, 2010.

[3] Central Statistical Agency and ICF Macro, *Ethiopia Demographic and Health Survey*, ICF Macro, Calverton, Md, USA, 2011.

[4] W. Deressa, A. Seme, A. Asefa, G. Teshome, and F. Enqusellassie, "Utilization of PMTCT services and associated factors among pregnant women attending antenatal clinics in Addis Ababa, Ethiopia," *BMC Pregnancy and Childbirth*, vol. 14, article 328, 2014.

[5] G. N. Nkuoh, D. J. Meyer, P. M. Tih, and J. Nkfusai, "Barriers to men's participation in antenatal and prevention of mother-to-child HIV transmission care in Cameroon, Africa," *Journal of Midwifery and Women's Health*, vol. 55, no. 4, pp. 363–369, 2010.

[6] WHO, *Preventing Mother-to-Child Transmission of HIV to Reach the UNGASS and MDGs Moving towards the Elimination of Pediatric HIV. PMTCT Strategic Vision 2010–2015*, WHO, Geneva, Switzerland, 2011.

[7] A. Adera, M. Wudu, Y. Yimam, S. Mengistie, M. Kidane, and A. Woreta, "Factors that affects male partner involvement in PMTCT services in africa: a review literature," *Science Journal of Public Health*, vol. 3, no. 4, pp. 460–467, 2015.

[8] F. Haile and Y. Brhan, "Male partner involvements in PMTCT: a cross sectional study, Mekelle, Northern Ethiopia," *BMC Pregnancy and Childbirth*, vol. 14, article 65, 2014.

[9] J. Homsy, J. Obonyo, J. Ojwang et al., "Routine intrapartum HIV counseling and testing for prevention of mother-to-child transmission of HIV in a rural Ugandan hospital," *Journal of Acquired Immune Deficiency Syndromes*, vol. 42, no. 2, pp. 149–154, 2006.

[10] I. Thior, S. Lockman, L. M. Smeaton et al., "Breastfeeding plus infant zidovudine prophylaxis for 6 months vs formula feeding plus infant zidovudine for 1 month to reduce mother-to-child HIV transmission in Botswana: a randomized trial: the Mashi Study," *The Journal of the American Medical Association*, vol. 296, no. 7, pp. 794–805, 2006.

[11] J. Orne-Gliemann, P. T. Tchendjou, M. Miric et al., "Couple-oriented prenatal HIV counseling for HIV primary prevention: An Acceptability Study," *BMC Public Health*, vol. 10, article 197, 2010.

[12] M. Tilahun and S. Mohamed, "Male partners' involvement in the prevention of mother-to-child transmission of HIV and associated factors in Arba Minch Town and Arba Minch Zuria Woreda, Southern Ethiopia," *BioMed Research International*, vol. 2015, Article ID 763876, 6 pages, 2015.

[13] A. Endawoke, T. Gebeyaw, and A. Amanuel, "Level of male partner involvement and associated factors in prevention of mother to child transmission of HIV/AIDS services in Debremarkos town, Northwest Ethiopia," *African Journal of AIDS and HIV Research*, vol. 1, no. 2, pp. 16–25, 2013.

[14] D. Getu, *Factors Related to Male Participation in Prevention of Mother-to-Child Transmission of Human Immunodeficiency Virus in Three Public Hospitals in Addis Ababa, Ethiopia*, University of South Africa, 2011.

[15] B. K. F. Mohlala, M.-C. Boily, and S. Gregson, "The forgotten half of the equation: randomized controlled trial of a male invitation to attend couple voluntary counselling and testing," *AIDS*, vol. 25, no. 12, pp. 1535–1541, 2011.

[16] I. T. Kamal, "Field experiences in involving men in safe motherhood," Report of the Meeting of WHO Regional Advisers in Reproductive Health, WHO, Washington, DC, USA, 2001.

[17] O. Shisana, T. Rehele, L. C. Simbayi et al., *South African National HIV Prevalence, HIV Incidence, Behavior and Communication Survey*, Cape Town HSRC Press, 2005.

[18] Z. Pemberai, C. Hope, S. Chiedzwa, and D. Rumbidzai, Understanding factors that cause low male involvement in Community HIV programs for effective design of gender inclusive programs, An operations research report submitted to the regional AIDS training network family and AIDS caring trust (fact) research and knowledge management Department, Zimbabwe, 2011.

[19] F. M. Bwambale, S. N. Ssali, S. Byaruhanga, J. N. Kalyango, and C. A. S. Karamagi, "Voluntary HIV counselling and testing among men in rural western Uganda: implications for HIV prevention," *BMC Public Health*, vol. 8, article 263, 2008.

[20] Department of Reproductive Health and Research, *Male Involvement in the Elimination of Mother-to-Child Transmission of HIV*, Department of Reproductive Health and Research, Geneva, Switzerland, 2011.

[21] D. A. Katz, J. N. Kiarie, G. C. John-Stewart, B. A. Richardson, F. N. John, and C. Farquhar, "Male perspectives on incorporating men into antenatal HIV counseling and testing," *PLoS ONE*, vol. 4, no. 11, Article ID e7602, 2009.

[22] T. Dinzela, *Factors influencing men's involvement in prevention of mother to child transmission (PMTCT) of HIV programmes in Mambwe District, Zambia [M.S. thesis]*, University of South Africa, 2006.

15

Posttraumatic Stress and Posttraumatic Stress Disorder after Termination of Pregnancy and Reproductive Loss

Viltė Daugirdaitė,[1] Olga van den Akker,[2] and Satvinder Purewal[3]

[1]*Department of General Psychology, Philosophy Faculty, Vilnius University, Universiteto 9/1, Vilnius, LT-01513, Lithuania*
[2]*Department of Psychology, Middlesex University, The Burroughs, Hendon, London NW4 4BT, UK*
[3]*Institute of Psychology, University of Wolverhampton, Wulfruna Street, Wolverhampton WV1 1LY, UK*

Correspondence should be addressed to Olga van den Akker; o.vandenakker@mdx.ac.uk

Academic Editor: Gian Carlo Di Renzo

Objective. The aims of this systematic review were to integrate the research on posttraumatic stress (PTS) and posttraumatic stress disorder (PTSD) after termination of pregnancy (TOP), miscarriage, perinatal death, stillbirth, neonatal death, and failed in vitro fertilisation (IVF). *Methods*. Electronic databases (AMED, British Nursing Index, CINAHL, MEDLINE, SPORTDiscus, PsycINFO, PubMEd, ScienceDirect) were searched for articles using PRISMA guidelines. *Results*. Data from 48 studies were included. Quality of the research was generally good. PTS/PTSD has been investigated in TOP and miscarriage more than perinatal loss, stillbirth, and neonatal death. In all reproductive losses and TOPs, the prevalence of PTS was greater than PTSD, both decreased over time, and longer gestational age is associated with higher levels of PTS/PTSD. Women have generally reported more PTS or PTSD than men. Sociodemographic characteristics (e.g., younger age, lower education, and history of previous traumas or mental health problems) and psychsocial factors influence PTS and PTSD after TOP and reproductive loss. *Conclusions*. This systematic review is the first to investigate PTS/PTSD after reproductive loss. Patients with advanced pregnancies, a history of previous traumas, mental health problems, and adverse psychosocial profiles should be considered as high risk for developing PTS or PTSD following reproductive loss.

1. Introduction

Posttraumatic stress (PTS) and posttraumatic stress disorder (PTSD) after reproductive loss have not been well recognised, despite the growing documentation of adverse psychological states associated with reproductive losses. Our focus is on PTS and PTSD but did not include acute stress disorder (ASD) because ASD is a separate disorder diagnosed only in the first month following the traumatic event. Although the classification of TOP and reproductive loss varies from country to country [1], TOP broadly refers to the *termination of a clinical pregnancy* and miscarriage to the *spontaneous loss* of a clinical pregnancy before 20 completed weeks of gestation. Perinatal death, on the other hand, refers to a fetal or neonatal death after 20+ weeks during pregnancy and childbirth or up to 7 days after birth, whereas stillbirth

denotes the death of a (20+ weeks of gestational age) baby before the complete expulsion/extraction from its mother. A neonatal death is said to have occurred when a live born baby dies within 28 days of birth [2]. Failed in vitro fertilisation (IVF) is also considered by some infertile couples as a reproductive loss [3], with some women reporting grief, sadness, and distress with IVF failures [4, 5] and, for those who do become pregnant, a more intense protective attachment to their fetus [6]. PTS and PTSD can evolve after any of these reproductive losses [7–10].

Further, TOP is different from other reproductive losses as it involves a "choice" of the woman to terminate a pregnancy or not, but the event itself is a stressful situation and can become traumatic for some women [11]. It is also important to separate nonmedical TOP (which is usually requested for social reasons) from medical TOP, which is usually requested when there is evidence of foetal abnormality which could lead to giving birth to a baby unlikely to survive long, or when the difficulties of rearing an affected child are perceived as too great to be acceptable to the couple [12]. The differences between medical and nonmedical TOP are further highlighted in societal/cultural acceptance and legal status. For instance, many African or Latin American countries will not allow nonmedical TOPs [13], although the World Health Organisation [14] reported that highly restrictive abortion laws did not lower TOP rates, stigmatising this illegal practice further. Specifically, the abortion rate is 29 per 1,000 women of childbearing age in Africa (where TOP is illegal under most circumstances in most countries) compared with 12 per 1000 in Western Europe (where abortion is permitted in many countries). Nonmedical TOP may not be recognized as a traumatic event by some women because they do not want the baby [15]. However, some of these women subsequently regret having had the abortion and can experience it as trauma [16]. Not all women experiencing a nonmedical TOP will experience posttraumatic consequences [17] but that is also true for medical TOP and all other reproductive losses. Nonetheless the psychological impact of nonmedical and medical TOP may be different, but the extent to which they differ needs further investigation.

Although mental health promotion following reproductive loss is underinvestigated [18], PTSD after childbirth and pregnancy loss has been distinguished from postnatal depression and complicated grief [19, 20]. Studies which have investigated PTS and/or PTSD following reproductive loss and TOP have reported mixed results [13, 21]. For example, high levels of PTSD following nonmedical TOP have been reported by some [22] but not all previous research [23]. At present, there is no systematically pooled research evidence on PTS and its disorder after TOP and reproductive loss. The rationale for this systematic review is therefore to reconcile previous research and deliver the first review that integrates research on PTS and PTSD after all reproductive losses (TOP, miscarriage, perinatal loss, stillbirth, neonatal death, and failed IVF) for women and men and investigate the prevalence and factors influencing the development of PTS/PTSD after each reproductive loss. TOP and other reproductive losses were included to provide a comprehensive account of the research literature, including a quality assessment and a direct examination of the differences between TOPS and reproductive losses in relation to PTS and PTSD.

2. Methods

2.1. Search Strategy.
The electronic databases (AMED, British Nursing Index, CINAHL, MEDLINE, SPORTDiscus, PsycINFO, PubMEd, and ScienceDirect) were searched for relevant articles and followed the PRISMA guidelines [24]. No restriction for time of publication was set and only English language peer-reviewed publications were included. The search was last updated in May 2012. In PubMEd, the following key words were used in title/abstract search: "miscarriage" or "stillbirth" or "abortion" or "neonatal death" or "perinatal loss" or "failed IVF" or "failed in vitro fertilization" or "failed in vitro fertilization" or "pregnancy loss" or "termination of

pregnancy" and "trauma" or "stress" or "PTSD" or "posttraumatic stress," or "posttraumatic stress disorder."

2.2. Study Selection.
All papers had to be published in peer-reviewed journals, available in English and presenting original data. Studies were selected if they investigated PTSD/PTS associated with TOP and/or other reproductive losses (miscarriage, perinatal loss, stillbirth, neonatal death, and failed IVF). Quantitative studies were selected if they used standardised measurements of PTS/PTSD and qualitative studies were selected if they investigated the trauma of TOP and reproductive loss in the interviews. Studies had to use standard criteria for PTS/PTSD to be included. For PTS the reaction to traumatic events is characterised with involuntary repetition in thought, emotion, and behaviour of stress relevant contents. PTS is a marker of possibly developing the disorder, which depends on the intensity of these and other symptoms and require other conditions to become a disorder [25]. We did not include ASD in our systematic review because ASD does not necessarily lead to PTSD and is more time limited. Further, PTSD (PTS's disorder) is the development of characteristic symptoms following exposure to an extreme traumatic stressor. The characteristic symptoms resulting from the exposure to the extreme trauma include persistent reexperiencing of the traumatic event, persistent avoidance of stimuli associated with the trauma and numbing of general responsiveness, and persistent symptoms of increased arousal [26].

Studies which investigated existing PTS/PTSD as a risk factor for TOP or reproductive loss were excluded because the focus was on reproductive loss as a risk factor for PTS/PTSD. Further, data were collected on whether the studies included controlled for pre-TOP or prereproductive loss of mental health in their data analyses. Clinical case studies with no research agenda, books, correspondence letters, discussions, book reviews, product reviews, editorials, publisher's notes, and errata were excluded from the review. To avoid multiple publication bias [27] only one paper was selected from multiple publications and selection was based upon highest quality, followed by largest number of participants, highest number of reproductive losses, longest length of follow-up, and the paper with most reported outcome measurement data. Numbers included and reasons for exclusion are shown in Figure 1.

2.3. Data Abstraction.
A data extraction sheet was used to collect relevant information. This included author's details, country of study, design, sample size, variables measured, results, quality of study evaluation. Data was extracted from relevant articles (VD) and cross-checked (OvdA and SP).

2.4. Screening and Quality Assessment.
Quality assessment of articles which met the inclusion criteria was determined by VD using Cochrane criteria adapted by Green et al. [28]. These were independently checked by OvdA and SP, and disagreements were resolved following discussion; criteria were

(i) adequate sample size,

(ii) representative of study population,

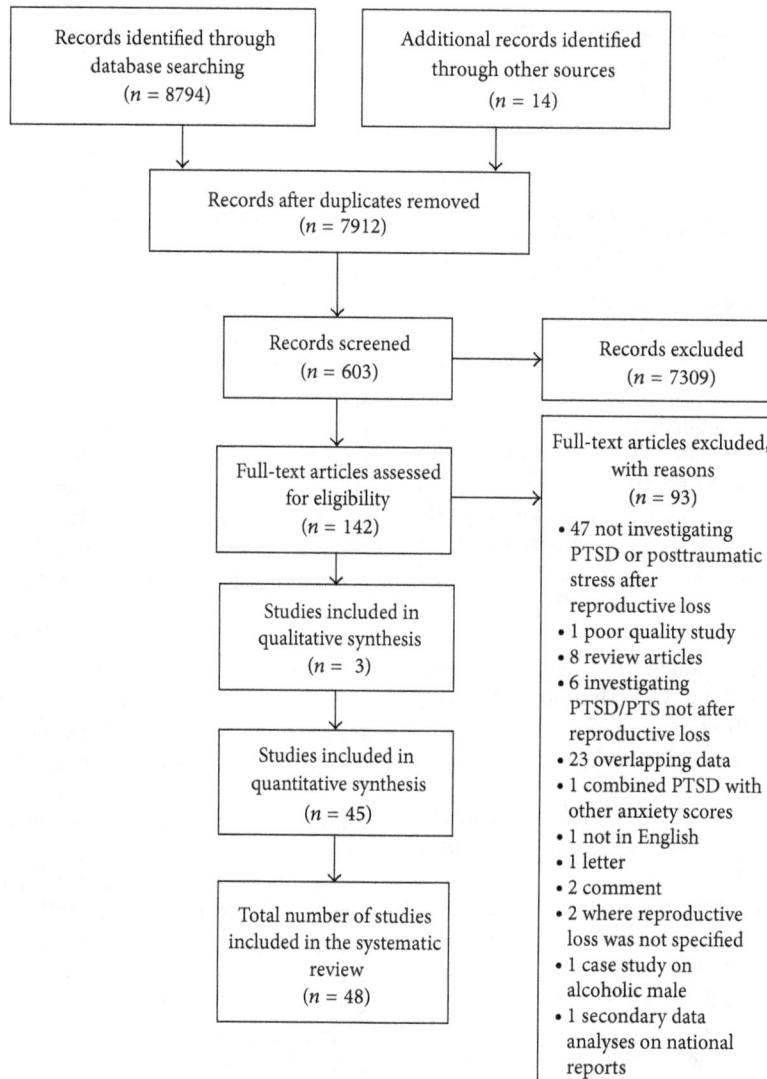

FIGURE 1: PRISMA flow diagram.

(iii) high response rate,

(iv) using mostly validated measures,

(v) mostly appropriate timing of measures,

(vi) measures consistent with aims,

(vii) conclusions consistent with results,

(viii) methodology is clear,

(ix) analysis is clear.

3. Results

As can be seen from the PRISMA flow chart (Figure 1), the search of the databases yielded 8794 titles of records and 14 records from searching reference lists. After duplicates were removed, 7912 records were left. Titles were reviewed and 7309 articles did not meet the inclusion criteria. Of the 603 abstracts reviewed, 461 failed to meet the inclusion criteria. Finally full texts of the remaining 142 papers were read and

48 studies were identified as meeting the inclusion criteria. As shown in Figure 1, 23 studies [29–51] were excluded for reporting overlapping data and 12 studies [22, 23, 52–61] from multiple reports were included. Further, one eligible study was removed [62] over serious reported methodological and statistical concerns over the study [63].

3.1. Study Characteristics. The study characteristics of the 48 included articles are shown in Tables 1–4; Table 1 includes TOP, Table 2 miscarriage, Table 3 perinatal loss, and Table 4 stillbirths. Each table is separated in two parts (a and b) with section a representing studies which have investigated the type of reproductive loss alone and section (b) presenting studies which have investigated that type with other losses.

As shown in Table 1, 20 studies examined PTS/PTSD after TOP (Table 1(a)); seven examined TOP with miscarriage, perinatal loss, or neonatal death (Table 1(b)). Eighteen reported nonmedical TOP [22, 23, 53, 61, 62, 64–76], one nonmedical TOP and medical TOP [77]; eight were medical TOP

TABLE 1: Characteristics of included studies for TOP (a) and TOP with miscarriage/perinatal loss/neonatal death (b).

Authors, year, country, and author listing in reference list	Methods	Reproductive loss, Participants, and control for Prereproductive loss	Outcomes measurements	Quality
(a) Termination of pregnancy (TOP). Numbers of participants are women, men, or couples and are noted separately.				
(1) Allanson (2007), Australia [64]	P, L	Nonmedical TOP $n = 96$ **Prereproductive loss mental health parameters statistically not controlled**	IES	5
(2) Cohen and Roth (1984), USA [65]	P	Nonmedical TOP $n = 55$ **Prereproductive loss mental health parameters statistically controlled**	IES	5
(3) Coyle et al. (2010) USA [22] *Note. This study was chosen over [32]; it had larger number of reported participants.*	R	Nonmedical TOP 374 women; 198 men **Prereproductive loss mental health parameters statistically controlled**	PTSD Checklist-Civilian Version	6
(4) Davies et al. (2005), UK [79]	P	Medical TOP 30; **Prereproductive loss mental health parameters statistically not controlled**	IES	5
(5) van Emmerik et al. (2008), The Netherlands [66]	P	Nonmedical TOP 67 **Prereproductive loss mental health parameters statistically not controlled**	IES	7
(6) Hemmerling et al. (2005), Germany [67]	P, I	Nonmedical TOP 219 **Prereproductive loss mental health parameters statistically not controlled**	IES	7
(7) Kelly et al. UK (2010) [68]	P, I	Nonmedical TOP 122 **Prereproductive loss mental health parameters statistically controlled**	IES	5
(8) Kersting et al. (2009), Germany [58] *Note. This study was chosen over [41] because of a higher quality rating and [42] because it reports more participants and relevant data.*	P, L	62 medical TOP; 43 preterm birth; 65 spontaneous delivery **Prereproductive loss mental health parameters statistically not controlled**	IES-R	7
(9) Korenromp et al. (2005a), The Netherlands [59] *Note. This study was chosen over [43] because of higher quality rating.*	R	Medical TOP 196 **Prereproductive loss mental health parameters statistically not controlled**	IES	8
(10) Korenromp et al. (2007), The Netherlands [60] *Note. This study was chosen over [44] because of a larger sample.*	P, L	Medical TOP 217 women; 169 men **Prereproductive loss mental health parameters statistically not controlled**	IES	9
(11) Layer et al. (2004), USA [69]	P, I	Nonmedical TOP 35 **Prereproductive loss mental health parameters statistically not controlled**	IES	7
(12) Major et al. (2000), USA [23] *Notes. This study was chosen over [45] because it reported more data.*	P, L	Nonmedical TOP 442 **Prereproductive loss mental health parameters statistically not controlled for PTSD**	Adapted PTSD measure-using DSM-III-R-used with Vietnam War veterans	7

TABLE 1: Continued.

Authors, year, country, and author listing in reference list	Methods	Reproductive loss, Participants, and control for Prereproductive loss	Outcomes measurements	Quality
(13) Mufel et al. (2002), Belarus, USA [61] *Note. This study was chosen over [475] because of a higher quality rating.*	R	Nonmedical TOP 150 **Prereproductive loss mental health parameters statistically not controlled**	IES-R	7
(14) Pope et al. (2001), USA [70]	P	Nonmedical TOP 96 **Prereproductive loss mental health parameters statistically not controlled** for PTS	IES	7
(15) Rousset et al. (2012), France [71]	P, I	Nonmedical TOP 70 **Prereproductive loss mental health parameters statistically not controlled**	IES-R	9
(16) Rue et al. (2004), USA [72]	R	Nonmedical TOP 331 Russian women; 217 American women **Prereproductive loss mental health parameters statistically not controlled**	Institute of Pregnancy Loss questionnaire-including criteria for PTSD on DSM-IV	4
(17) Slade et al. (1998), UK [73]	P, I	Nonmedical TOP 275 **Prereproductive loss mental health parameters statistically not controlled** for PTS	IES	9
(18) Suliman et al. (2007), South Africa [74]	P, I	Nonmedical TOP 151 **Prereproductive loss mental health parameters statistically controlled**	Clinician-administered PTSD scale (CAPS-I)	7
(19) Trybulski (2006), USA [75]	Q	Nonmedical TOP 16	Qualitative interview.	5
(20) Walters and Oakley (2002), UK [76]	CS	Nonmedical TOP 1 **Prereproductive loss mental health parameters statistically not controlled**	The Post-Traumatic Stress Diagnostic Scale	7
(b) TOP and miscarriage/perinatal loss/neonatal death				
(21) Broen et al. (2005b), Norway [53] *Note. This study was chosen over [31]; it has a higher quality rating/longer follow-up time [30].*	P, L	40 miscarriages; 80 Nonmedical TOP **Prereproductive loss mental health parameters statistically controlled**	IES	7
(22) Canário et al. (2011), Portugal [77]	P	Nonmedical TOP (30); medical TOP (10); miscarriage (10). **Prereproductive loss mental health parameters statistically not controlled**	IES-R	6
(23) Cowchock et al. (2011), USA [78]	P	7 medical TOP, 8 miscarriages **Prereproductive loss mental health parameters statistically not controlled**	IES	6
(24) Fernandez et al. (2011), Canada [80]	Q	2 medical TOP; 5 miscarriages	Qualitative interviews	5
(25) Hamama et al. (2010), USA [55] *Note. This study was chosen over [46] because of more relevant PTSD data.*	P	405 prior pregnancies; 221 prior nonmedical TOP; 206 miscarriages; 22 reported both **Prereproductive loss mental health parameters statistically not controlled**	Interview (National Women's Study PTSD Module (NWS-PTSD)).	9

TABLE 1: Continued.

Authors, year, country, and author listing in reference list	Methods	Reproductive loss, Participants, and control for Prereproductive loss	Outcomes measurements	Quality
(26) Kroth et al. (2004), USA [81]	R	Medical TOP, miscarriage, perinatal loss, and neonatal death 37 women **Prereproductive loss mental health parameters statistically not controlled**	IES	▰▰▱▱ 4
(27) Salvesen et al. (1997), Norway [82]	P	24 medical TOP, 29 perinatal losses/neonatal deaths **Prereproductive loss mental health parameters statistically not controlled**	IES	▰▰▰▰ 9

Notes: CS = case study; I = intervention design; IES = Impact of Event Scale; IES-R = Revised; L = longitudinal; P = prospective; Q = qualitative; R = retrospective.

[58–60, 77–82]. Table 2 shows 10 studies examining PTS/PTSD after miscarriage (Table 2(a) [54, 83–91]), five miscarriages with perinatal loss, stillbirth, and neonatal death (Table 2(b) [92–96]). Table 3 shows that one study examined PTS/PTSD after perinatal loss (Table 3(a) [52]) and two studies examined perinatal loss with neonatal death (Table 3(b) [57, 97]). Finally, Table 4 reports two studies investigating PTS/PTSD after stillbirth (Table 4(a) [56, 98]) and one stillbirth with neonatal death (Table 4(b) [99]). No study investigated PTS or PTSD after failed IVF.

Some studies did not distinguish between reproductive types in their data analyses (e.g., [57, 81, 82, 93, 94, 99]) and gestational ages were not reported for $n = 10/48$ studies. The majority of studies used prospective designs, and sample sizes were generally small. PTS was consistently measured ($n = 33/49$) with the Impact of Event Scale (IES), the Revised IES (IES-R), or Perinatal Event Scale-adapted from Impact of Events Scale. The IES includes two subscales, intrusion and avoidance, and the IES-R also includes hyperarousal. Diagnoses of PTSD were done using diagnostic interviews ($n = 4$) or questionnaires ($n = 10$). Timing of outcome measurements or time since reproductive loss ranged from immediately after ($n = 7/48$) up to one year postloss ($n = 25/48$). Most quantitative studies did not control for pre-TOP or prereproductive loss of mental health parameters in their statistical analyses (33/48). Data from 6379 women and men who experienced TOP or reproductive loss and 573 controls were included in the review. The majority of studies were conducted either in Europe ($n = 24/48$) or the USA ($n = 18/48$), most participants were white, and postloss support in Western countries is likely to be better resourced than in developing countries [8]. The quality of the studies was mostly good. See the Appendix more detailed information on each study.

3.2. Prevalence of PTS and PTSD after TOP and Reproductive Loss. Where more than one type of reproductive loss is reported ($n = 16/48$), studies are only discussed with the TOP or reproductive loss they are presented with, as demonstrated on Tables 1–4. Further, only observational studies are presented here; intervention studies (i.e., therapy or TOP procedure type, nonsurgical versus surgical) are discussed later.

3.2.1. Nonmedical TOP. For nonmedical TOP 12.6% met PTSD criteria, similar to rates for women with a prior miscarriage (12.5%) but higher than women without prior reproductive loss (6.3%) [55]. Data from online surveys estimated much higher rates of PTSD (54.9% women and 43.4% of men) up to 15 years after the TOP [22]. However, recruitment was through online resources including abortion support groups suggesting that the sample may not be representative.

Studies from abortion clinics reported moderate levels (19.4%) of PTS at two months post-TOP decreasing over time [66], and few cases of PTSD (1% $n = 441$) were reported at two years' post-TOP [23]. Adolescents also report low scores on intrusion four weeks post-TOP (719), and one study reported that PTS was high before TOP but decreased within 5 hours postoperation [65] or reported initially high PTS reducing to "negligible levels of distress" at 3 months post-TOP [64].

No differences between men and women or at 1 and 6 months were found for nonmedical TOP or medical TOP and miscarriage [77]. Before nonmedical TOP, women were less likely to report PTS intrusion than women before miscarriage ($n = 40$) and less PTS avoidance at 2 years and 5 years post-TOP compared to post miscarriage [53]. American women (14.3%) are more likely to meet full diagnostic criteria for PTSD compared to Russian women (0.9%) [72].

3.2.2. Medical TOP. Following medical TOP, reports of PTS are high (64.5%) [58], with PTS reducing from 67% to 41% at 12 months. Second trimester medical TOP is more likely to result in PTS at six weeks than first trimester medical TOP but this difference disappeared at 12 months [79]. In a retrospective study of medical TOP, 33% continued to report PTS up to a mean time of 4 years since the loss [59]. Women (44%) report higher rates of PTS than men (21.6%) [60]; pregnant women who had a previous medical TOP are less likely to report PTS than pregnant women with previous miscarriage [78] and significantly lower PTS is reported after medical TOP than perinatal/neonatal death [82].

3.2.3. Miscarriage. One study found that PTSD is infrequently reported three months after miscarriage [90]. Of

TABLE 2: Characteristics of included studies for miscarriage (a) and miscarriage with perinatal loss/stillbirth/neonatal death (b).

Authors year, country, and author listing in reference list	Methods	Reproductive loss, Participants, and control for Prereproductive loss	Outcomes measurements	Quality
(a) Characteristics of included studies for miscarriage				
(28) Alderman et al. (1998), USA [83]	R	Miscarriage 19 couples **Prereproductive loss mental health parameters statistically not controlled**	IES	5
(29) Bowles et al. (2006), USA [84]	P, L	Miscarriage 25 **Prereproductive loss mental health parameters statistically not controlled**	Posttraumatic Stress Diagnostic Scale	6
(30) Engelhard et al. (2003a), The Netherlands [54] *Note. This study was chosen over [33–37] because of the largest number of reported participants/reported the most data.*	P, L	Miscarriage 118 **Prereproductive loss mental health parameters statistically controlled**	Posttraumatic Symptom Scale	9
(31) Johnson and Puddifoot (1996), UK [85]	P	Miscarriage 126 men **Prereproductive loss mental health parameters statistically not controlled**	IES	7
(32) Lee et al. (1996), UK [86]	P, I	Miscarriage 39 **Prereproductive loss mental health parameters statistically controlled**	IES	5
(33) Rowsell et al. (2001), UK [87]	P, I	Miscarriage 37 **Prereproductive loss mental health parameters statistically not controlled**	IES	6
(34) Séjourné et al. (2010), France [88]	P, I	Miscarriage 134 **Prereproductive loss mental health parameters statistically not controlled for PTS**	IES-R	9
(35) Serrano and Lima (2006), Portugal [89]	R	Miscarriage 30 women and 30 men **Prereproductive loss mental health parameters statistically not controlled**	IES	7
(36) Sham et al. (2010), Hong Kong [90]	P, L	Miscarriage 161 **Prereproductive loss mental health parameters statistically controlled**	Structural clinical interview for DSM-IV	9
(37) Walker and Davidson (2001), UK [91]	P	Miscarriage 40 **Prereproductive loss mental health parameters statistically controlled**	IES	9
(b) Miscarriage and perinatal/stillbirth/neonatal death				
(38) Armstrong (2004), USA [92]	P	Miscarriage and Perinatal loss 40 expectant couples **Prereproductive loss mental health parameters statistically not controlled**	IES	7
(39) Forray et al. (2009), USA [93]	P	Miscarriage; perinatal loss/neonatal loss/other complications 76 pregnant women, of which 18 underwent interviews **Prereproductive loss mental health parameters statistically not controlled**	(Modified Clinical administered PTSD Scale (m-CAPS))	7

TABLE 2: Continued.

Authors year, country, and author listing in reference list	Methods	Reproductive loss, Participants, and control for Prereproductive loss	Outcomes measurements	Quality	
(40) Jind (2001), Denmark [94]	R	Miscarriage/perinatal, stillbirth, and neonatal death/infant loss 602 parents **Prereproductive loss mental health parameters statistically not controlled**	IES, Harvard trauma Questionnaire	▬▬▬▬□□	5
(41) Jind (2003), Denmark [95]	P, L	Miscarriage, perinatal loss, stillbirth, and neonatal death/infant loss; 93 parents at the first measurement, 65 parents at the second measurement **Prereproductive loss mental health parameters statistically not controlled**	The Harvard Trauma Questionnaire	▬▬▬▬▬□	7
(42) O'leary (2005), USA [96]	Q	Miscarriage, perinatal loss, stillbirth and infant loss; 12 expecting mothers and 9 expecting fathers	Qualitative Interviews.	▬▬▬▬□	6

TABLE 3: Characteristics of included studies for perinatal loss (a) and perinatal loss with neonatal death (b).

Authors year, country, and author listing in reference list	Methods	Reproductive loss, Participants and control for Prereproductive loss	Outcomes measurements	Quality	
(a) Perinatal loss					
(43) Armstrong et al. (2009), USA [52] *Note. This study was chosen over [29] because it had a higher quality rating.*	P, L	Perinatal loss 36 couples **Prereproductive loss mental health parameters statistically not controlled**	IES	▬▬▬▬▬□	7
(b) Perinatal loss and neonatal death					
(44) Hunfeld et al. (1993), Netherlands [57] *Note. This study was chosen over [39, 40] because of a higher quality rating and [38] because of more relevant PTSD data.*	P, L	Perinatal loss and neonatal death; 46 **Prereproductive loss mental health parameters statistically not controlled**	Perinatal Event Scale –adapted from Impact of Event Scale	▬▬▬▬▬▬	9
(45) Hutti et al. (2011), USA [97]	P, L	Perinatal loss and neonatal death; 106 women **Prereproductive loss mental health parameters statistically not controlled**	IES	▬▬▬▬▬□	7

studies reporting PTS after miscarriage, a reduction is reported after 3 [91] to 4 months [54], although an increase in PTSD over time has also been reported [84]. Other reports find higher levels with 67.9% of pregnant women with prior miscarriage or perinatal loss meeting partial or full criteria for PTSD [93]. Similar high numbers (82% PTS; 80% PTSD) were reported in men and women after miscarriage, perinatal, stillbirth, or neonatal death/infant death three years previously [94]. However, data was not separated for reproductive loss type and the sample was recruited from a support group and may not be representative. Hospital samples record lower numbers (11% with PTSD) which reduced still further (2.8%) 4–12 months follow-up [95].

Women who experienced recurrent miscarriage were more likely to report intrusion [83] or intrusion and avoidance than their partners [89]. Pregnant women who had a previous miscarriage or perinatal loss scored high on avoidance and men scored high on intrusion with 88% of women and 90% of men meeting the cut-off for PTS [92], confirming other reports of clinical levels of PTS in men [85].

TABLE 4: Characteristics of included studies for stillbirth (a) and stillbirth with neonatal death (b).

Authors year, country, and author listing in reference list	Methods	Reproductive loss, Participants and control for Prereproductive loss	Outcomes measurements	Quality
(a) Stillbirth				
(46) Cacciatore (2007), USA [98]	R	Stillbirth 47 **Prereproductive loss mental health parameters statistically not controlled**	IES-R	6
(47) Hughes et al. (2002), UK [56] *Note. This study was chosen over [48–51] because of the highest quality rating/reported more participants/data.*	P	65 pregnant women, with prior stillbirth, 60 controls **Prereproductive loss mental health parameters statistically controlled**	PTSD-1 Interview	9
(b) Stillbirth and neonatal death				
(48) Uren and Wastell (2002), Australia [99]	R	Stillbirth and neonatal loss; 109 women **Prereproductive loss mental health parameters statistically not controlled**	IES-R	5

3.2.4. Perinatal Loss. PTS is initially high [52, 97] and decreases to moderate levels 8 months postpartum in couples with a history of perinatal loss who subsequently had a healthy infant [52]. Specifically intrusion increased more in women and avoidance remained stable in both [52], or PTS remained high and unchanged from the first diagnosis to three months after delivery/death [57].

3.2.5. Stillbirth. One longitudinal study of 65 pregnant women who had a prior stillbirth reported 21% PTSD in the third trimester and 4% at one year after birth [56].

3.3. Factors Influencing PTS and/or PTSD after TOP and Reproductive Loss

3.3.1. Nonmedical TOP. Having a TOP predicted a diagnosis of PTSD and sociodemographic variables (younger age, poverty, poor education, poor housing, and race), history of sexual trauma, and illness or medical trauma are other risk factors independently predicting PTSD [55]. A history of sexual or medical trauma doubled the risk for PTSD [55], whereas harsh discipline as a child, adult rape, and physical or emotional abuse were associated with PTSD [72], and a history of major depression also predicted PTSD [23]. Peritraumatic dissociation and difficulties in describing feelings were significant predictors of PTS [66].

Relationship stability as a reason to continue the pregnancy is a strong predictor of intrusion symptoms [64]. Couple's disagreement towards having a TOP and inadequate before abortion counselling significantly predicted PTSD in women and men [22] and in women, knowing others who have not coped with TOP [64], attachment to the foetus, recognition of life, time since abortion, and increased maternal age predicted PTSD [61]. Higher levels of perceived quality in couple's relationship [77] and active coping influence short term PTS after nonmedical TOP [65]. Spiritual

group therapy reduces PTS for women experiencing post-TOP grief, although no control group was used [69] and hypnosis with psychological therapy successfully reduced symptoms of PTSD in a case study [76]. Recurrent thoughts continued to affect and traumatise women's lives up to 15 years post-TOP in a qualitative study [75].

Research considering type of TOP procedure reporting nonsurgical TOP predicts PTSD [68, 71], surgical TOP is associated with PTS [67], or no differences between nonsurgical or surgical TOP on PTS [72]. No differences between local anaesthesia and intravenous sedation in surgical TOP were reported either [74].

3.3.2. Medical TOP. PTS in women was also predicted by sociodemographic factors [79] (low education, younger maternal age, and advanced gestation) and low levels of partner support [59, 60], whereas, for men, being religious and doubt over decision predicted PTS [60]. PTS is also associated with perinatal grief, depression, and anxiety for pregnant women with prior medical TOP or miscarriage [78]. In women with medical TOP, miscarriage, stillbirth, and neonatal death, recruited through support groups, PTS was correlated with low levels of social support, perinatal grief, emotional pain, emotional expression, and, less strongly, dream frequency [81]. Depression had also been associated with high intrusion scores for women who experienced medical TOP and perinatal loss/neonatal death [82]. Difficult physical symptoms of miscarriage and TOP and having to make the decision to have a medical TOP were experienced as traumatic in a qualitative investigation [80].

3.3.3. Miscarriage. A diagnosis of acute stress disorder [84], peritraumatic dissociation, and neuroticism [54] leads to PTSD one to 4 months after loss. Unplanned pregnancies are significantly related to PTS [91]. Both men and women have clinical levels of PTS although sociodemographic variables and quality of relationship do not predict PTS for either [89]. However, for men, PTS was more likely to be associated with perinatal grief and older gestational age and viewing the ultrasound scan were significantly associated with PTS [85], whereas, for women, viewing scans and early warning signs for miscarriage were not associated with PTS [91]. Psychological therapy to reduce PTS is ineffective; it usually declines spontaneously over time [86–88].

Depression, and pregnancy related anxiety, but not prenatal attachment related to PTS in couples with prior miscarriage or perinatal loss [92]. Depression, anxiety, and poly substance disorders cooccurred for some women with full or partial PTSD diagnosis after miscarriage and other reproductive losses [93]. PTSD is also associated with feelings of doubt [94] and attribution of blame [95]. Ultrasound of the current pregnancy triggered flashbacks and symptoms of PTSD for some women with prior miscarriage, perinatal loss, stillbirth, and infant loss [96].

3.3.4. Perinatal Loss. Depression was significantly correlated with PTS during a current pregnancy and eight months following delivery for women and men with prior perinatal losses [52]. For women, anxiety was associated with PTS during pregnancy but, for men, anxiety was associated with PTS during and after delivery [52]. For pregnant women with a history of perinatal loss and neonatal death, intrusion was associated with an increase of women's healthcare use [97]. For women experiencing a neonatal death, those who delivered early were more likely to experience intrusion than women who delivered after 34 weeks [57].

3.3.5. Stillbirth. At one year postdelivery, seeing and holding the stillborn infant was significantly associated with PTSD in pregnant women with a previous history of stillbirth [56]. Attending support groups significantly predicted lower PTS [98]. Finally, in women who experienced a stillbirth or neonatal death, intrusion and hyperarousal predicted perinatal grief [99].

4. Conclusion

Systematic research evidence on the prevalence of PTS or PTSD associated with failed IVF is nonexistent, and few studies reported on PTS/PTSD following perinatal loss, neonatal death, or stillbirth, usually alongside other reproductive losses. There were more studies on PTS/PTSD after miscarriage and TOP for nonmedical and medical reasons. However, the research is inconsistent with regards to prevalence rates which depended on how participants were recruited. In some cases, no prevalence rates, reproductive loss type, or gestational age of the loss were recorded, reflecting the lack of research into the mental health of patients following reproductive loss [18].

Overall, this review has demonstrated that PTSD occurs after nonmedical and medical TOP, miscarriage, perinatal loss, and stillbirth, although it is much less commonly reported than PTS. Length of gestational age is associated with an increased likelihood for diagnosis of PTS or PTSD.

The percentage of PTS and its disorder is highest during the first weeks after TOP or reproductive loss and decreases significantly over time for most but not all women and men. Women generally report more PTS or PTSD symptoms but clinical levels of distress are also reported for men.

Research has generally demonstrated that PTS or PTSD after TOP and reproductive losses are complex and a variety of factors play an influencing role. Studies which have investigated the impact of sociodemographic characteristics (TOP and miscarriage studies) and the experience of other previous traumas on PTS and PTSD have found that demographic factors such as maternal age, gestational age, lower education, and a history of previous physical or sexual trauma are significant risk factors for the development of PTS or PTSD after loss. Prior history of mental health problems and current depression, anxiety, and perinatal grief are also risk factors, confirming previous research [100], although it is not clear if the mental health or the known lack of health seeking behaviour is responsible for the reproductive loss [101]. Time has generally been found to be the most influential protective factor in reducing levels of PTS/PTSD. The evidence for the effectiveness of "individual" psychological therapy is mixed and generally suggest therapy is ineffective at reducing PTS or PTSD anymore than time does by itself. The quality of relationship between the couple has also been found to act as a protective factor, as is found more generally in research reporting coping with reproductive disorders [3].

The quality of studies included in the review was generally good, reaching average scores of 7/9, but the samples are often small, select, and nonrepresentative. Most studies report data for one year after TOP or loss and no inferences can be drawn about the long term consequences. This is a serious limitation because the time since the loss occurred is an important factor that influences PTS and PTSD. Further, most of the studies included did not control for pre-TOP or prereproductive loss mental health in their statistical analyses. This is potentially another significant limitation of existing research because a recent Danish population based cohort study found evidence that the incidence of pre-TOP psychiatric contacts up to 9 months preabortion (14.6%) was similar to the incidence at 12 months post-TOP (15.2%) among the large cohort of girls and women included in the analysis [102]. The lack of research on perinatal loss, stillbirth, and neonatal death is also of concern because a longer gestation predicts an increasing likelihood of PTS or PTSD. Evidence of PTS and reproductive loss of men, nonwhite, single women, adolescent girls, and women past the age of natural childbearing is meagre and nonexistent on failure of infertility treatment needing further attention. Finally, most of the studies that have examined TOP have come from countries that permit nonmedical TOP. Restrictive TOP laws are not associated with lower TOP rates, indeed the opposite appears to be true [13, 14]. Therefore, the findings from this review cannot easily be transferred to those countries where TOP is illegally practiced, particularly where unsafe TOP's are carried out.

To sum, this systematic review investigated PTS/PTSD after TOP and reproductive loss. The prevalence of PTS was greater than PTSD and both decreased over time. However, the more advanced the pregnancy is, the more PTS and

PTSD are likely to be reported. Women generally report more PTS/PTSD but men also report clinical rates of PTS/PTSD. Time since TOP and loss, demographic characteristics and psychosocial factors influence the development and maintenance of PTS and PTSD after TOP and reproductive loss.

Appendix

See Tables 1, 2, 3, and 4.

Conflict of Interests

There are no competing interests.

Funding

Viltė Daugirdaitė received an ERASMUS Internship scholarship.

References

[1] O. B. A. van den Akker, "The psychological and social consequences of miscarriage," *Expert Review of Obstetrics and Gynecology*, vol. 6, no. 3, pp. 295–304, 2011.

[2] F. Zegers-Hochschild, G. D. Adamson, J. de Mouzon et al., "International Committee for Monitoring Assisted Reproductive Technology (ICMART) and the World Health Organization (WHO) revised glossary of ART terminology, 2009," *Fertility and Sterility*, vol. 92, no. 5, pp. 1520–1524, 2009.

[3] O. B. A. van den Akker, *Reproductive Health Psychology*, Wiley-Blackwell, 2012.

[4] A. L. Greil, "Infertility and psychological distress: a critical review of the literature," *Social Science and Medicine*, vol. 45, no. 11, pp. 1679–1704, 1997.

[5] B. D. Peterson, M. Pirritano, U. Christensen, J. Boivin, J. Block, and L. Schmidt, "The longitudinal impact of partner coping in couples following 5 years of unsuccessful fertility treatments," *Human Reproduction*, vol. 24, no. 7, pp. 1656–1664, 2009.

[6] J. R. W. Fisher, K. Hammarberg, and G. H. W. Baker, "Antenatal mood and fetal attachment after assisted conception," *Fertility and Sterility*, vol. 89, no. 5, pp. 1103–1112, 2008.

[7] W. Bandenhorst and P. Hughes, "Psychological aspects of perinatal loss," *Best Practice & Research Clinical Obstetrics & Gynaecology*, vol. 21, pp. 249–259, 2007.

[8] S. M. Bennett, B. S. Lee, B. T. Litz, and S. Maguen, "The scope and impact of perinatal loss: current status and future directions," *Professional Psychology: Research and Practice*, vol. 36, no. 2, pp. 180–187, 2005.

[9] P. A. Geller, D. Kerns, and C. M. Klier, "Anxiety following miscarriage and the subsequent pregnancy: a review of the literature and future directions," *Journal of Psychosomatic Research*, vol. 56, no. 1, pp. 35–45, 2004.

[10] D. A. Bagarozzi, "Identification, assessment and treatment of women suffering from post traumatic stress after abortion," *Journal of Family Psychotherapy*, vol. 5, no. 3, pp. 25–54, 1994.

[11] J. Condon, "Women's mental health: a 'wish-list' for the DSM V," *Archives of Women's Mental Health*, vol. 13, no. 1, pp. 5–10, 2010.

[12] S. Iles, "The loss of early pregnancy," *Bailliere's Clinical Obstetrics and Gynaecology*, vol. 3, no. 4, pp. 769–790, 1989.

[13] G. Sedgh, S. Singh, I. H. Shah, E. Åhman, S. K. Henshaw, and A. Bankole, "Induced abortion: incidence and trends worldwide from 1995 to 2008," *The Lancet*, vol. 379, no. 9816, pp. 625–632, 2012.

[14] World Health Organisation (WHO), "Facts on induced abortion worldwide," April 2014, http://www.guttmacher.org/pubs/fb_IAW.html.

[15] N. F. Russo and K. L. Zierk, "Abortion, childbearing, and women's well-being," *Professional Psychology: Research and Practice*, vol. 23, no. 4, pp. 269–280, 1992.

[16] S. M. Stanford-Rue, *Will I Cry Tomorrow? Healing Post-Abortion Trauma*, Fleming H. Revell, 1999.

[17] B. Major, M. Appelbaum, L. Beckman, M. A. Dutton, N. F. Russo, and C. West, "Abortion and mental health: evaluating the evidence," *American Psychologist*, vol. 64, no. 9, pp. 863–890, 2009.

[18] J. Astbury, "Overview of key issues," in *Mental Health Aspects of Women's Reproductive Health. A Global Review of Literature*, pp. 1–7, World Health Organization, 2009, http://whqlibdoc.who.int/publications/2009/9789241563567_eng.pdf.

[19] D. Carter, S. Misri, and L. Tomfohr, "Psychologic aspects of early pregnancy loss," *Clinical Obstetrics and Gynecology*, vol. 50, no. 1, pp. 154–165, 2007.

[20] C. Lee and P. Slade, "Miscarriage as a traumatic event: a review of the literature and new implications for intervention," *Journal of Psychosomatic Research*, vol. 40, no. 3, pp. 235–244, 1996.

[21] A. Horsch, "Post-traumatic stress disorder following childbirth and pregnancy loss," in *Clinical Psychology in Practice*, H. Beinart, P. Kennedy, and S. Llewelyn, Eds., pp. 274–287, Blackwell Publishing, West Sussex, UK, 2009.

[22] C. T. Coyle, P. K. Coleman, and V. M. Rue, "Inadequate preabortion counseling and decision conflict as predictors of subsequent relationship difficulties and psychological stress in men and women," *Traumatology*, vol. 16, no. 1, pp. 16–30, 2010.

[23] B. Major, C. Cozzarelli, M. L. Cooper et al., "Psychological responses of women after first-trimester abortion," *Archives of General Psychiatry*, vol. 57, no. 8, pp. 777–784, 2000.

[24] D. Moher, A. Liberati, J. Tetzlaff, and D. Altman, "Preferred reporting items for systematic reviews and meta-analyses: the PRISMA statement," *Journal of Clinical Epidemiology*, vol. 62, pp. 1006–1012, 2009.

[25] M. J. Horowitz, *Stress Response Syndromes*, Jason Aronson, Northvale, NJ, USA, 2001.

[26] American Psychiatric Association, *Diagnostic and Statistical Manual of Mental Disorders*, American Psychiatric Press, Washington, DC, USA, 5th edition, 2013, http://www.dsm5.org/Pages/Default.aspx.

[27] J. P. T. Higgins and S. Green, *Cochrane Handbook for Systematic Reviews of Interventions*, 2011, http://handbook.cochrane.org/.

[28] J. M. Green, J. Hewison, H. L. Bekker, L. D. Bryant, and H. S. Cuckle, "Psychosocial aspects of genetic screening of pregnant women and newborns: a systematic review," *Health Technology Assessment*, vol. 8, no. 33, pp. 1–128, 2004.

[29] D. S. Armstrong, "Perinatal loss and parental distress after the birth of a healthy infant," *Advances in Neonatal Care*, vol. 7, no. 4, pp. 200–206, 2007.

[30] A. N. Broen, T. Moum, A. S. Bödtker, and Ö. Ekeberg, "Psychological impact on women of miscarriage versus induced abortion: a 2-year follow-up study," *Psychosomatic Medicine*, vol. 66, no. 2, pp. 265–271, 2004.

[31] A. N. Broen, T. Moum, A. S. Bödtker, and Ö. Ekeberg, "Reasons for induced abortion and their relation to women's emotional distress: a prospective, two-year follow-up study," *General Hospital Psychiatry*, vol. 27, no. 1, pp. 36–43, 2005.

[32] P. K. Coleman, C. T. Coyle, and V. M. Rue, "Late-term elective abortion and susceptibility to posttraumatic stress symptoms," *Journal of Pregnancy*, vol. 2010, Article ID 130519, 10 pages, 2010.

[33] I. M. Engelhard, M. A. van den Hout, and A. Arntz, "Posttraumatic stress disorder after pregnancy loss," *General Hospital Psychiatry*, vol. 23, no. 2, pp. 62–66, 2001.

[34] I. M. Engelhard, M. A. van den Hout, and M. Kindt, "The relationship between neuroticism, pre-traumatic stress, and posttraumatic stress: a prospective study," *Personality and Individual Differences*, vol. 35, no. 2, pp. 381–388, 2003.

[35] I. M. Engelhard, M. A. van den Hout, and J. W. S. Vlaeyen, "The sense of coherence in early pregnancy and crisis support and posttraumatic stress after pregnancy loss: a prospective study," *Behavioral Medicine*, vol. 29, no. 2, pp. 80–84, 2003.

[36] I. M. Engelhard, M. A. van den Hout, and E. G. W. Schouten, "Neuroticism and low educational level predict the risk of posttraumatic stress disorder in women after miscarriage or stillbirth," *General Hospital Psychiatry*, vol. 28, no. 5, pp. 414–417, 2006.

[37] M. A. van den Hout and I. M. Engelhard, "Pretrauma neuroticism, negative appraisals of intrusions, and severity of PTSD symptoms," *Journal of Psychopathology and Behavioral Assessment*, vol. 26, no. 3, pp. 181–183, 2004.

[38] J. A. M. Hunfeld, J. W. Wladimiroff, F. Verhage, and J. Passchier, "Previous stress and acute psychological defence as predictors of perinatal grief—an exploratory study," *Social Science and Medicine*, vol. 40, no. 6, pp. 829–835, 1995.

[39] J. A. M. Hunfeld, J. W. Wladimiroff, and J. Passchier, "Prediction and course of grief four years after perinatal loss due to congenital anomalies: a follow-up study," *British Journal of Medical Psychology*, vol. 70, no. 1, pp. 85–91, 1997.

[40] J. A. M. Hunfeld, J. W. Wladimiroff, and J. Passchier, "The grief of late pregnancy loss," *Patient Education and Counseling*, vol. 31, no. 1, pp. 57–64, 1997.

[41] A. Kersting, M. Dorsch, C. Kreulich et al., "Trauma and grief 2–7 years after termination of pregnancy because of fetal anomalies—a pilot study," *Journal of Psychosomatic Obstetrics and Gynecology*, vol. 26, no. 1, pp. 9–14, 2005.

[42] A. Kersting, K. Kroker, J. Steinhard et al., "Complicated grief after traumatic loss: a 14-month follow up study," *European Archives of Psychiatry and Clinical Neuroscience*, vol. 257, no. 8, pp. 437–443, 2007.

[43] M. J. Korenromp, G. C. M. L. Page-Christiaens, J. van den Bout et al., "Psychological consequences of termination of pregnancy for fetal anomaly: similarities and differences between partners," *Prenatal Diagnosis*, vol. 25, no. 13, pp. 1226–1233, 2005.

[44] M. J. Korenromp, G. C. M. L. Page-Christiaens, J. van den Bout, E. J. H. Mulder, and G. H. A. Visser, "Adjustment to termination of pregnancy for fetal anomaly: a longitudinal study in women at 4, 8, and 16 months," *American Journal of Obstetrics and Gynecology*, vol. 201, no. 2, pp. 160.e1–160.e7, 2009.

[45] B. Major and R. H. Gramzow, "Abortion as stigma: cognitive and emotional implications of concealment," *Journal of Personality and Social Psychology*, vol. 77, no. 4, pp. 735–745, 1999.

[46] J. S. Seng, L. K. Low, M. Sperlich, D. L. Ronis, and I. Liberzon, "Prevalence, trauma history, and risk for posttraumatic stress disorder among nulliparous women in maternity care," *Obstetrics and Gynecology*, vol. 114, no. 4, pp. 839–847, 2009.

[47] A. Speckhard and N. Mufel, "Universal responses to abortion? Attachment, trauma, and grief responses in women following abortion," *The Journal of Prenatal and Perinatal Psychology and Health*, vol. 18, pp. 3–7, 2003.

[48] P. Turton, W. Badenhorst, P. Hughes, J. Ward, S. Riches, and S. White, "Psychological impact of stillbirth on fathers in the subsequent pregnancy and puerperium," *British Journal of Psychiatry*, vol. 188, pp. 165–172, 2006.

[49] P. Turton, C. Evans, and P. Hughes, "Long-term psychosocial sequelae of stillbirth. Phase II of a nested case-control cohort study," *Archives of Women's Mental Health*, vol. 12, no. 1, pp. 35–41, 2009.

[50] P. Turton, P. Hughes, C. D. H. Evans, and D. Fainman, "Incidence, correlates and predictors of post-traumatic stress disorder in the pregnancy after stillbirth," *British Journal of Psychiatry*, vol. 178, pp. 556–560, 2001.

[51] P. Turton, P. Hughes, P. Fonagy, and D. Fainman, "An investigation into the possible overlap between PTSD and unresolved responses following stillbirth: an absence of linkage with only unresolved status predicting infant disorganization," *Attachment and Human Development*, vol. 6, no. 3, pp. 241–253, 2004.

[52] D. S. Armstrong, M. H. Hutti, and J. Myers, "The influence of prior perinatal loss on parents' psychological distress after the birth of a subsequent healthy infant," *Journal of Obstetric, Gynecologic, and Neonatal Nursing*, vol. 38, no. 6, pp. 654–666, 2009.

[53] A. N. Broen, T. Moum, A. S. Bødtker, and Ø. Ekeberg, "The course of mental health after miscarriage and induced abortion: a longitudinal, five-year follow-up study," *BMC Medicine*, vol. 3, article 18, 2005.

[54] I. M. Engelhard, M. A. van den Hout, M. Kindt, A. Arntz, and E. Schouten, "Peritraumatic dissociation and posttraumatic stress after pregnancy loss: a prospective study," *Behaviour Research and Therapy*, vol. 41, no. 1, pp. 67–78, 2003.

[55] L. Hamama, S. A. M. Rauch, M. Sperlich, E. Defever, and J. S. Seng, "Previous experience of spontaneous or elective abortion and risk for posttraumatic stress and depression during subsequent pregnancy," *Depression and Anxiety*, vol. 27, no. 8, pp. 699–707, 2010.

[56] P. Hughes, P. Turton, E. Hopper, and C. D. H. Evans, "Assessment of guidelines for good practice in psychosocial care of mothers after stillbirth: a cohort study," *The Lancet*, vol. 360, no. 9327, pp. 114–118, 2002.

[57] J. A. M. Hunfeld, J. W. Wladimiroff, J. Passchier, M. Uniken Venema-Van Uden, P. G. Frets, and F. Verhage, "Emotional reactions in women in late pregnancy (24 weeks or longer) following the ultrasound diagnosis of a severe or lethal fetal malformation," *Prenatal Diagnosis*, vol. 13, no. 7, pp. 603–612, 1993.

[58] A. Kersting, K. Kroker, J. Steinhard et al., "Psychological impact on women after second and third trimester termination of pregnancy due to fetal anomalies versus women after preterm birth—a 14-month follow up study," *Archives of Women's Mental Health*, vol. 12, no. 4, pp. 193–201, 2009.

[59] M. J. Korenromp, G. C. M. L. Christiaens, J. Van Den Bout et al., "Long-term psychological consequences of pregnancy termination for fetal abnormality: a cross-sectional study," *Prenatal Diagnosis*, vol. 25, no. 3, pp. 253–260, 2005.

[60] M. J. Korenromp, G. C. M. L. Page-Christiaens, J. van den Bout et al., "A prospective study on parental coping 4 months after termination of pregnancy for fetal anomalies," *Prenatal Diagnosis*, vol. 27, no. 8, pp. 709–716, 2007.

[61] N. Mufel, A. Speckhard, and S. Sivuha, "Predictors of post-traumatic stress disorder following abortion in a former Soviet Union country," *The Journal of Prenatal and Perinatal Psychology and Health*, vol. 17, pp. 41–61, 2002.

[62] P. K. Coleman, C. T. Coyle, M. Shuping, and V. M. Rue, "Induced abortion and anxiety, mood, and substance abuse disorders: isolating the effects of abortion in the national comorbidity survey," *Journal of Psychiatric Research*, vol. 43, no. 8, pp. 770–776, 2009.

[63] J. R. Steinberg and L. B. Finer, "Examining the association of abortion history and current mental health: a reanalysis of the National Comorbidity Survey using a common-risk-factors model," *Social Science and Medicine*, vol. 72, no. 1, pp. 72–82, 2011.

[64] S. Allanson, "Abortion decision and ambivalence: insights via an abortion decision balance sheet," *Clinical Psychologist*, vol. 11, no. 2, pp. 50–60, 2007.

[65] L. Cohen and S. Roth, "Coping with abortion," *Journal of Human Stress*, vol. 10, no. 3, pp. 140–145, 1984.

[66] A. A. P. van Emmerik, J. H. Kamphuis, and P. M. G. Emmelkamp, "Prevalence and prediction of re-experiencing and avoidance after elective surgical abortion: a prospective study," *Clinical Psychology & Psychotherapy*, vol. 15, no. 6, pp. 378–385, 2008.

[67] A. Hemmerling, F. Siedentopf, and H. Kentenich, "Emotional impact and acceptability of medical abortion with mifepristone: a German experience," *Journal of Psychosomatic Obstetrics and Gynecology*, vol. 26, no. 1, pp. 23–31, 2005.

[68] T. Kelly, J. Suddes, D. Howel, J. Hewison, and S. Robson, "Comparing medical versus surgical termination of pregnancy at 13–20weeks of gestation: a randomised controlled trial," *British Journal of Obstetrics and Gynaecology*, vol. 117, no. 12, pp. 1512–1520, 2010.

[69] S. D. Layer, C. Roberts, K. Wild, and J. Walters, "Postabortion grief: evaluating the possible efficacy of a spiritual group intervention," *Research on Social Work Practice*, vol. 14, no. 5, pp. 344–350, 2004.

[70] L. M. Pope, N. E. Adler, and J. M. Tschann, "Postabortion psychological adjustment: are minors at increased risk?" *Journal of Adolescent Health*, vol. 29, no. 1, pp. 2–11, 2001.

[71] C. Rousset, C. Brulfert, N. Séjourné, N. Goutaudier, and H. Chabrol, "Posttraumatic stress disorder and psychological distress following medical and surgical abortion," *Journal of Reproductive and Infant Psychology*, vol. 29, no. 5, pp. 506–517, 2012.

[72] V. M. Rue, P. K. Coleman, J. J. Rue, and D. C. Reardon, "Induced abortion and traumatic stress: a preliminary comparison of American and Russian women," *Medical Science Monitor*, vol. 10, no. 10, pp. SR5–SR16, 2004.

[73] P. Slade, S. Heke, J. Fletcher, and P. Stewart, "A comparison of medical and surgical termination of pregnancy choice, psychological consequences and satisfaction with care," *British Journal of Obstetrics and Gynaecology*, vol. 105, no. 12, pp. 1288–1295, 1998.

[74] S. Suliman, T. Ericksen, P. Labuschgne, R. de Wit, D. J. Stein, and S. Seedat, "Comparison of pain, cortisol levels, and psychological distress in women undergoing surgical termination of pregnancy under local anaesthesia versus intravenous sedation," *BMC Psychiatry*, vol. 7, article 24, 2007.

[75] J. Trybulski, "Women and abortion: the past reaches into the present," *Journal of Advanced Nursing*, vol. 54, no. 6, pp. 683–690, 2006.

[76] V. J. Walters and D. A. Oakley, "Hypnosis in post-abortion distress: an experimental case study," *Contemporary Hypnosis*, vol. 19, no. 2, pp. 85–99, 2002.

[77] C. Canário, B. Figueiredo, and M. Ricou, "Women and men's psychological adjustment after abortion: a six months prospective pilot study," *Journal of Reproductive and Infant Psychology*, vol. 29, no. 3, pp. 262–275, 2011.

[78] F. S. Cowchock, S. E. Ellestad, K. G. Meador, H. G. Koenig, E. G. Hooten, and G. K. Swamy, "Religiosity is an important part of coping with grief in pregnancy after a traumatic second trimester loss," *Journal of Religion and Health*, vol. 50, no. 4, pp. 901–910, 2011.

[79] V. Davies, J. Gledhill, A. McFadyen, B. Whitlow, and D. Economides, "Psychological outcome in women undergoing termination of pregnancy for ultrasound-detected fetal anomaly in the first and second trimesters: a pilot study," *Ultrasound in Obstetrics and Gynecology*, vol. 25, no. 4, pp. 389–392, 2005.

[80] R. Fernandez, D. Harris, and A. Leschied, "Understanding grief following pregnancy loss: a retrospective analysis regarding women's coping responses," *Illness Crisis and Loss*, vol. 19, no. 2, pp. 143–163, 2011.

[81] J. Kroth, M. Garcia, M. Hallgren, E. LeGrue, M. Ross, and J. Scalise, "Perinatal loss, trauma, and dream reports," *Psychological Reports*, vol. 94, no. 3, pp. 877–882, 2004.

[82] K. A. Salvesen, L. Øyen, N. Schmidt, U. F. Malt, and S. H. Eik-Nes, "Comparison of long-term psychological responses of women after pregnancy termination due to fetal anomalies and after perinatal loss," *Ultrasound in Obstetrics and Gynecology*, vol. 9, no. 2, pp. 80–85, 1997.

[83] L. Alderman, J. Chisholm, F. Denmark, and S. Salbod, "Bereavement and stress of a miscarriage: as it affects the couple," *Omega*, vol. 37, no. 4, pp. 317–327, 1998.

[84] S. V. Bowles, R. S. Bernard, T. Epperly et al., "Traumatic stress disorders following first-trimester spontaneous abortion: a pilot study of patient characteristics associated with these disorders," *Journal of Family Practice*, vol. 55, no. 11, pp. 969–973, 2006.

[85] M. P. Johnson and J. E. Puddifoot, "The grief response in the partners of women who miscarry," *Psychology and Psychotherapy: Theory, Research and Practice*, vol. 69, no. 4, pp. 313–327, 1996.

[86] C. Lee, P. Slade, and V. Lygo, "The influence of psychological debriefing on emotional adaptation in women following early miscarriage: a preliminary study," *The British Journal of Medical Psychology*, vol. 69, no. 1, pp. 47–58, 1996.

[87] E. Rowsell, G. Jongman, M. Kilby, R. Kirchmeier, and J. Orford, "The psychological impact of recurrent miscarriage, and the role of counselling at a pre-pregnancy counselling clinic," *Journal of Reproductive and Infant Psychology*, vol. 19, no. 1, pp. 33–45, 2001.

[88] N. Séjourné, S. Callahan, and H. Chabrol, "The utility of a psychological intervention for coping with spontaneous abortion," *Journal of Reproductive and Infant Psychology*, vol. 28, no. 3, pp. 287–296, 2010.

[89] F. Serrano and M. L. Lima, "Recurrent miscarriage: psychological and relational consequences for couples," *Psychology and Psychotherapy: Theory, Research and Practice*, vol. 79, no. 4, pp. 585–594, 2006.

[90] A. K.-H. Sham, M. G.-C. Yiu, and W. Y.-B. Ho, "Psychiatric morbidity following miscarriage in Hong Kong," *General Hospital Psychiatry*, vol. 32, no. 3, pp. 284–293, 2010.

[91] T. M. Walker and K. M. Davidson, "A preliminary investigation of psychological distress following surgical management of

early pregnancy loss detected at initial ultrasound scanning: a trauma perspective," *Journal of Reproductive and Infant Psychology*, vol. 19, no. 1, pp. 7–16, 2001.

[92] D. S. Armstrong, "Impact of prior perinatal loss on subsequent pregnancies," *JOGNN—Journal of Obstetric, Gynecologic, and Neonatal Nursing*, vol. 33, no. 6, pp. 765–773, 2004.

[93] A. Forray, L. C. Mayes, U. Magriples, and C. N. Epperson, "Prevalence of post-traumatic stress disorder in pregnant women with prior pregnancy complications," *Journal of Maternal-Fetal and Neonatal Medicine*, vol. 22, no. 6, pp. 522–527, 2009.

[94] L. Jind, "Do traumatic events influence cognitive schemata?" *Scandinavian Journal of Psychology*, vol. 42, no. 2, pp. 113–120, 2001.

[95] L. Jind, "Parents' adjustment to late abortion, stillbirth or infant death: the role of causal attributions," *Scandinavian Journal of Psychology*, vol. 44, no. 4, pp. 383–394, 2003.

[96] J. O'Leary, "The trauma of ultrasound during a pregnancy following perinatal loss," *Journal of Loss and Trauma*, vol. 10, no. 2, pp. 183–204, 2005.

[97] M. H. Hutti, D. S. Armstrong, and J. Myers, "Healthcare utilization in the pregnancy following a perinatal loss," *MCN The American Journal of Maternal/Child Nursing*, vol. 36, no. 2, pp. 104–111, 2011.

[98] J. Cacciatore, "Effects of support groups on post traumatic stress responses in women experiencing stillbirth," *Omega: Journal of Death and Dying*, vol. 55, no. 1, pp. 71–90, 2007.

[99] T. H. Uren and C. A. Wastell, "Attachment and meaning-making in perinatal bereavement," *Death Studies*, vol. 26, no. 4, pp. 279–308, 2002.

[100] K. J. Gold and S. M. Marcus, "The effect of maternal mental illness on pregnancy outcomes," *Expert Review of Obstetrics and Gynecology*, vol. 3, no. 3, pp. 391–401, 2008.

[101] L. Bonari, N. Pinto, E. Ahn, A. Einarson, M. Steiner, and G. Koren, "Perinatal risks of untreated depression during pregnancy," *Canadian Journal of Psychiatry*, vol. 49, no. 11, pp. 726–735, 2004.

[102] T. Munk-Olsen, T. M. Laursen, C. B. Pedersen, Ø. Lidegaard, and P. B. Mortensen, "Induced first-trimester abortion and risk of mental disorder," *The New England Journal of Medicine*, vol. 364, no. 4, pp. 332–339, 2011.

16

Foetal Macrosomia and Foetal-Maternal Outcomes at Birth

Sahruh Turkmen ⓘ,[1,2] **Simona Johansson,**[1] **and Marju Dahmoun**[2]

[1]*Department of Clinical Sciences, Obstetrics and Gynecology, Sundsvalls Research Unit, Umeå University, Umeå 90185, Sweden*
[2]*Department of Obstetrics and Gynecology, Sundsvall County Hospital, Sundsvall 85186, Sweden*

Correspondence should be addressed to Sahruh Turkmen; sahruh.turkmen@umu.se

Academic Editor: Fabio Facchinetti

To investigate how macrosomia affects foetal-maternal birth outcomes, we conducted a retrospective cohort study of singleton pregnant women who gave birth at gestational age ≥37+0 weeks. The patients were divided into three groups according to birth weight: "macrosomia" group, ≥4500 g, n=285; "upper-normal" group, 3500–4499 g, n=593; and "normal" group, 2500–3499 g, n=495. Foetal-maternal and delivery outcomes were compared among the three groups after adjustment for confounders. Caesarean section was more frequent in the macrosomia group than in upper-normal and normal groups. The duration of labour ($p < 0.05$) and postpartum care at the hospital ($p < 0.001$) were the highest in the macrosomia group. Increased birth weight was associated with higher risks of shoulder dystocia ($p < 0.001$), increased bleeding volume ($p < 0.001$), and perineal tear ($p < 0.05$). The Apgar score at 5 minutes ($p < 0.05$), arterial cord pH ($p < 0.001$), and partial pressure of O_2 ($p < 0.05$) were lower, while the arterial cord partial pressure of CO_2 was higher ($p < 0.001$), in the macrosomia group. Macrosomia has potentially serious impacts for neonate and mother as a result of a complicated and occasionally traumatic delivery.

1. Introduction

Macrosomia is a term used to describe an estimated foetal weight or birthweight of more than 4500 g, but a birthweight above 4000 g is also commonly used to define this condition. The term is often used as a synonym for large-for-gestational-age foetuses (birthweight > 90th percentile), and nearly 10% of all pregnancies are affected by macrosomia [1, 2]. The factors associated with this condition include a history of macrosomia, multiparity, maternal obesity prior to conception, excessive weight gain during pregnancy, advanced gestational age, and maternal diabetes as the strongest risk factor; however, in many high-birthweight cases, the cause is unknown [3, 4]. Earlier studies have shown that macrosomia can increase the risk of unfavourable delivery outcomes, including instrumental and/or caesarean deliveries, postpartum haemorrhage, shoulder dystocia, collarbone fracture, brachial plexus injury, and asphyxia [5–7]. Some authors have suggested that the complications during delivery caused by macrosomia can be prevented by delivery via elective caesarean section [8]. This strategy is considered justified only when the estimated foetal weight is over 4500 g in women with diabetes or over 5000 g in women without diabetes [9]. Another strategy to overcome the negative impacts of macrosomia is early induction of labour to reduce the likelihood of foetal growth; however, the increased risks of maternal and neonatal morbidity and mortality associated with induction should be taken into consideration [10, 11]. Several studies have suggested that labour induction is associated with an increased risk of caesarean section delivery, with no reduction in the number of birth-related injuries [12–14]. A recent randomized control study suggested that labour induction for macrosomic foetuses at gestational age 37–39 weeks reduces the risks of dystocia and collarbone fracture while increasing the likelihood of spontaneous vaginal birth [15].

Although accurate estimation of birthweight prior to labour and identification of foetuses at risk are challenges, there are no existing common guidelines as to how to manage macrosomia. In this retrospective study, we attempted to determine the effects of birth weight on labour, foetal-maternal outcomes, and obstetric complications. The purpose of this study is to increase the knowledge and nursing care preparedness of the emergency obstetric staff in managing macrosomia.

2. Materials and Methods

A retrospective cohort study was undertaken of all singleton pregnant women who gave birth at gestational age ≥ 37 weeks + 0 days in the maternity unit of a county hospital in Sundsvall, Sweden, over a 5-year period (from January 1, 2011 to December 31, 2015). The patients were divided into three groups according to foetal birth weight: ≥ 4500 g (macrosomia group), 3500–4499 g (upper-normal group), and 2500–3499 g (normal group). The maternal and foetal outcomes were evaluated and compared among the three groups.

The aim of the study was to evaluate the associations between birthweight and foetal-maternal outcomes. The patients who met the criteria detailed below were identified by searching our hospital medical records using Obstetrix (Siemens Corporation, Upplands Väsby, Sweden), a Swedish electronic medical record system that is specialised for prenatal care and childbirth. In Obstetrix, the pregnancy is followed in a logical and structured manner, from enrolment in the prenatal health care centre to arrival to the maternity unit and the time of delivery. This study was approved by the Regional Ethical Review Board of Umeå, Sweden.

Patients with a singleton pregnancy who gave birth at gestational age ≥ 37 weeks + 0 days to a foetus with a birthweight ≥ 2500 g were included in the study. Since the risk of morbidity for newborn and women increases drastically, when the birth weight is more than 4500 g [16], macrosomia was defined as a birthweight >4500 g. Patients were excluded for the following reasons: a multiple pregnancy, infection or contagious disease, history of psychiatric care, more than one delivery by caesarean section, or premature birth (before gestational age 37 weeks). Maternal hypothyroidism and asthma were not considered exclusion criteria.

Maternal demographic characteristics (age, body mass index [BMI], parity, previous caesarean section, and systemic disease) and the following outcomes were assessed: time from the start of delivery (cervical dilation ≥ 4 cm) to birth, period of postpartum care at the hospital (time from delivery to discharge), delivery method, shoulder dystocia, genital tract injury (vaginal or perineal rupture), anal sphincter injury, and bleeding volume at birth.

The following foetal outcomes were assessed: neonatal complications attributed to macrosomia in terms of the Apgar score at 5 minutes and umbilical cord arterial blood parameters (pH, partial pressure of O2 [pO2], partial pressure of CO2 [pCO2], and a base excess [BE]).

Statistical Analysis. All statistical analyses were performed using Statistical Package for Social Sciences version 23 (SPSS Inc., Chicago, IL, USA). Descriptive statistics were used to present the data, which were divided into categorical, ordinal, and continuous variables. The normality of the distribution of the data was tested using Shapiro–Wilks test. Continuous nonparametric variables were evaluated by the Kruskal–Wallis and Mann–Whitney U tests and presented as medians (range), while categorical/ordinal variables were evaluated by chi-square test. The relationships between variables were determined by adjusting for confounders in multiple logistic regression analyses. Stepwise linear regression analyses were performed for continuous variables and binary logistic regression analyses for categorical variables.

3. Results

A total of 7362 women delivered at the maternity unit of a county hospital in Sundsvall, Sweden, from January 1, 2011 to December 31, 2015. The patients' medical records were checked, and those with incomplete data records were excluded. After applying the inclusion and exclusion criteria and randomization, 1373 women were included in the study (Figure 1). The patients were divided into three groups according to birth weight: macrosomia group, ≥ 4500 g (n = 285); upper-normal group, 3500–4499 g (n = 593); and normal group, 2500–3499 g (n = 495). As the sample sizes of groups were highly unequal and the number of macrosomic neonates differed substantially from the numbers of newborns in the other two groups, to preclude a general loss of statistical power, we reduced the number of patients in upper-normal and normal groups using simple randomization. The randomization was performed in the Excel program (Microsoft® Office, 2013), by providing an arbitrary number from 0 to 1 in both upper-normal and normal groups. After sorting the patients in ascending order in one and each group, the first 600 respective 500 patients were selected in upper-normal and normal groups, respectively, and included in study. The number of patients in macrosomia group remained unchanged. 16 patients with incomplete documentation in clinical records were excluded afterwards from the three groups, and the number of patients who were analyzed decreased to 1373.

Overall differences were found among the three groups in terms of maternal age (p < 0.001), gestational age at birth (p = 0.001), maternal BMI (p < 0.001), and diabetes during pregnancy (p < 0.01); however, the number of previous caesarean section deliveries did not differ among the groups (Table 1). The mode of starting delivery (p = 0.001), delivery method (p = 0.001), labour duration (p = 0.013), length of postpartum care at the hospital (p < 0.001), bleeding volume (p < 0.001), and number of shoulder dystocia events (p < 0.001) were also different among the groups (Table 2). Neonatal outcomes, including the Apgar score at 5 minutes (p = 0.001), arterial cord pH (p < 0.001), arterial cord pO2 (p = 0.002), and arterial cord pCO2 (p < 0.001), also showed differences among the groups (Table 3).

In comparisons of macrosomia and upper-normal groups, women in macrosomia group had a greater BMI (p < 0.001), gestational age at birth (p < 0.001), and bleeding volume (p < 0.001) and a longer labour duration (p = 0.004) and postpartum care period (p < 0.001). The neonates of macrosomia group had a higher umbilical cord pCO2 (p < 0.001) but a lower pO2 (p < 0.001), Apgar score at 5 minutes (p = 0.044), and arterial pH (p = 0.017). The results suggest that the neonates were more stressed in macrosomia group than in upper-normal group during labour. Maternal age and umbilical cord arterial BE were not different between macrosomia and upper-normal groups (Tables 2 and 3).

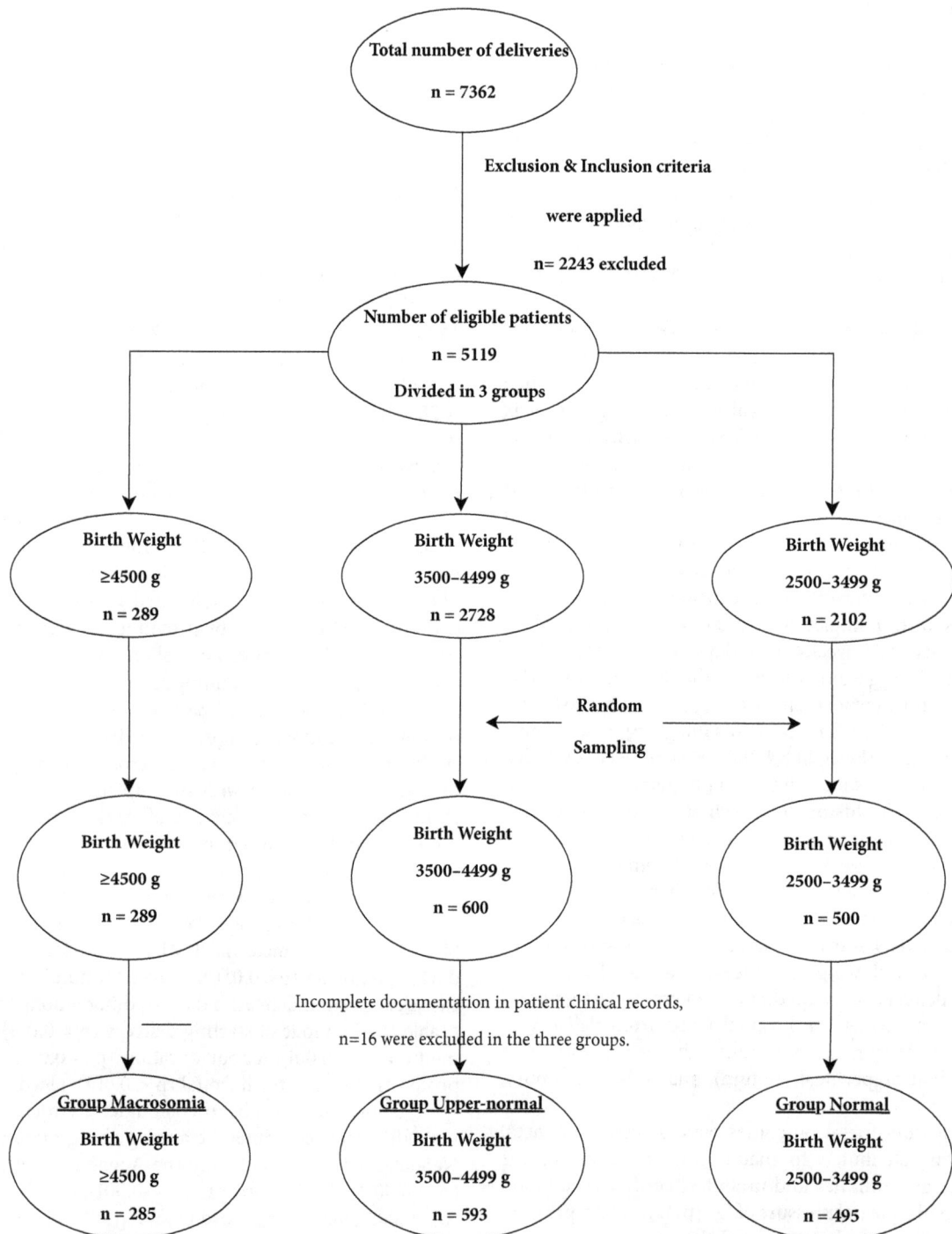

FIGURE 1: Flowchart. A visual representation of the sequence of steps and decisions made to include patients.

Comparison between macrosomia and normal groups showed significant differences suggestive of a complicated labour for both the mothers and neonates of macrosomia group. Maternal age (p < 0.001), gestational age at birth (p < 0.001), maternal BMI (p < 0.001), and bleeding volume (p < 0.001) were greater and the labour duration (p = 0.017) and postpartum care period (p < 0.001) longer in macrosomia group than in normal group. Regarding the neonatal outcomes, the Apgar score at 5 minutes (p = 0.001), pO2 (p = 0.007), and umbilical cord arterial pH (p < 0.001) were lower, and pCO2 (p < 0.001) was higher in macrosomia group than in normal group. Umbilical artery BE was not different between the groups.

Comparisons of upper-normal and normal groups revealed that the patients in upper-normal group had a significantly greater maternal age (p = 0.004), gestational age

TABLE 1: Demographic and baseline characteristics of the patients.

	G Macrosomia (n = 285)	G Upper-normal (n = 593)	G Normal (n = 495)	G comparisons
Maternal age (years)	30 (26)	30 (33)	29 (33)	b, c, c
BMI (kg/m^2)	26.8 (53.5)	24.5 (54.9)	23.5 (41.2)	a, b, c
Gestational age (weeks)	41 (5)	40 (6)	39 (5)	a, b, c
Previous caesarean, n (%)	26 (9.1%)	51 (8.6%)	38 (7.7%)	

Data are presented as numbers (%) or medians (range). G, group; a, $p < 0.01$ for G1 versus G2; b, $p < 0.01$ for G1 versus G3; c, $p < 0.01$ for G 2 versus G3; and n, number of patients.

TABLE 2: Maternal and delivery outcomes.

	G Macrosomia (n = 285)	G Upper-normal (n = 593)	G Normal (n = 495)	G comparisons
Diabetes, n (%)	12 (4.2%)	7 (1.2%)	1 (0.2%)	a, b
Labour duration (h)	6 (84)	5 (101)	5 (109)	a, b
Postpartum care (h)	49 (306)	18 (162)	26 (221)	a, b, c
Bleeding at birth (mL)	400 (2700)	300 (2450)	300 (2750)	a, b, c
Shoulder dystocia	7 (2.5%)	3 (0.5%)	0 (0%)	a, b
Tearing				
Vaginal	17 (6%)	32 (5.4%	32 (6.5)	
Cervical	1 (0.4%)	1 (0.2%)	1 (0.2%)	
Perineal				a
Grade II	7 (2.5%)	17 (2.9%)	18 (3.6%)	
Grade III	10 (3.5%)	21 (3.5%)	11 (2.2%)	
Grade IV	4 (1.4%)	0 (0%)	1 (0.2%)	
Anal sphincter				
< half	5 (1.8%)	13 (2.2%)	7 (1.4%)	
> half	2 (0.7%)	4 (0.7%)	2 (0.4%)	
Total	7 (2.5%)	3 (0.5%)	3 (0.6%)	
Delivery start				a, b
Spontaneous	185 (64.9%)	467 (78.8%)	382 (77.2%)	
Induction	74 (26%)	83 (14%)	79 (16%)	
Caesarean	26 (9.1%)	43 (7.3%)	34 (6.9%)	
Delivery method				a, b, c
Normal vaginal	190 (66.7%)	456 (76.9%)	369 (74.5%)	
Forceps	0 (0%)	1 (0.2%)	1 (0.2%)	
Vacuum	15 (5.3%)	39 (6.6%)	60 (12%)	
Caesarean	80 (28.1%)	97 (16.4%)	65 (13.1%)	

Mann–Whitney U, Kruskal–Wallis, and chi-square tests were used for the statistical analyses. Data are presented as the number (%) or the median (range). G, group; a, $p < 0.05$ for G1 versus G2; b, $p < 0.01$ for G1 versus G3; c, $p < 0.01$ for G 2 versus G3; and n, number of patients.

at birth ($p < 0.001$), maternal BMI ($p < 0.001$), and bleeding volume ($p = 0.001$) and a longer postpartum care period ($p = 0.005$). Cord arterial pH ($p = 0.049$) and pCO2 ($p = 0.018$) were also different between the groups (lower pH and higher pCO2 level in upper-normal group), suggesting more stress among neonates in upper-normal group; however, the Apgar score at 5 minutes, arterial cord pO2, BE, and duration of delivery were not different between the two groups (Tables 2 and 3).

To compare the observed and expected data among the three groups, we performed chi-square tests with Bonferroni correction of the p-values. Among the women in macrosomia group, diabetes ($x^2 = 20.801$, df = 2, $p < 0.001$) was more frequent, delivery was started mainly by induction ($x^2 = 23.286$, df = 4, $p < 0.001$), and caesarean section was the most common delivery method ($x^2 = 41.155$, df = 6, $p < 0.001$). Shoulder dystocia ($x^2 = 15.805$, df = 2, $p < 0.001$) and perineal tear ($x^2 = 13.727$, df = 6, $p = 0.033$) were also more frequent in this group. However, the numbers of cervical, vaginal, and anal sphincter tears and previous caesarean section deliveries were not significantly different among the groups. Comparisons of two groups showed

TABLE 3: Neonatal outcomes.

	G Macrosomia (n = 285)	G Upper-normal (n = 593)	G Normal (n = 495)	G comparisons
Birthweight (g)	4674 (4568 to 4840 g)	3816 (3657 to 4050)	3210 (3032 to 3358 g)	a, b, c
Apgar score at 5 min	10 (8)	10 (10)	10 (7)	a, b
Umbilical artery pH	7.2 (0.5)	7.2 (0.6)	7.2 (0.4)	a, b, c
pO2	2.6 (7.2)	3 (17.5)	3 (6.4)	a, b
pCO2	8.1 (12.5)	7.5 (14.2)	7.2 (9.2)	a, b, c
BE	−4.7 (23.8)	−5.2 (26.2)	−5.3 (19.9)	

Mann–Whitney U and Kruskal–Wallis tests were used for the statistical analyses. Data are presented as the number (%) or the median (range). Variation in birthweight showed by interquartile range (Q3-Q1). G, group; a, $p < 0.05$ for G1 versus G2; b, $p < 0.01$ for G1 versus G3; c, $p < 0,05$ for G 2 versus G3; n, number of patients; pO2, partial pressure of O2; pCO2, partial pressure of CO2; and BE, base excess.

differences between macrosomia and upper-normal groups in terms of the frequencies of diabetes ($x^2 = 8.348$, df = 1, p = 0.004), shoulder dystocia ($x^2 = 6.502$, df = 1, p = 0.016), and perineal tear ($x^2 = 8.461$, df = 3, p = 0.037) and in the mode of starting delivery ($x^2 = 21.242$, df = 2, p < 0.001) and the delivery method ($x^2 = 16.858$, df = 3, p = 0.001). Macrosomia and normal groups differed in terms of the mode of starting delivery ($x^2 = 11.214$, df = 3, p = 0.011) and delivery method ($x^2 = 11.214$, df = 3, p = 0.011). Upper-normal and normal groups differed in the frequencies of diabetes ($x^2 = 17.733$, df = 1, p < 0.001) and shoulder dystocia ($x^2 = 12.268$, df = 1, p < 0.001), mode of starting delivery ($x^2 = 14.165$, df = 2, p = 0.001), and delivery method ($x^2 = 32.702$, df = 3, p < 0.001) (Table 2).

Multiple logistic regression analyses were performed to identify correlations and confounders, and the results were shown in Table 4. The analysis revealed that birth weight was associated with diabetes (p < 0.005) and positively correlated with maternal BMI (p ≤ 0.001), gestational age at birth (p ≤ 0.001), and maternal age (p = 0.020). The total bleeding volume at birth was positively correlated with birth weight, delivery method (vaginal deliveries being associated with the least and caesarean section with the most bleeding), and vaginal and cervical tears. The total bleeding volume at birth was also affected by the mode of starting delivery; bleeding volume was the highest for caesarean section and induction (both p < 0.001). The duration of labour was positively correlated with maternal age and was associated with the mode of starting delivery and delivery method (p < 0.05). The period of postpartum care at the hospital appeared to be influenced by the delivery method, which increased with instrumental and caesarean section deliveries; the mode of starting delivery (hospitalization time was shorter when delivery started spontaneously); and by labour duration, gestational age at birth, bleeding volume, the grades of vaginal and anal sphincter tears, and diabetes (hospitalization time was twice as long for women with diabetes) (p < 0.05). Birth weight (p = 0.003) and diabetes (p = 0.048) were predictor of shoulder dystocia. The Apgar score at 5 minutes was negatively associated with shoulder dystocia, maternal BMI, vaginal tears, delivery method, and diabetes (p < 0.05). The cord arterial pH was negatively associated with the hospitalization stay after birth, birth weight, vaginal tearing,

total bleeding volume, and delivery method (p < 0.05). The cord pO2 was correlated with the delivery method, diabetes, and vaginal tearing (p < 0.05), while the cord pCO2 value was correlated with maternal BMI, birth weight, and diabetes (p < 0.05).

4. Discussion

The results of this study suggest that macrosomia is associated with increased risks of caesarean section and trauma to the birth canal and the foetus. Advanced maternal age and gestational age at birth, high BMI, and the presence of diabetes emerged as predisposing factors for macrosomia. As the rate of caesarean section delivery was higher among women with macrosomic foetuses, birth weight may influence the delivery method. The number of patients with grade 4 perineal tear, as a labour-associated injury, was also higher in this group. Macrosomia can increase the rate of shoulder dystocia and maternal bleeding volume at birth.

The risk of morbidity for newborn and women increases drastically when the birth weight is more than 4500 g [1, 4, 17]. In another trial, the authors studied birth weight categories to determine predictive thresholds of adverse outcomes. The study results suggested that a definition of macrosomia as >4000 g may be useful for the identification of increased risks of labour and newborn complications, >4500 g may be more predictive of neonatal morbidity, and >5000 g may be a better indicator of infant mortality risk [2]. Our results confirm partly their findings that adverse outcomes such as labour complications, delivery method, mode of delivery start, and neonatal morbidity differ across varying birth weight thresholds, but we have not observed any difference in rate of neonatal mortality between weight categories, and moreover, many outcomes were similar in two groups with birth weight <4500 g (see Tables 2 and 3). Differences between two studies may be explained by the fact that the sample size in our study was smaller and the study conducted in a geographically limited population.

In the macrosomia group, the incidence of spontaneous delivery was lower, but the rates of elective caesarean section and labour induction were higher, compared with the other two groups. These results are in accordance with other studies showing that the rate of caesarean section delivery was

TABLE 4: Regression analysis.

	Birth weight OR (95% CI)	Shoulder dystocia OR (95% CI)	Anal Sphinct. tears OR (95% CI)	Duration of Labour (B)	Bleeding Volume (B)	Apgar 5 min (B)	PPPC (B)
				Dependent variable			
Age (years)	1.0 (0.9-1.0) *	0.9 (0.8 – 1.1)	1.0 (0.9 – 1.0)	(0.2) * * *	(-2.6)	(0.01)	(-0.6)
BMI (kg/m2)	0.9 (0.9 – 1.0) **	0.9 (0.8 – 1.1)	1.0 (0.9 – 1.0)	(0.1)	(1.4)	(0.01) *	(0.2)
Diabetes (yes/no)	10.2 (3.5 - 29.4) **	26.5 (1.0 - 684) *	0.7 (0.8 – 5.1)	(-6.8)	(-16.7)	(0.4) *	(8.1) *
Gestational age at birth (week)	0.5 (0.4-0.6) * * *	2.1 (0.7 – 6.0)	1.1 (0.9 – 1.4)	(-0.2)	(1.2)	(0.01)	(-2.2) **
Birth weight (g)	-	1.0 (0.9 – 1.0) **	1.0 (1.0 - 1.1) *	(-0.01)	(0.1) *	(-0.6)	(-0.01)
Apgar score at 5 min	-	0.3 (0.1 – 0.6)	0.9 (0.7 – 1.2)	(0.2)	(5.0)	-	(-2.0)
Shoulder dystocia	-	-	7.5 (1.5 - 36.3) *	(-2.2)	(-31.3)	(1.7) * * *	(14.3)
Delivery method	-	0.7 (0.2 – 2.0)	0.9 (0.7 – 1.1)	(2.1) * * *	(52.2) * * *	(0.9) * * *	(8.1) * * *
Mode of starting labour	-	1.8 (0.6 – 5.7)	1.1 (0.8 – 1.6)	(7.1) * * *	(37.3) * * *	(0.01)	(6.0) * * *
Vaginal tears	-	13 (2.2 - 78.5) **	37.2 (18.6 - 74.3) * * *	(1.7)	(146.7) **	(0.2) **	(11.9) *
Cervical tears	-	0.01 (0.01 – 0.1)	0.4 (0.2 – 0.9)	(-4.6)	(503.5) **	(0.1)	(-0.7)
Anal Sphincter tears	-	9.7 (0.5 – 178)	-	(0.3)	(65.1)	(0.2)	(10.3) *
Bleeding volume (ml)	-	1.0 (0.9 – 1.0)	0.9 (0.3 – 2.6)	(-0.01)	-	(0.01)	(0.01) * * *
Duration of labour (h)	-	0.9 (0.8 – 1.0)	1.0 (0.9 – 1.0)	-	(-0.9)	(0.01)	(0.7) * * *
Postpartum care at the hospital (h)	-	1.0 (0.9 – 1.0)	1.0 (1.0 – 1.1)	(0.05) **	(1.5)	(-0.01)	-

OR, odds ratio; CI, confidence interval; B, B-coefficient; and PPPC, period of postpartum care at hospital. * = p < 0.05; ** = p < 0.01; * * * = p < 0.001.

increased among women who delivered macrosomic foetuses after labour induction [5, 18, 19]. Surprisingly, we found that normal group (the lowest birthweight neonates) had the highest rate of instrumental delivery via vacuum. Although the rate of complications during labour in nonmacrosomic neonates is not generally expected to be high, it is probable that conditions other than stress that required delivery assistance or acceleration (e.g., a prolonged second phase of delivery) were more common in this group. Foetal distress and/or the threat of asphyxia were rare in this group, as indicated by the higher Apgar score at 5 minutes and cord arterial pH in group 3 than in the other two groups.

Some studies have suggested that macrosomia is associated with a higher rate of injuries during labour [4, 5]. Although the number of patients with perineal injuries was low in all groups of our study, there was an overall difference among the three groups (see Table 2). There were twice as many patients with anal sphincter tears in the macrosomic group compared with the other two groups. An earlier study suggested a positive association between cervical and/or vaginal lacerations and macrosomia [19]; however, our results showed that the number of vaginal tears in the macrosomia group was less than half those in the other two groups, and the number of cervical tears did not differ among groups. An explanation for this may be that macrosomic neonates are commonly delivered via caesarean section, whereas normal vaginal and instrumental deliveries are more frequent in the other two groups.

Earlier studies have shown that macrosomia increases the risk of shoulder dystocia [15, 18, 20]. Some studies have suggested that offspring born to women with diabetes are at higher risk of experiencing shoulder dystocia, but this risk was decreased when labour was induced at 38–39 weeks of gestation [20–22]. Our finding that the risk of shoulder dystocia was higher among macrosomic neonates is consistent with the above-mentioned studies, but we did not find an association between diabetes and shoulder dystocia. We found that a higher foetal weight was associated with the presence of diabetes and advanced gestational age; other studies have also suggested an increased prevalence of large-for-gestational-age neonates in women with diabetes [21]. The inconsistency regarding the association between diabetes and shoulder dystocia may result from differences in study populations and/or policies regarding the management of pregnancy in diabetic women, as labour may be induced at an earlier gestational age in women with diabetes. Prophylactic caesarean delivery may also be considered for suspected macrosomia with an estimated foetal weight of at least 4500 g in women with diabetes and at least 5000 g in women without diabetes, but the clinical effectiveness of a prophylactic caesarean delivery is controversial [23–25]. Analysis of our data shows that, in the group of women with diabetes, the delivery method has no effect on the Apgar score at 5 min and the risk of shoulder dystocia ($p > 0.05$, OR 0.133), although the results need to be interpreted cautiously, due to low number of diabetes patients in our study.

We evaluated the impact of macrosomia on foetal outcomes. Macrosomic neonates had a lower arterial cord pH, pO_2, and Apgar score at 5 minutes and a higher pCO_2 compared with the neonates of the other groups. These parameters are accepted indicators of the vitality and well-being of newborns. We found that instrumental/surgical deliveries and diabetes are negatively associated with the Apgar score at 5 minutes. Moreover, the number of shoulder dystocia cases among macrosomic neonates was higher, and the Apgar score at 5 minutes of the shoulder dystocia cases was lower. Lower Apgar scores are seen more frequently in macrosomic neonates when the delivery is complicated by shoulder dystocia [26], although other studies were unable to demonstrate any difference in the Apgar score between normal-birthweight and macrosomic neonates [27]. According to our findings, macrosomia seems to increase the risk of foetal impairment, and the low Apgar score at 5 minutes in the macrosomic group may be a consequence of the complications associated with macrosomia.

We also evaluated the impact of birthweight on delivery outcomes. The postpartum care period in the hospital was longer in women with diabetes and/or macrosomic neonates. This finding can be explained by the high frequencies of caesarean section deliveries and perineal tears in this group. It has been suggested that labour induction for foetal macrosomia can increase the risk of complications such as genital tract injuries, thereby increasing the hospital stay for recovery of these women [18]. In addition, the risk of foetal-maternal complications increases in women with diabetes. The postpartum control of diabetes is a very important issue for the well-being of the mother and newborn because of the increased incidence of hypoglycaemia, indicating a need for close monitoring and prolonged care in the hospital.

We identified four variables (maternal age, maternal BMI prior to pregnancy, gestational age at delivery, and maternal diabetes) as potential predisposing factors and predictors of macrosomia. Many previous studies have also suggested that diabetes is the strongest predisposing factor for macrosomia [28, 29]. It has also been shown that women with diabetes are more likely to be obese and to gain more weight during pregnancy; furthermore, maternal BMI is a predictor of diabetes and is therefore considered a risk factor for macrosomia [30, 31]. Diabetes during pregnancy elevates the mother's blood glucose and insulin levels, causing insulin to circulate from the mother to baby, which can lead to excessive fat deposits and macrosomia. Our findings are in line with those of other studies that showed positive correlations among maternal BMI, maternal diabetes, and foetal macrosomia. Because the weight of the foetus increases with gestational age, it is not unusual that foetal macrosomia is associated with a higher gestational age. In addition, we found a positive association between increased maternal age and macrosomia, although a previous study showed no such effect [28].

In conclusion, macrosomia may place the mother and neonate at risk for adverse outcomes. Our findings suggest that the delivery of a macrosomic neonate has potentially serious impacts for neonates and mothers in terms of a difficult and occasionally traumatic delivery. We identified maternal BMI, maternal age, gestational age at birth, and maternal diabetes as risk factors that influence the development of macrosomia in pregnant women. Furthermore, an earlier induction of labour in pregnant women with presumed foetal macrosomia may reduce the risks of caesarean section and trauma to the birth canal and foetus.

However, because earlier trials to investigate the negative effects of macrosomia have shown contradictory results, more studies are needed to determine a safe and effective method for proper management of macrosomia. The purpose of this study was to increase the knowledge and nursing care preparedness of the emergency obstetric staff in managing macrosomia. The results of this study are of course not decisive, but it can still illustrate circumstances to perceive the complications and situations that may occur during the delivery of a foetus with macrosomia.

Conflicts of Interest

The authors have no conflicts of interest to declare in connection with this article.

Acknowledgments

The authors are particularly grateful to midwife Valborg Nordlander for her help with the data collection. This work was supported by an "SKL-Medel" grant from "Sverige Kommuner och Landsting".

References

[1] "Practice Bulletin No. 173 Summary: Fetal Macrosomia," *Obstetrics and Gynecology*, vol. 128, pp. 1191-1192, 2016.

[2] S. L. Boulet, G. R. Alexander, H. M. Salihu, and M. Pass, "Macrosomic births in the United States: Determinants, outcomes, and proposed grades of risk," *American Journal of Obstetrics & Gynecology*, vol. 188, no. 5, pp. 1372-1378, 2003.

[3] P. M. Catalano, "Management of obesity in pregnancy," *Obstetrics & Gynecology*, vol. 109, no. 2, pp. 419-433, 2007.

[4] W. N. Spellacy, S. Miller, A. Winegar, and P. Q. Peterson, "Macrosomia–maternal characteristics and infant complications," *Obstetrics & Gynecology*, vol. 66, no. 2, pp. 158-161, 1985.

[5] J. R. King, L. M. Korst, D. A. Miller, and J. G. Ouzounian, "Increased composite maternal and neonatal morbidity associated with ultrasonographically suspected fetal macrosomia," *The Journal of Maternal-Fetal & Neonatal Medicine : The Official Journal of the European Association of Perinatal Medicine, the Federation of Asia and Oceania Perinatal Societies, the International Society of Perinatal Obstet*, vol. 25, pp. 1953-1959, 2012.

[6] H. Vidarsdottir, R. T. Geirsson, H. Hardardottir, U. Valdimarsdottir, and A. Dagbjartsson, "Obstetric and neonatal risks among extremely macrosomic babies and their mothers," *American Journal of Obstetrics & Gynecology*, vol. 204, no. 5, pp. 423.e1-423.e6, 2011.

[7] E. L. Barber, L. S. Lundsberg, K. Belanger, C. M. Pettker, E. F. Funai, and J. L. Illuzzi, "Indications contributing to the increasing cesarean delivery rate," *Obstetrics & Gynecology*, vol. 118, no. 1, pp. 29-38, 2011.

[8] D. J. Rouse, J. Owen, R. L. Goldenberg, and S. P. Cliver, "The effectiveness and costs of elective cesarean delivery for fetal macrosomia diagnosed by ultrasound," *Journal of the American Medical Association*, vol. 276, no. 18, pp. 1480-1486, 1996.

[9] R. J. Sokol, S. C. Blackwell, American College of Obstetricians and Gynecologists, and Committee on Practice Bulletins-Gynecology, "ACOG practice bulletin: Shoulder dystocia. Number 40, November 2002. (Replaces practice pattern number 7, October 1997)," *International Journal of Gynaecology and Obstetrics*, vol. 80, pp. 87-92, 2003.

[10] R. De Luca, M. Boulvain, O. Irion, M. Berner, and R. E. Pfister, "Incidence of early neonatal mortality and morbidity after late-preterm and term cesarean delivery," *Pediatrics*, vol. 123, no. 6, pp. e1064-e1071, 2009.

[11] K. Ghartey, J. Coletta, L. Lizarraga, E. Murphy, C. V. Ananth, and C. Gyamfi-Bannerman, "Neonatal respiratory morbidity in the early term delivery," *American Journal of Obstetrics & Gynecology*, vol. 207, no. 4, pp. 292.e1-292.e4, 2012.

[12] C. A. Combs, N. B. Singh, and J. C. Khoury, "Elective induction versus spontaneous labor after sonographic diagnosis of fetal macrosomia," *Obstetrics & Gynecology*, vol. 81, no. 4, pp. 492-496, 1993.

[13] O. Gonen, D. J. D. Rosen, Z. Dolfin, R. Tepper, S. Markov, and M. D. Fejgin, "Induction of labor versus expectant management in macrosomia: A randomized study," *Obstetrics & Gynecology*, vol. 89, no. 6, pp. 913-917, 1997.

[14] T. K. Parissenti, G. Hebisch, W. Sell, P. E. Staedele, V. Viereck, and M. K. Fehr, "Risk factors for emergency caesarean section in planned vaginal breech delivery," *Archives of Gynecology and Obstetrics*, vol. 295, no. 1, pp. 51-58, 2017.

[15] M. Boulvain, M.-V. Senat, F. Perrotin et al., "Induction of labour versus expectant management for large-for-date fetuses: A randomised controlled trial," *The Lancet*, vol. 385, no. 9987, pp. 2600-2605, 2015.

[16] American College of O Gynecologists' Committee on Practice B-O, "Practice Bulletin No. 173: Fetal Macrosomia," *Obstetrics and gynecology*, vol. 128, pp. e195-e209, 2016.

[17] T. S. Nesbitt, W. M. Gilbert, and B. Herrchen, "Shoulder dystocia and associated risk factors with macrosomic infants born in California," *American Journal of Obstetrics & Gynecology*, vol. 179, no. 2, pp. 476-480, 1998.

[18] O. Irion and M. Boulvain, "Induction of labour for suspected fetal macrosomia," *Cochrane Database of Systematic Reviews*, no. 2, 2000.

[19] M. Najafian and M. Cheraghi, "Occurrence of Fetal Macrosomia Rate and Its Maternal and Neonatal Complications: A 5-Year Cohort Study," *ISRN Obstetrics and Gynecology*, vol. 2012, Article ID 353791, 5 pages, 2012.

[20] S. Lurie, V. Insler, and Z. J. Hagay, "Induction of labor at 38 to 39 weeks of gestation reduces the incidence of shoulder dystocia in gestational diabetic patients class A2," *American Journal of Perinatology*, vol. 13, no. 5, pp. 293-296, 1996.

[21] S. L. Kjos, O. A. Henry, M. Montoro, T. A. Buchanan, and J. H. Mestman, "Insulin-requiring diabetes in pregnancy: A randomized trial of active induction of labor and expectant management," *American Journal of Obstetrics & Gynecology*, vol. 169, no. 3, pp. 611-615, 1993.

[22] O. Langer, M. D. Berkus, R. W. Huff, and A. Samueloff, "Shoulder dystocia: should the fetus weighing greater than or equal to 4000 grams be delivered by cesarean section?" *American Journal of Obstetrics & Gynecology*, vol. 165, no. 4, pp. 831-837, 1991.

[23] K. D. Gregory, O. A. Henry, E. Ramicone, L. S. Chan, and L. D. Platt, "Maternal and infant complications in high and normal weight infants by method of delivery," *Obstetrics & Gynecology*, vol. 92, no. 4 I, pp. 507–513, 1998.

[24] J. L. Ecker, J. A. Greenberg, E. R. Norwitz, A. S. Nadel, and J. T. Repke, "Birth weight as a predictor of brachial plexus injury," *Obstetrics & Gynecology*, vol. 89, no. 5, pp. 643–647, 1997.

[25] S. M. Menticoglou, F. A. Manning, I. Morrison, and C. R. Harman, "Must macrosomic fetuses be delivered by a caesarean section? A review of outcome for 786 babies greater than or equal to 4,500 g," *Australian and New Zealand Journal of Obstetrics and Gynaecology*, vol. 32, no. 2, pp. 100–103, 1992.

[26] L. Raio, F. Ghezzi, E. Di Naro et al., "Perinatal outcome of fetuses with a birth weight greater than 4500 g: An analysis of 3356 cases," *European Journal of Obstetrics & Gynecology and Reproductive Biology*, vol. 109, no. 2, pp. 160–165, 2003.

[27] A. Weissmann-Brenner, M. J. Simchen, E. Zilberberg et al., "Maternal and neonatal outcomes of macrosomic pregnancies," *Medical Science Monitor*, vol. 18, no. 9, pp. PH77–PH81, 2012.

[28] A. Mohammadbeigi, F. Farhadifar, N. Soufi Zadeh, N. Mohammadsalehi, M. Rezaiee, and M. Aghaei, "Fetal macrosomia: risk factors, maternal, and perinatal outcome," *Annals of Medical and Health Sciences Research*, vol. 3, pp. 546–550, 2013.

[29] M. Mathew, L. Machado, R. Al-Ghabshi, and R. Al-Haddabi, "Fetal macrosomia. Risk factor and outcome," *Saudi Medical Journal*, vol. 26, no. 1, pp. 96–100, 2005.

[30] Z. Wang, L. Kanguru, J. Hussein, A. Fitzmaurice, and K. Ritchie, "Incidence of adverse outcomes associated with gestational diabetes mellitus in low- and middle-income countries," *International Journal of Gynecology and Obstetrics*, vol. 121, no. 1, pp. 14–19, 2013.

[31] S. A. Feresu, Y. Wang, and S. Dickinson, "Relationship between maternal obesity and prenatal, metabolic syndrome, obstetrical and perinatal complications of pregnancy in Indiana, 2008-2010," *BMC Pregnancy and Childbirth*, vol. 15, no. 1, p. 266, 2015.

17

Prevalence and Determinants of Complete Postnatal Care Service Utilization in Northern Shoa, Ethiopia

Mohammed Akibu (ID),[1] **Wintana Tsegaye,**[2] **Tewodros Megersa,**[3] **and Sodere Nurgi**[1]

[1]*Department of Midwifery, Institute of Medicine and Health Sciences, Debre Berhan University, Debre Berhan, Ethiopia*
[2]*Concordia University, Montreal, Quebec, Canada*
[3]*Obstetrics Unit, Gandhi Maternal Specialized Hospital, Addis Ababa, Ethiopia*

Correspondence should be addressed to Mohammed Akibu; mahammedakibu@gmail.com

Academic Editor: Fabio Facchinetti

Background. Postnatal period presents the highest risk of death for mothers and newborns. Although progress has been made in expanding the coverage for most of maternal health services, national prevalence of postnatal care service utilization in Ethiopia is still extremely limited. Hence, this study aims to determine the prevalence and factors associated with complete postnatal care service utilization in Northern Shoa, Ethiopia. *Methods.* Community based cross-sectional survey was conducted between November 2016 and February 2017. A total of 510 mothers were included in the study using multistage sampling technique. The data were collected through face-to-face interview. Bivariate and multivariate logistic regression models were fitted to identify factors associated with complete postnatal care utilization at p value of < 0.05. SPSS version 20 was used to analyze the data. *Results.* The prevalence of complete postnatal care utilization was found to be 28.4% in the study area. Mode of delivery (AOR=5.7, 95% CI = 3.9, 19), number of children (AOR= 2.5 95% CI, 1.4, 14.2), and level of education (AOR=3.2 95% CI, 1.1, 9.2) were the factors statistically associated with complete postnatal service uptake. Being healthy was the major (48.8%) reason mentioned for not complying with the recommended three postnatal visits. *Conclusion.* The prevalence of complete postnatal care service in the study area was found to be low, and it is far less than the targeted zonal and regional plan. Reinforcing the existing policies and strategies to increase women level of awareness about postnatal care and intensive counseling during antenatal care and delivery are the recommendations based upon the current finding.

1. Background

The postnatal period (PNP) is the time beginning immediately following the delivery of the placenta and extending through the six weeks (42 days) of birth. This period represents a critical phase in determining the health and survival of the mother and her newborn [1]. The wellbeing and chance of staying free of morbidity or mortality are much dependent upon the care given during pregnancy, delivery, and most importantly after delivery, the time when many maternal and neonatal deaths take place. Therefore, lack of care during postnatal period may end up in death or morbidity as well as missed opportunities to various healthy behaviors benefiting the mother and her newborn [2, 3]

For both newborns and mothers, the highest risk of death occurs at delivery, followed by the first hours and days after childbirth. It has been shown that more than two-thirds of newborn deaths would occur by the end of the first week after delivery, with up to one-half of all newborn deaths occurring in the first 24 hours. Similarly, approximately two-thirds of all maternal deaths occur in the postnatal period [4, 5].

Although some countries have made a dramatic progress, half of the maternal deaths in the world still take place in Sub-Saharan Africa where little or no progress has been made. Even though there is no single, simple, straightforward intervention that will significantly decrease maternal mortality, several studies have shown that majority of these maternal and neonatal problems could be reduced if women receive appropriate postnatal care [6–9]. In spite of proven benefits of postnatal care on maternal and neonatal health, most newborns and mothers do not receive this service from a skilled healthcare provider during the first few days after delivery; thus, this is the most neglected period for the provision of quality care. Similarly, rates of provision of skilled care are much lower during postnatal period when compared to rates before and during childbirth [3, 10] Likewise, the coverage of postnatal care (PNC) in Ethiopia remains alarmingly limited with only 7% increment over the last one and half decade [11, 12]. Hence, this study aimed at providing a contemporary evidence about the level of PNC coverage and various determinant factors in Northern Shoa, Ethiopia.

2. Methods

2.1. Study Design and Population. Community based cross-sectional study was conducted from November 2016 to February 2017 with 520 mothers who gave birth within the last ten months preceding the survey. The study was conducted at Debre Berhan town, the capital city of Northern Shoa zone of Amhara regional state located about 130 kilometers to the North East of Addis Ababa (the capital of Ethiopia). Debre Berhan town contains nine urban and five rural kebeles according to administrative classification with estimated population size of 84, 944. More than half 43, 696 (51.4%) of the population in the town are represented by females. Of total females, 26,876 of them are found within reproductive age (15-49) group.

2.2. Inclusion and Exclusion Criteria. All women who have given birth within the last ten months preceding the survey were included. Women admitted for much of postnatal periods, those who gave birth greater than ten months ago, and women with still births were excluded from the study.

2.3. Sample Size and Sampling Procedure. The sample size for the current study was calculated using single population proportion formula with the assumption of 95% confidence level, 20.2% prevalence of postnatal care utilization [13], 5% marginal error, and design effect of 2. The final sample size (520) was obtained after 5% adjustment for nonresponse rate. The sample size was distributed proportionally for each selected kebeles (the smallest administrative unit in Ethiopia). Finally, systematic random sampling with k^{th} value of five was used to obtain the study subjects in each selected kebele.

2.4. Variables and Measurements. The outcome variable was complete postnatal care service utilization which refers to postnatal care service uptake within 24 hours of delivery, the first 3-7 days after delivery, and 7-14th days subsequently. Women who have received the service during all three periods were considered to have complete utilization. The independent variables comprised various sociodemographic (age, educational status, income, and marital status), obstetrics (parity, mode of delivery, ANC use, course of pregnancy, and plan for the current pregnancy), and other health service related characteristics (autonomy, distance from health facility).

The outcome variable was measured by asking the practice and timing of postnatal care visit with three possible responses (i.e., (1) only received postnatal care once after delivery, (2) received twice within the recommended postnatal schedule (successive or interrupted), and (3) received thrice subsequent postnatal care within the recommended time frame). This self-reported visit was cross-confirmed by reviewing postnatal registration records. Finally, the outcome variable was dichotomized as 1: complete PNC utilization and 0: sporadic PNC utilization.

2.5. Data Collection and Quality Control. The data were collected using a structured questionnaire via a face-to-face interview at the participant's home. The questionnaire was first prepared in English and then translated into local language (Amharic) and back to English to ensure consistency. The pretest was done on 5% of the total sample size and a necessary adjustment was made. Six midwives and two nurses who are fluent in speaking the local language were involved in the data collection. Two-day training was given to the data collectors and supervisors.

2.6. Operational Definition

Complete Postnatal Visit. It is for mothers who have stayed in the hospital for 24 hours after delivery and returned for checkup between 3-7 days and 7–14 days subsequently.

Seclusion. It is a cultural/social practice that forbids mothers from going out and/or joining peoples for 40 days starting from the day of delivery.

2.7. Data Analysis. The data were described using frequency and/or cross-tabulation for categorical variables and mean (standard deviation (SD)) for continuous variables. Binary and multiple logistic regression tests were carried out to identify associated factors at p value threshold < 0.05. The data were coded, cleaned, and entered using EPI-INFO version 7 and analyzed with SPSS version 20. The result was reported strictly following Strengthening the Reporting of Observational Studies in Epidemiology (STROBE) Statement (Supplementary File (available here)).

3. Results

3.1. Sociodemographic Characteristics. A total of 510 mothers participated in the study making a response rate of 98%. Nearly one-third (31.8%) of respondents were found within the age group of 25–29. Majority of the participants were from Amhara (79.4%) ethic group and orthodox (72.5%) religious background. One-quarter (26.9%) of the mothers attended at least secondary level education and a significant number of women (21.4%) had no any graded education but can read and write (Table 1).

3.2. Obstetrics Characteristics. More than half (56.7%) of participants were low multiparous (with children between two and four), whereas nearly third of (29.2%) mothers were primiparous. Some (11.6%) of the mothers reported

TABLE 1: Sociodemographic characteristics of women who gave birth within the last ten months preceding the survey, Northern Shoa, Ethiopia 2017.

Sociodemographic characteristics	Frequency (n)	Percent (%)
Age		
15 – 19	44	8.6
20 -24	150	29.4
25-29	162	31.8
30 -34	94	18.4
35 and above	60	11.8
Marital Status		
Unmarried	30	5.9
Married	456	89.4
Divorced	24	4.7
Ethnicity		
Amhara	405	79.4
Tigree	37	7.3
Oromo	39	7.6
Gurage	26	5.1
Others[a]	3	.6
Religion		
Orthodox	370	72.5
Muslim	86	16.9
Protestant	41	8.0
Catholic	9	1.8
Others[b]	4	.8
Educational Status		
Illiterate	26	5.1
Read and write	109	21.4
Primary Education	125	24.5
Secondary Education	137	26.9
Higher Education	113	22.2
Husband Education		
Illiterate	54	10.6
Read and write	72	14.1
Primary Education	111	21.7
Secondary Education	98	19.3
Higher Education	175	34.3
Household Income		
< $25	248	48.6
$26 -$99	173	33.9
$100 or more	89	17.5
Mother occupation		
House Wife	252	49.4
Self-Employee	100	19.6
Government Employee	114	22.4
Maid servant	32	6.3
Student	12	2.4

[a] Afar and Wolayita; [b] Bhai and apostolic.

that the most recent pregnancy was complicated and most (39%) of this problem was attributed to premature rupture of membrane. Cesarean section accounted for 18% of these deliveries and 3.9% of babies born were twins. More than half (53.7%) of participants received the recommended four or more antenatal care service (ANC) (Table 2).

3.3. Postnatal Care Service. Only 28.4% of participants received the recommended three postnatal care visits within six weeks of delivery. Among mothers who have visited antenatal care clinic, the majority (58.4%) of these women did not receive counseling about postnatal care. Similarly, only 18.4% of these women initially had information about postnatal care service from different sources. About two-thirds (76.3%) of mothers suggested that there was a social and cultural norm called "Seclusion" which forbids them from coming out of home after delivery. Most importantly almost half (49.1%) of these women respond that this event was more important and valuable than any outdoor visit (Table 3).

3.4. Factors Associated with Complete Postnatal Care Utilization. In multivariate logistic regression model, mothers who have given birth through cesarean section were 5.7 [AOR=5.7 95% CI = 3.9 - 19] times more likely to receive complete postnatal care service than those who delivered through spontaneous vaginal delivery. Similarly, mothers having one child (primiparous) were 4.5 more likely to have full postnatal care [AOR= 2.5 95% CI 1.4 – 14.2] than multiparous women. Level of education [AOR=3.2 95% CI, 1.1, 9.2] was another factor which is statistically significant with complete postnatal care utilization (Table 4).

4. Discussion

The current study revealed that only 145 (28.4%) of mothers have received complete postnatal care as per the standard recommendation. This finding was slightly higher compared to the reports from other studies [13, 14]. This discrepancy may be attributed to the time gap difference as there would be an improvement on access to healthcare and awareness about the service through time. However, a study conducted in Addis Ababa city administrative by Senait Berhanu and Berhanu wordofa indicated that the postnatal care prevalence was twice of this report (65.6%) [15]. This disparity might be explained by the sociodemographic variation between the study participants such as educational level and living standard as well as nature of the study area including better access to healthcare.

The current study has shown that mothers who attended higher education were three times more likely to receive complete postnatal care service than illiterate women [AOR=3.2 95% CI, 1.1, 9.2]. This finding was in agreement with results from Dembecha district, North west Ethiopia, Nepal, Nigeria, and one more study in Ethiopia [16–19]. This could be explained by the notion that education is a key factor in empowering maternal decision making towards healthcare service, increasing awareness of basic health services, and being informed about health risks, with all of these eventually leading to the improved health seeking behavior.

TABLE 2: Distribution of obstetrics history of women who gave birth within the last ten months preceding the survey, in Northern Shoa, Ethiopia 2017.

Obstetrics characteristics	Frequency (n)	Percent (%)
Number of children alive		
One	149	29.2
Two – four	290	56.7
Five and above	71	13.9
ANC in recent pregnancy	454	89
Yes	56	11
No		
Number of visits		
One	38	8.4
Two	54	11.9
Three	88	19.4
Four and above	274	60.4
Course of Pregnancy		
Complicated	59	11.6
Uncomplicated	451	88.4
Type of conditions faced		
Hypertensive disorders	10	16.9
PROM	23	39.0
Post Term	14	23.7
Anemia	7	11.9
Bleeding during pregnancy	5	8.5
Mode of delivery		
SVD	356	69.8
SVD assisted with Instrument	62	12.2
Cesarean section	92	18.0
Number of babies born		
Single	490	96.1
Twins	20	3.9
Autonomy on Heath care seeking		
It's up to me to decide	424	83.1
It's not only me	86	16.9

∗ANC: antenatal care; ∗SVD: spontaneous vaginal delivery; ∗ PROM: premature rupture of membranes.

Cesarean section delivery resulted in increased odds of having complete postnatal service. This finding has also been supported by different studies from Ethiopia and Tanzania [20–22]. This could be because mothers who had operative delivery are tending to have greater perceived susceptibility to a wide range of postoperative complications; therefore, frequent return to the health institution would be the strategy to minimize these perceived risks. Primiparity was another obstetrics determinant for full postnatal care service attendance. Studies in Ethiopia and Nepal have shown consistent finding [19, 20, 23]. This might be justified by the fact that first time mothers are usually dependent upon the support of health professionals and their family on infant care and feeding practice. Similarly, they would be very curious about the health of their newborn baby; thus, these needs might be satisfied through frequent contact with health professionals.

5. Limitation of the Study

The result of this study must be interpreted cautiously considering the following inevitable limitations. Though the study has included mothers who gave birth in the last ten months, there might be a possibility of some recall bias. Causality cannot be inferred due to the cross-sectional nature of the study. Moreover, the external validity of the finding might be limited. However, it is the first study which tried to assess the level of complete postnatal care visit in the study area.

6. Conclusion

The coverage of full postnatal care service in the study was found to be lower than the targeted zonal and regional plan. Maternal educational status, parity, and mode of delivery

TABLE 3: Coverage of postnatal care services and related information's among women who gave birth in the last ten months preceding this survey, Northern Shoa, Ethiopia, 2017.

Variables	Frequency (n)	Percent (%)
Postnatal care utilization		
Complete PNC (3 or more visits)	145	28.4
Sporadic PNC (2 or less PNC)	365	71.6
Reason for not complying with PNC recommendation		
I didn't know about its importance	124	33.9
It's a waste of time once we get birth	39	10.7
I waited long time to get the service	57	15.6
Baby and I were completely healthy	178	48.8
Social reasons	84	23
Counseling about PNC		
Yes	189	41.6
No	265	58.4
Previous Information about PNC		
Had information	94	18.4
Never had information	416	81.6
Source of Information		
Media	19	20.2
Magazines or other reading materials	30	31.9
Health extension workers	57	60.6
Friends	13	13.8
Postdelivery seclusion		
Yes	389	76.3
No	121	23.7
Postnatal care vs seclusion		
It's more important than any clinic visit	191	49.1
No difference to me	103	26.5
No, the visit would be more important	95	24.4

*PNC: postnatal care.

were factors significantly associated with postnatal acre service utilization. Reinforcing the existing policies and strategies to increase mother's level of awareness about postnatal care, intensive counseling during antenatal and delivery, and scheduling mothers based on the national postnatal care follow-up protocol to increase postnatal care service utilization were recommended.

Ethical Approval

Ethical approval was obtained from the Institutional Review Board (IRB) of Debre Berhan University, Institute of Medicine and Health Science.

Consent

Both written and verbal consent were taken from the study subjects after explaining the purpose and procedures of the study. Information obtained was kept confidential.

Conflicts of Interest

The authors declare that they have no conflicts of interest.

Authors' Contributions

Mohammed Akibu conceived and designed the study. Mohammed Akibu, Tewodros Megersa, and Sodere Nurgi supervised the data collection and prepared the manuscript. Mohammed Akibu and Wintana Tsegaye performed analysis and interpretation of the data. All authors read and approved the final manuscript.

Acknowledgments

The authors would like to pass their gratitude to the University of Debre Berhan for its ethical approval. Their appreciation also extends to all mothers who took part in the study.

TABLE 4: Bivariate and multivariate analysis of factors associated with complete postnatal care service utilization, Northern Shoa, Ethiopia, 2017.

Variables		PNC		Crude OR (95%, CI)	Adjusted OR (95%, CI)
		Complete	Sporadic		
Husband education	Illiterate	15	39	1	1
	Read and Write	15	57	.684 (.300,1.559)	.431 (.151, 1.226)
	Primary education	16	95	.438 (.196,.972)	.254 (.091, .706)
	Secondary education	26	72	.939 (.446, 1.98)	.807 (.316, 2.061)
	Higher education	73	102	1.861 (1.25, 3.62)*	1.253 (.531, 2.956)
Maternal Education	Illiterate	2	24	1	1
	Read and write	27	82	3.9 (.876, 17.83)	3.1 (.597, 16.9)
	Primary Education	30	95	3.7 (.846, 16.9)	2.5 (.476,13.1)
	Secondary Education	35	102	4.1 (.925, 18.32)	2.02 (.387,10.5)
	Higher education	51	62	6.8 (2.226, 14.34)	3.2 (1.19, 9.2)*
Parity	Primiparous	58	91	2.08 (1.2, 7.8)	2.5 (1.42,14.2)*
	Multiparous	88	202	1.7 (.692, 4.37)	1.76 (.575, 5.39)
	Grande multiparous	24	47	1	1
Information about PNC	Had information	32	62	1.34 (1.08,2.23)*	1.98(.553,3.74)
	Had no information	113	303	1	1
Autonomy on health care	Self-decision	117	307	1.79 (1.479, 6.30)*	1.27 (.362, 2.261)
	Collaborative decision	28	58	1	1
Mode of delivery	SVD	88	268	1	1
	SVD with instrumentation	19	43	3.27 (.927, 4.3)	4.27 (.82,6.2)
	Cesarean section	38	54	2.35 (1.45, 3.81)*	5.7 (3.96, 18.3)*
Number of babies born	Singleton	140	350	1	1
	Twins	5	15	.833 (.297, 2.336)	1.025 (.295, 3.558)
Counseling on PNC	Received	48	141	.709 (.467, 1.075)	.737 (.446, 1.217)
	Not received	86	179	1	1

*Statistically significant variable; 1 reference category; COR: crude odds ratio; AOR: adjusted odds ratio.

References

[1] X. F. Li, J. A. Fortney, M. Kotelchuck, and L. H. Glover, "The postpartum period: The key to maternal mortality," *International Journal of Gynecology and Obstetrics*, vol. 54, no. 1, pp. 1–10, 1996.

[2] J. E. Lawn, S. Cousens, and J. Zupan, "4 Million neonatal deaths: when? Where? Why?" *The Lancet*, vol. 365, no. 9462, pp. 891–900, 2005.

[3] The Partnership for Maternal Newborn and Child Health. Opportunities for Africa's newborns: Practical data, policy and programmatic support for newborn care in Africa. world health organization 2006 (cited 2017 February); Available from: http://www.who.int/pmnch/knowledge/publications/africanewborns/en/.

[4] Joy E. Lawn analysis based on 38 DHS datasets (2000 to 2004) with 9,022 neonatal deaths, using MEASURE DHS STAT compiler (https://dhsprogram.com/). Used in: Save the Children-U.S., State of the World's Mothers 2006 (Washington, DC: Save the Children-U.S., 2006).

[5] R. Carine and J. G. Wendy, "Maternal mortality: who, when, where, and why," *The Lancet*, vol. 368, no. 9542, pp. 1189–1200, 2006.

[6] World Health Organization. WHO technical consultation on postpartum and postnatal care. 2010 (cited 2017 March); Available from: http://www.who.int/maternal_child_adolescent/documents/WHO_MPS_10_03/en/.

[7] P. K. Singh, C. Kumar, R. K. Rai, and L. Singh, "Factors associated with maternal healthcare services utilization in nine high focus states in India: A multilevel analysis based on 14 385 communities in 292 districts," *Health Policy and Planning*, vol. 29, no. 5, pp. 542–559, 2014.

[8] R. Pattinson, K. Kerber, E. Buchmann et al., "Stillbirths: How can health systems deliver for mothers and babies?" *The Lancet*, vol. 377, no. 9777, pp. 1610–1623, 2011.

[9] A. Blank, H. Prytherch, J. Kaltschmidt et al., "'Quality of prenatal and maternal care: bridging the know-do gap' (QUALMAT study): an electronic clinical decision support system for rural Sub-Saharan Africa," *BMC Medical Informatics and Decision Making*, vol. 13, article 44, 2013.

[10] World Health Organization. WHO recommendations on postnatal care of the mother and newborn. 2013 (cited 2017 May); Available from: http://www.who.int/maternal_child_adolescent/documents/postnatal-care-recommendations/en/.

[11] Central Statistical Authority [Ethiopia] and ORC Macro. 2001. Ethiopia Demographic and Health Survey 2000. Addis Ababa, Ethiopia and Calverton, Maryland, USA: Central Statistical Authority and ORC Macro.

[12] Central Statistical Agency (CSA) [Ethiopia] and ICF. 2016. Ethiopia Demographic and Health Survey 2016: Key Indicators

Report. Addis Ababa, Ethiopia, and Rockville, Maryland, USA. CSA and ICF.

[13] Y. Gebeyehu Workineh, "Factors Affecting Utilization of Postnatal Care Service in Amhara Region, Jabitena District, Ethiopia," *Science Journal of Public Health*, vol. 2, no. 3, pp. 169–176, 2014.

[14] H. Alemayeh, H. Assefa, and Y. Adama, "Prevalence and Factors Associated with Post Natal Care Utilization in Abi-Adi Town, Tigray, Ethiopia: A Cross Sectional Study," *International Journal of Pharmaceutical and Biological Sciences Fundamentals*, vol. 8, no. 1, 2014.

[15] S. Berhanu, Y. Asefa, and B. W. Giru, "Prevalence of Postnatal Care Utilization and Associated Factors among Women Who Gave Birth and Attending Immunization Clinic in Selected Government Health Centers in Addis Ababa, Ethiopia," *Journal of Health, Medicine and Nursing*, vol. 26, 2016.

[16] M. Ayana Hordofa, S. S. Almaw, M. G. Berhanu, and H. B. Lemiso, "Postnatal Care Service Utilization and Associated Factors Among Women in Dembecha District, Northwest Ethiopia," *Science Journal of Public Health*, vol. 3, no. 5, pp. 686–692, 2015.

[17] K. Vishnu, M. Adhikari, R. Karkee, and T. Gavidia, "Factors associated with the utilisation of postnatal care services among the mothers of Nepal: Analysis of Nepal Demographic and Health Survey 2011," *BMC Women's Health*, vol. 14, no. 19, 2014.

[18] O. D. Somefun and L. Ibisomi, "Determinants of postnatal care non-utilization among women in Nigeria," *BMC Research Notes*, vol. 9, no. 1, article no. 21, 2016.

[19] S. M. Tarekegn, L. S. Lieberman, and V. Giedraitis, "Determinants of maternal health service utilization in Ethiopia: analysis of the 2011 Ethiopian Demographic and Health Survey," *BMC Pregnancy and Childbirth*, vol. 14, no. 1, article 161, 2014.

[20] K. Mehari and E. Wencheko, "Factors affecting maternal health care services utilization in rural Ethiopia: a study based on the 2011 EDHS data," *Ethiopian Journal of Health Development*, vol. 27, no. 1, pp. 16–24, 2013.

[21] M. A. Limenih, Z. M. Endale, and B. A. Dachew, "Postnatal Care Service Utilization and Associated Factors among Women Who Gave Birth in the Last 12 Months prior to the Study in Debre Markos Town, Northwestern Ethiopia: A Community-Based Cross-Sectional Study," *International Journal of Reproductive Medicine*, vol. 2016, Article ID 7095352, 7 pages, 2016.

[22] D. Mohan, S. Gupta, A. LeFevre, E. Bazant, J. Killewo, and A. H. Baqui, "Determinants of postnatal care use at health facilities in rural Tanzania: Multilevel analysis of a household survey," *BMC Pregnancy and Childbirth*, vol. 15, no. 282, 2015.

[23] S. Dhakal, G. N. Chapman, P. P. Simkhada, E. R. van Teijlingen, J. Stephens, and A. E. Raja, "Utilisation of postnatal care among rural women in Nepal," *BMC Pregnancy and Childbirth*, vol. 7, no. 1, p. 19, 2007.

18

Association between Breastfeeding Duration and Type of Birth Attendant

Jordyn T. Wallenborn ⓘ **and Saba W. Masho** ⓘ

School of Medicine, Division of Epidemiology, Department of Family Medicine and Population Health,
Virginia Commonwealth University, 830 East Main Street, Suite 821, P.O. Box 980212, Richmond, VA, USA

Correspondence should be addressed to Jordyn T. Wallenborn; wallenbornjt@vcu.edu

Academic Editor: Fabio Facchinetti

Introduction. Healthcare providers play an integral role in breastfeeding education and subsequent practices; however, the education and support provided to patients may differ by type of provider. The current study aims to evaluate the association between type of birth attendant and breastfeeding duration. *Methods*. Data from the prospective longitudinal study, Infant Feeding Practices Survey II, was analyzed. Breastfeeding duration and exclusive breastfeeding duration were defined using the American Academy of Pediatrics' national recommendations. Type of birth attendant was categorized into obstetricians, other physicians, and midwife or nurse midwife. If mothers received prenatal care from a different type of provider than the birth attendant, they were excluded from the analysis. Multinomial logistic regression was conducted to obtain crude and adjusted odds ratios and 95% confidence intervals. *Results*. Compared to mothers whose births were attended by an obstetrician, mothers with a family doctor or midwife were twice as likely to breastfeed at least six months. Similarly, mothers with a midwife birth attendant were three times as likely to exclusively breastfeed less than six months and six times more likely to exclusively breastfeed at least six months compared to those who had an obstetrician birth attendant. *Conclusions*. Findings from the current study highlight the importance of birth attendants in breastfeeding decisions. Interventions are needed to overcome barriers physicians encounter while providing breastfeeding support and education. However, this study is limited by several confounding factors that have not been controlled for as well as by the self-selection of the population.

1. Introduction

While the majority of births are attended by obstetricians, the proportion of midwife attended vaginal births in the United States reached an all-time high (11.4%) in 2009 [1]. However, these rates vary drastically by state. For example, certified nurse-midwifes attended almost a quarter (23.9%) of all births in New Mexico whereas they attended only 0.8% of births in Arkansas. Despite these variations, the prevalence of midwife attended births has increased in almost all states since 1990 [1].

Literature has shown that births attended by midwives have improved outcomes. A large study conducted in Canada reported that mothers with a home-birth attended by a midwife had a reduced risk of birth trauma and resuscitation at birth compared to mothers with a planned hospital birth attended by a physician [2]. Midwives have also been reported to manage the third stage of labor based on the patient's preference whereas physicians were more likely to actively manage this stage of labor [3].

Research has also shown that midwives have greater knowledge of breastfeeding benefits and higher self-confidence when managing breastfeeding problems [4]. For example, over half of certified nurse midwives report being "well" or "very well" prepared to assist breastfeeding women. Also, 9 out of 10 midwives reported encouraging mothers to breastfeed more if mothers were concerned about insufficient milk supply [4], a major reason women prematurely cease breastfeeding [5].

In contrast to favorable outcomes shown among midwives, literature provides insight into physicians deteriorating attitudes and commitment to breastfeeding support [6–8].

A study that assessed practicing obstetrics/gynecologists, pediatricians, and family member physicians reported a significant deficit in the knowledge of breastfeeding benefits and clinical management [7]. In fact, a survey of pediatricians showed that 20% made no breastfeeding recommendation, 13% recommended breastfeeding with formula, and 2% recommended formula feeding only [9].

Numerous studies have assessed healthcare professional's knowledge of breastfeeding outcomes and attitudes and commitment to providing breastfeeding support [4, 6–9]. However, knowledge may not directly translate to clinical practice. Healthcare professionals may not have the skills, expertise, or time to provide adequate breastfeeding support to mothers. Nevertheless, these attributes may differ between types of healthcare professional. To better understand the ability of healthcare providers in providing breastfeeding counseling, the current study aims to investigate the association between type of birth attendant and breastfeeding duration.

2. Materials and Methods

Data from the prospective longitudinal Infant Feeding Practices Survey (IFPS) II was analyzed. IFPS II was conducted by the Food and Drug Administration and Centers for Disease Control and Prevention from May 2005 through June 2007. Information on maternal and child health, infant feeding behaviors, and a mother's diet was collected through questionnaires and a short telephone interview. To be included in the study, mothers were at least 18 years old at the time of the prenatal survey, had a full-term or nearly full-term singleton infant, and had good maternal and child health at birth. Good maternal and child health at birth was defined as "neither the mother nor the infant could have a medical condition at birth that would affect feeding and that the infant had to have been born after at least 35 weeks' gestation, weigh at least 5 lb, be a singleton, and not have stayed in the intensive care for >3 days" [10]. Additional information on IFPS II methodology can be found elsewhere [10].

The current study also applied exclusion criteria. Mothers were excluded if women received prenatal care from a different type of provider and then the birth attendant or reported no healthcare provider at birth ($N = 15$) or another type of healthcare provider ($N = 34$) due to small numbers or if women had missing information on breastfeeding duration and healthcare provider at birth, leaving 2,979 women for analysis. This study was approved as exempt by the Virginia Commonwealth University Institutional Review Board.

The main outcome variable, breastfeeding duration, was categorized as "never breastfed," "breastfed less than 6 months," and "breastfed at least 6 months" which is consistent with national recommendations [11]. Breastfeeding duration was based on three self-report survey items: "Did you ever breastfeed this baby (or feed this baby your pumped milk)?" If mothers responded "yes," they were asked "Have you completely stopped breastfeeding and pumping milk for your baby?" every month until breastfeeding cessation

occurred. To establish duration of breastfeeding after cessation, participants were asked, "How old was your baby when you completely stopped breastfeeding and pumping milk?" If mothers were still breastfeeding at the time of the last interview (at 12 months postpartum) ($N = 917$), the following question was asked at the six-year follow-up: "How old was your 6-year-old when the following happened? He or she stopped being fed breast milk, including pumped breast milk." The current study also investigated excusive breastfeeding, which was defined as an infant's consumption of "no other food or drink, not even water, except breast milk (including milk expressed or from a wet nurse) . . . but allows the infant to receive oral rehydration solution (ORS), drops and syrups (vitamins, minerals and medicines)" [12].

Birth attendant, the main exposure variable, was based on the question, "Which type of health professional was your birth attendant?" which was assessed during the neonatal questionnaire. Healthcare provider at birth was categorized as "obstetrician," "family doctor, general practitioner, internist, or other physicians," and "midwife or nurse midwife."

A variety of factors that were available in the dataset were considered as potential confounders. Demographic factors included marital status (married; not married), maternal race (White; Black; Hispanic; others including Asian/pacific islander), maternal age (18–24 years; 25–29 years; 30–34 years; 35–45 years), maternal education (less than high school; high school graduate; 1–3 years of college; college graduate), income (less than $20,000; $20,000–49,999; at least $50,000), and prepregnancy body mass index (underweight ($<18.5 \, kg/m^2$); normal weight ($18.5–24.9 \, kg/m^2$); overweight ($25.0–29.9 \, kg/m^2$); obese ($30.0+ \, kg/m^2$)). Healthcare variables included prenatal participation in the Special Supplemental Nutrition Program from Women, Infants, and Children (WIC) program (yes; no), postnatal participation in WIC, health insurance (yes; no), and mode of delivery (vaginally, not induced; vaginally, induced; planned Cesarean section; unplanned or emergency Cesarean section). Other factors included breastfeeding intention (breastfeed only; formula feed; or combination) and smoking during pregnancy (yes; no).

Descriptive statistics with frequencies and percentages were calculated to assess the distribution of characteristics by type of healthcare provider at birth. Separate bivariate multinomial logistic regression models produced crude odds ratio (COR) and 95% confidence intervals (CI) to show factors associated with breastfeeding duration. Effect modification for breastfeeding intention, marital status, race/ethnicity, education, and mode of delivery were assessed; however, they were not statistically significant. Therefore, all factors were considered as potential confounders. Multicollinearity was tested between pre- and post-WIC utilization and did not reach a variance inflation factor (VIF) of 5. A final parsimonious model including all factors that resulted in at least a 10% change in the crude estimate was used to generate adjusted odds ratios (AOR) and 95% CI. All analyses were conducted using SAS version 9.4 statistical software (SAS, Cary, NC). Virginia Commonwealth University Institutional Review Board determined the current study to be exempt.

3. Results

The majority of study participants were married (79.8%) and non-Hispanic white (85.6%), had at least some college education (80.2%), had health insurance (95.6%), had a vaginal delivery (71.4%), and initiated breastfeeding (85.4%) (Table 1). Over three quarters (86.9%) of mothers had an obstetrician as their birth attendant while 5.6% had a family doctor, and 7.5% utilized a midwife (not shown in Tables 1–4). Approximately 1 in 12 (8.2%) mothers exclusively breastfed for six months. Among mothers who used a midwife for their birth, more women were aged 25–29 years (37.4%), were normal weight (52.9%), intended to breastfeed only (78.1%), and gave birth vaginally (93.4%). Bivariate analyses demonstrated significant associations between all demographic, reproductive, and lifestyle factors and breastfeeding duration, except health insurance (Table 2).

Compared to mothers with an obstetrician birth attendant, those with a midwife were twice as likely (crude odds ratio (COR) = 2.32; 95% CI = 1.22–4.42) to breastfeed less than six months and almost four times (COR = 3.99; 95% CI = 2.12–7.49) more likely to breastfed at least six months. After adjusting for marital status, education, race, income, age, mode of delivery, breastfeeding intention, and prenatal and postpartum WIC participation, mothers with a family doctor, general practitioner, internist, or other physicians were twice as likely to breastfeed at least six months (AOR = 2.04; 95% CI = 1.04–4.00) compared to those who had an obstetrician birth attendant. Similarly, mothers with a midwife birth attendant were more than twice as likely to breastfeed at least six months (AOR = 2.43; 95% CI = 1.12–5.25) compared to those who had an obstetrician birth attendant (Table 3).

Similar results were obtained when investigating exclusive breastfeeding duration. Compared to mothers with an obstetrician birth attendant, those with a midwife were four times (COR = 4.01; 95% CI = 2.13–7.55) more likely to exclusively breastfeed less than six months and almost ten times (COR = 9.96; 95% CI = 4.78–20.75) more likely to exclusively breastfed at least six months. After adjusting for marital status, income, age, mode of delivery, and prenatal and postpartum WIC participation, estimates remained significant but slightly attenuated. Mothers with a midwife birth attendant were more likely to exclusively breastfeed less than six months (AOR = 3.11; 95% CI = 1.62–5.98) and exclusively breastfeed at least six months (AOR = 6.65; 95% CI = 3.05–14.50) compared to those who had an obstetrician birth attendant. No association was found among women whose birth was attended by obstetrician and family doctor, general practitioner, internist, or other physicians (Table 4).

4. Discussion

The current study found a relationship between type of birth attendant and breastfeeding duration. Specifically, mothers whose births were attended by midwives were more likely to breastfeed six months or more compared to mothers whose births were attended by obstetricians. Similarly, mothers whose birth was attended by midwives were more likely to exclusively breastfeed a longer duration compared to mothers whose birth was attended by obstetricians.

While no research, to our knowledge, has investigated the relationship between birth attendant and breastfeeding duration, the findings can be explained by the clinical management practices healthcare professionals utilize during the postpartum period. For example, recent literature has demonstrated that nurse midwives are more attentive and have more control over the education mothers receive [13]. Due to constraints of the current healthcare system, physicians spend limited time with their patients [14]. This could lead to (1) a lack of support while staying in the hospital or (2) a provision of inadequate information about breastfeeding to patients, all of which has the potential to influence breastfeeding practices. For example, a prospective cohort study reported that appraisal of the breastfeeding experience while in the hospital was significantly associated with breastfeeding success, defined as the mother successfully breastfeeding the duration planned at the mother's initial estimate [15]. Because physicians' time with patients is limited, nurses play a major role in postpartum care and breastfeeding education. Furthermore, studies have shown that nurses directly impact breastfeeding success through emotional, informational, and tangible support [16]. In fact, nurses' breastfeeding knowledge was the best predictor of breastfeeding support [14]. However, deficits in nurse's knowledge, attitudes, and commitment to breastfeeding have been reported [14].

Strengths of this study include the longitudinal prospective study design which allows temporality to be established. IFPS II also utilized a standardized data collection protocol that minimizes the potential for information bias. Other strengths include the ability to account for breastfeeding factors such as breastfeeding intention that can potentially affect breastfeeding outcomes. Further, the definition of breastfeeding duration includes breastfeeding exclusivity, which measures in full compliance with national recommendations [11].

Despite the numerous strengths, this study is not without limitations. Because a consumer opinion panel was used to identify participants, the study population disproportionately represents women who are white, are of higher socioeconomic status, can read English, and have stable mailing addresses. Therefore, results are not generalizable. Breastfeeding duration is self-report and subject to social desirability bias which could bias results towards the null; however, self-report of breastfeeding duration has been demonstrated as a reliable measurement [17]. Potential confounding factors such as facility where mother gave birth, labor and delivery staffing at the hospital where the mother delivered, if the mother self-selected the type of birth attendant and if hospitals had initiatives or policies that increase breastfeeding success (e.g., Baby-Friendly hospital policies), self-efficacy, and alcohol use were not available and may have impacted the effect size. Current literature lacks information on midwifery in hospitals. Future research should investigate correlates of midwifery practice within hospitals. Further, researchers should investigate if midwives are more likely to assist "skin-to-skin care." Lastly, literature surrounding midwife and

TABLE 1: Distribution of maternal characteristics by healthcare provider at birth.

Characteristic	Total Percent N = 2,651	Obstetrician Percent N = 2,304	Family or other MD Percent N = 149	Midwife Percent N = 198	Chi square (p value)
Age					**0.0046**
18–24 years	22.1	21.4	26.4	27.8	
25–29 years	33.7	33.4	33.8	37.4	
30–34 years	27.9	27.9	31.8	24.2	
35–45 years	16.3	17.3	8.1	10.6	
Marital status					0.3323
Not married	20.2	19.8	24.1	22.5	
Maternal race					**0.0477**
White, NH	85.6	84.8	90.9	90.8	
Black, NH	4.4	4.6	4.2	2.0	
Hispanic	5.8	6.1	4.9	3.6	
Others	4.2	4.5	0.0	3.6	
Maternal education					**0.001**
Less than high school	3.0	2.6	5.1	6.5	
High school	16.8	16.3	24.8	16.7	
1–3 years of college	40.0	39.8	41.6	40.9	
College graduate	40.2	41.3	28.5	36.0	
Income					**0.0004**
<$20,000	13.0	12.2	19.5	17.2	
$20,000–$49,999	42.4	41.6	49.0	46.0	
≥$50,000	44.6	46.1	31.5	36.9	
Prepregnancy BMI					**0.0286**
Underweight	4.8	4.8	3.4	6.2	
Normal weight	45.3	45.1	39.2	52.9	
Overweight	25.5	25.1	33.8	23.8	
Obese	24.4	25.1	23.7	17.1	
Health insurance					**0.0005**
No	4.4	3.8	7.4	9.1	
Postnatal WIC					**0.0153**
Yes	38.9	37.9	48.3	43.4	
Prenatal WIC					**0.0494**
Yes	28.8	27.9	34.9	33.8	
Mode of delivery					**<0.0001**
Vaginally, not induced	37.4	33.6	53.0	69.7	
Vaginally, induced	34.0	35.0	31.5	23.7	
Planned C-section	16.5	18.3	8.1	2.0	
Unplanned or emergency C-section	12.2	13.2	7.4	4.6	
Breastfeeding duration (any)					**<0.0001**
Never	14.6	15.5	14.1	5.6	
<6 months	44.1	44.8	43.6	37.4	
≥6 months	41.2	39.8	42.3	57.1	
Breastfeeding duration (exclusive)					**<0.0001**
Never	25.3	27.3	23.9	7.6	
<6 months	66.5	65.7	68.2	73.1	
≥6 months	8.2	7.0	8.0	19.3	
Breastfeeding intention					**<0.0001**
Breastfeed only	60.1	59.1	53.0	78.1	
Formula or combination	39.9	40.9	47.0	21.9	
Smoked during pregnancy					0.6304
Yes	9.6	9.4	10.7	11.2	

NH = non-Hispanic; WIC = women; infants and children; BMI = body mass index; C-section = Cesarean section. *Note.* Not all percentages sum to 100% due to rounding.

TABLE 2: Factors associated with breastfeeding duration.

Characteristic	Breastfed < 6 months OR (95% CI)	Breastfed ≥ 6 months OR (95% CI)
Age		
18–24 years	**1.45 (1.07–1.96)**	**0.41 (0.29–0.57)**
25–29 years	**1.77 (1.30–2.41)**	**1.37 (1.01–1.85)**
30–34 years	1.00	1.00
35–45 years	1.15 (0.80–1.67)	1.29 (0.90–1.83)
Marital status		
Married	1.00	1.00
Not married	1.12 (0.85–1.48)	**0.39 (0.28–0.53)**
Maternal race		
White, NH	1.00	1.00
Black, NH	1.31 (0.77–2.20)	**0.53 (0.29–0.96)**
Hispanic	**2.48 (1.36–4.49)**	1.38 (0.74–2.57)
Others	**5.36 (1.93–14.89)**	**4.03 (1.44–11.29)**
Maternal education		
Less than high school	**0.47 (0.26–0.83)**	**0.11 (0.06–0.22)**
High school	**0.55 (0.39–0.77)**	**0.20 (0.14–0.29)**
1–3 years of college	1.07 (0.79–1.45)	**0.46 (0.34–0.62)**
College graduate	1.00	1.00
Income		
<$20,000	**0.69 (0.49–0.96)**	**0.35 (0.24–0.49)**
$20,000–$49,999	0.83 (0.64–1.07)	**0.68 (0.53–0.88)**
≥$50,000	1.00	1.00
Prepregnancy BMI		
Underweight	0.73 (0.44–1.20)	**0.48 (0.28–0.81)**
Normal weight	1.00	1.00
Overweight	1.10 (0.81–1.48)	0.89 (0.66–1.20)
Obese	0.77 (0.58–1.03)	**0.58 (0.44–0.78)**
Health insurance		
No	1.04 (0.58–1.89)	1.32 (0.74–2.36)
Yes	1.00	1.00
Postnatal WIC		
No	1.00	1.00
Yes	**0.77 (0.61–0.97)**	**0.30 (0.24–0.38)**
Prenatal WIC		
No	1.00	1.00
Yes	**0.76 (0.60–0.97)**	**0.33 (0.25–0.42)**
Mode of delivery		
Vaginally, not induced	1.00	1.00
Vaginally, induced	1.05 (0.79–1.39)	**0.72 (0.54–0.95)**
Planned C-section	**0.62 (0.44–0.86)**	**0.60 (0.44–0.83)**
Unplanned or emergency C-section	1.18 (0.81–1.73)	**0.64 (0.43–0.95)**
Breastfeeding intention		
Breastfeed only	1.00	1.00
Formula or combination	**0.01 (0.01–0.27)**	**0.003 (0.001–0.007)**
Smoked during pregnancy		
No	1.00	1.00
Yes	**0.56 (0.41–0.76)**	**0.15 (0.10–0.22)**

OR = odds ratio; CI = confidence interval; NH = non-Hispanic; WIC = women; infants and children; BMI = body mass index; C-Section = Cesarean section.
Note. Bold estimates are significant.

TABLE 3: Association between healthcare provider at birth and breastfeeding duration.

	Unadjusted COR (95% CI)		Parsimonious model[a] AOR (95% CI)	
	Breastfed < 6 months	Breastfed ≥ 6 months	Breastfed < 6 months	Breastfed ≥ 6 months
Family Physician/other Physicians	1.07 (0.64–1.77)	1.17 (0.70–1.94)	1.52 (0.82–2.79)	**2.04 (1.04–4.00)**
Midwife/nurse midwife	**2.32 (1.22–4.42)**	**3.99 (2.12–7.49)**	1.43 (0.68–3.01)	**2.43 (1.12–5.25)**
Obstetrician	Reference			

COR = crude odd ratio; CI = confidence interval; AOR = adjusted odd ratio. *Note.* Never breastfeeding is the reference category. [a]Parsimonious model controlling for marital status, education, race, income, age, prenatal WIC participation, postpartum WIC participation, mode of delivery, and breastfeeding intention.

TABLE 4: Association between healthcare provider at birth and exclusive breastfeeding duration.

	Unadjusted COR (95% CI)		Parsimonious model[a] AOR (95% CI)	
	Breastfed < 6 months	Breastfed ≥ 6 months	Breastfed < 6 months	Breastfed ≥ 6 months
Family or other physicians	1.19 (0.71–1.99)	1.30 (0.54–3.16)	1.13 (0.65–1.98)	1.30 (0.51–3.31)
Midwife/nurse midwife	**4.01 (2.13–7.55)**	**9.96 (4.78–20.75)**	**3.11 (1.62–5.98)**	**6.65 (3.05–14.50)**
Obstetrician	Reference			

COR = crude odd ratio; CI = confidence interval; AOR = adjusted odd ratio. *Note.* Bold estimates are significant. Never breastfeeding is the reference category. [a]Parsimonious model controlling for marital status, income, age, mode of delivery, prenatal WIC participation, and postpartum WIC participation.

physician breastfeeding education and support is outdated. Additional research is needed to understand current breastfeeding knowledge among healthcare providers.

5. Conclusions

A woman's birth attendant was found to be significantly associated with breastfeeding duration and exclusivity. Despite the numerous health benefits and potential to improve maternal and child health, women are not receiving adequate support to breastfeed the recommended six-month duration. This is evident through a recent report from the Centers for Disease Control and Prevention which stated that mothers may not be receiving the breastfeeding support needed from healthcare providers [18]. Future studies are needed to understand the reasons for the low rates of breastfeeding among mothers attended by physicians. Current literature lacks information on midwifery in hospitals. Future research should investigate correlates of midwifery practice within hospitals. Further, researchers should investigate if midwives are more likely to assist skin-to-skin care. Interventions are also needed to overcome barriers encountered by physicians. Moreover, providers should be aware of the impact they can have on women's breastfeeding practices.

Conflicts of Interest

The authors declare that there are no conflicts of interest regarding the publication of this paper.

References

[1] E. Declercq, "Trends in Midwife-Attended Births in the United States, 1989-2009," *Journal of Midwifery & Women's Health*, vol. 57, no. 4, pp. 321–326, 2012.

[2] P. A. Janssen, L. Saxell, L. A. Page, M. C. Klein, R. M. Liston, and S. K. Lee, "Outcomes of planned home birth with registered midwife versus planned hospital birth with midwife or physician," *Canadian Medical Association Journal*, vol. 181, no. 6-7, pp. 377–383, 2009.

[3] W. M. Tan, M. C. Klein, L. Saxell, S. E. Shirkoohy, and G. Asrat, "How do physicians and midwives manage the third stage of labor?" *Women and Birth*, vol. 35, no. 3, pp. 220–229, 2008.

[4] P. Hellings and C. Howe, "Assessment of breastfeeding knowledge of nurse practitioners and nurse-midwives," *Journal of Midwifery & Women's Health*, vol. 45, no. 3, pp. 264–270, 2000.

[5] R. Li, S. B. Fein, J. Chen, and L. M. Grummer-Strawn, "Why mothers stop breastfeeding: Mothers' self-reported reasons for stopping during the first year," *Pediatrics*, vol. 122, no. 2, pp. S69–S76, 2008.

[6] L. B. Feldman-Winter, R. J. Schanler, K. G. O'Connor, and R. A. Lawrence, "Pediatricians and the promotion and support of breastfeeding," *JAMA Pediatrics*, vol. 162, no. 12, pp. 1142–1149, 2008.

[7] G. L. Freed, S. J. Clark, J. Sorenson, J. A. Lohr, R. Cefalo, and P. Curtis, "National assessment of physicians' breast-feeding knowledge, attitudes, training, and experience," *The Journal of the American Medical Association*, vol. 273, no. 6, pp. 472–476, 1995.

[8] B. L. Philipp, A. Merewood, and S. O'Brien, "Physicians and breastfeeding promotion in the united states: A call for action," *Pediatrics*, vol. 107, no. 3, pp. 584–588, 2001.

[9] R. J. Schanler, K. G. O'Connor, and R. A. Lawrence, "Pediatricians' practices and attitudes regarding breastfeeding promotion." *Pediatrics*, vol. 103, no. 3, p. E35, 1999.

[10] S. B. Fein, J. Labiner-Wolfe, K. R. Shealy, R. Li, J. Chen, and L. M. Grummer-Strawn, "Infant feeding practices study II: Study methods," *Pediatrics*, vol. 122, Supplement 2, pp. 28–35, 2008.

[11] "Section on Breastfeeding. Breastfeeding and the use of human milk," *Pediatrics*, vol. 129, no. 3, pp. e827–e841, 2012.

[12] World Health Organization, UNICEF. Global strategy for infant and young child feeding. 2003.

[13] K. B. Kozhimannil, L. B. Attanasio, Y. T. Yang, M. D. Avery, and E. Declercq, "Midwifery Care and Patient–Provider Communication in Maternity Decisions in the United States," *Maternal and Child Health Journal*, vol. 19, no. 7, pp. 1608–1615, 2015.

[14] L. W. Bernaix, "Nurses' Attitudes, Subjective Norms, and Behavioral Intentions Toward Support of Breastfeeding Mothers," *Journal of Human Lactation*, vol. 16, no. 3, pp. 201–209, 2000.

[15] L. W. Kuan, M. Britto, J. Decolongon, P. J. Schoettker, H. D. Atherton, and U. R. Kotagal, "Health system factors contributing to breastfeeding success.," *Pediatrics*, vol. 104, no. 3, p. e28, 1999.

[16] T. M. Hong, L. C. Callister, and R. Schwartz, "First-time mothers' views of breastfeeding support from nurses," *MCN, The American Journal of Maternal/Child Nursing*, vol. 28, no. 1, pp. 10–15, 2003.

[17] R. Li, K. S. Scanlon, and M. K. Serdula, "The validity and reliability of maternal recall of breastfeeding practice," *Nutrition Reviews*, vol. 63, no. 4, pp. 103–110, 2005.

[18] Centers for Disease Control and Prevention. Breastfeeding report card https://www.cdc.gov/breastfeeding/data/reportcard.htm.

19

Pregnancy and Birth Outcomes among Women with Idiopathic Thrombocytopenic Purpura

Diego F. Wyszynski,[1] **Wendy J. Carman,**[2] **Alan B. Cantor,**[3] **John M. Graham Jr.,**[4]
Liza H. Kunz,[5] **Anne M. Slavotinek,**[6] **Russell S. Kirby,**[7] **and John Seeger**[2,8]

[1]*Pregistry, Los Angeles, CA 90045, USA*

[2]*Epidemiology, OptumInsight, Waltham, MA 02451, USA*

[3]*Children's Hospital Boston, Boston, MA 02115, USA*

[4]*Medical Genetics Institute, Cedars Sinai Medical Center, Los Angeles, CA 90048, USA*

[5]*Palo Alto Medical Foundation, Mountain View, CA 94040, USA*

[6]*Department of Pediatrics, Division of Genetics, University of California, San Francisco, San Francisco, CA 94115, USA*

[7]*College of Public Health, University of South Florida, Tampa, FL 33612, USA*

[8]*Department of Medicine, Division of Pharmacoeconomics and Pharmacoepidemiology, Brigham & Women's Hospital, Harvard Medical School, Boston, MA 02120, USA*

Correspondence should be addressed to Diego F. Wyszynski; diegow@pregistry.com

Academic Editor: Albert Fortuny

Objective. To examine pregnancy and birth outcomes among women with idiopathic thrombocytopenic purpura (ITP) or chronic ITP (cITP) diagnosed before or during pregnancy. *Methods*. A linkage of mothers and babies within a large US health insurance database that combines enrollment data, pharmacy claims, and medical claims was carried out to identify pregnancies in women with ITP or cITP. Outcomes included preterm birth, elective and spontaneous loss, and major congenital anomalies. *Results*. Results suggest that women diagnosed with ITP or cITP prior to their estimated date of conception may be at higher risk for stillbirth, fetal loss, and premature delivery. Among 446 pregnancies in women with ITP, 346 resulted in live births. Women with cITP experienced more adverse outcomes than those with a pregnancy-related diagnosis of ITP. Although 7.8% of all live births had major congenital anomalies, the majority were isolated heart defects. Among deliveries in women with cITP, 15.2% of live births were preterm. *Conclusions*. The results of this study provide further evidence that cause and duration of maternal ITP are important determinants of the outcomes of pregnancy.

1. Introduction

Immune (idiopathic) thrombocytopenic purpura (ITP) is an autoimmune disorder characterized by persistent thrombocytopenia due to antibody binding to platelet antigen(s) and causing their premature destruction by the reticuloendothelial system, particularly in the spleen. The American Society for Hematology guidelines [1] define ITP as "isolated thrombocytopenia with no clinically apparent associated conditions or other causes of thrombocytopenia." Therefore, ITP is a condition generally diagnosed by exclusion of the numerous other causes of thrombocytopenia, such as infections, medications, hematological malignancies, disseminated intravascular coagulation, and other autoimmune conditions. In ITP, persistent thrombocytopenia is associated with an otherwise normal full blood count [2]. Chronic ITP is defined as ITP persisting for more than 6 months [3].

It is estimated that thrombocytopenia (defined as a platelet count less than 150×10^9/L) occurs in approximately 7% of pregnant women, with 74% of those with low platelet counts having incidental thrombocytopenia of pregnancy that can be managed routinely and in which the platelet count remains more than $70 \times 10^9/L$ [4]. Additional causes of thrombocytopenia include complications of hypertensive disorders in pregnancy (21%) and immunological disorders of pregnancy, including ITP, systemic lupus erythematosus, and other secondary causes of immune thrombocytopenia (4%) [4]. ITP occurs in 1 to 2 of every 1000 pregnancies, which in the United States represents about 3000 to 6000 cases of ITP in pregnancy per year [5].

Several studies have examined pregnancy outcomes for women with ITP and found that most pregnancies were uneventful, with successful outcomes for both mothers and children [6–8]. The majority of studies used data from single medical centers [6, 9, 10], by employing retrospective analyses of medical charts [10–15]. Most studies have not differentiated between incidental thrombocytopenia, ITP, and cITP in women who have low platelet counts during pregnancy, and, to our knowledge, there are few published reports regarding the outcomes of pregnant women with cITP.

The primary objective of this study was to examine the pregnancy and birth outcomes of women with ITP and cITP identified from medical claims and abstracted medical records from a large health plan in the United States. Our hypothesis was that there would be no significant difference in adverse pregnancy outcomes, including congenital anomalies, between the two groups of women (ITP versus cITP). The method of data ascertainment enabled the inclusion of data from multiple medical centers, thus increasing the size of the patient cohort and extending the study to a broader population.

2. Materials and Methods

2.1. Study Design. We studied pregnancy and birth outcomes among women with ITP or cITP over 16 years of age from 1994 to 2009 inclusive. The data for this study were derived from a large US health insurance database based on eligibility, pharmacy claims, and medical claims data.

2.2. Data Source. This study utilized STORK (Systematic Tracking of Real Kids) to identify pregnancies and link the health experience of mothers with that of their infants within an administrative claims database in order to study the effects of maternal exposures and health conditions on pregnancy outcomes [16, 17]. Further details about STORK are provided in Supplementary Material available online at http://dx.doi.org/10.1155/2016/8297407. After obtaining institutional review board (IRB) approval and waiver of patient authorization from the affiliated privacy board, medical records were accessed and reviewed to ascertain covariate information and to confirm outcomes.

2.3. Study Population. The study population consisted of women with at least one diagnostic claim for ITP (ICD-9 code 287.31 or 287.3 if used before 01/12/2005) and at least one diagnostic or procedure code related to pregnancy (live birth, spontaneous abortion, stillbirth, or therapeutic abortion) in the database between 1995 and 2009. To be eligible for the study, women with at least one claim for ITP

had to fulfill the following criteria: have complete medical and pharmacy benefit coverage, have at least 280 days of continuous enrollment before the pregnancy outcome date, and have a 9-month baseline period prior to the estimated date of conception. If a woman had more than one pregnancy during the study period, analyses included the first pregnancy after the first ITP claim, ignoring any subsequent pregnancies. If a woman's first ITP claim was later than the end date of her last pregnancy, she was not eligible for this study. The database was then searched for infants associated with the deliveries and linked them to the mother's claims. Linkage between mother's and newborn's claims could not be performed if the infant was enrolled in another health insurance plan, as may happen if the partner has a different health insurer.

2.4. Definition of cITP and Timing of Diagnosis Relative to Pregnancy. Patients were classified as having cITP if they met at least one of these requirements: two or more claims for ITP separated by at least 6 months; a claim for ITP and treatment occurring at least 6 months later with one or more of these medications: corticosteroids, anti-D antibody, rituximab, danazol, colchicine, and dapsone; and/or a claim for splenectomy after the first diagnostic ITP claim. Indicators for the timing of the ITP or cITP diagnosis relative to pregnancy were based on the estimated date of conception and the end of pregnancy. Patients were classified as having ITP or cITP before pregnancy if they met the full diagnostic criteria before the estimated date of conception. Patients were classified as having ITP or cITP during pregnancy if they met the full diagnostic criteria before the end of the pregnancy. Women who had an initial claim for ITP prior to delivery or termination of pregnancy but met the full diagnostic criteria for cITP after pregnancy were considered to have ITP during pregnancy, but not cITP, since they did not meet the full criteria until after the pregnancy ended.

2.5. Outcomes. The primary outcome of interest was the prevalence of major congenital anomalies (MCAs) at birth (i.e., anomalies that cause significant functional or cosmetic impairment, require surgery, or are life-limiting). Other birth outcomes evaluated included 3 or more minor congenital anomalies, preterm birth (<37 weeks of gestation), low birthweight (<2,500 grams), and measurements consistent with small for gestational age (SGA) status (weight, length, or head circumference below the 10th percentile for sex and gestational age) among infants born to mothers with ITP or cITP. Pregnancy outcomes in this study included live born infant, spontaneous abortion, elective termination, and stillbirth. Potential outcomes were identified by a search for the qualifying diagnosis and procedure codes. If the claims search did not identify a pregnancy outcome, the pregnancy outcome was classified as "unknown." Claims were reviewed to identify medical providers and facilities to query from them medical records to confirm pregnancy outcomes and to collect additional data on pregnancy characteristics and infant follow-up for the first year of life.

2.6. Chart Abstraction. Each patient's pregnancy medical records were abstracted to obtain relevant covariate data from their prenatal and pregnancy outcome history, including estimated date of conception and date and type of pregnancy outcome. For infants with evidence of a congenital anomaly diagnosed within the first 12 months after birth, as identified through ICD-9 diagnosis or procedure codes in the medical claims, the medical record was sought from the physician or hospital where the anomaly was diagnosed. A standardized medical record abstraction form was used to record elements from each mother's chart, including the reported estimated date of conception, type of pregnancy outcome, and other pregnancy characteristics from relevant clinician notes, inpatient records, and/or hospital discharge summaries.

2.7. Adjudication of Infant Outcomes. Patient information drawn directly (without abstraction) from deidentified medical records of infants with claims-based congenital anomalies was combined with claims data and reviewed by a dysmorphologist to validate the diagnosis.

2.8. Maternal Characteristics and Comorbidities. Following medical record review, all pregnancies were classified according to covariates describing maternal characteristics, pregnancy characteristics, and maternal comorbidities and according to whether they were identified through claims or medical chart abstraction. Maternal characteristics included age and year at conception, geographic region of health plan, and ethnicity. Pregnancy characteristics included use of prenatal vitamins, amniocentesis, chorionic villus sampling, fetal monitoring, ultrasonography, alpha-fetoprotein (AFP) testing, obstetric panel, multiple gestation, high-risk pregnancy supervision, antepartum hemorrhage, abruptio placentae, placenta previa, excessive vomiting, early or threatened labor, late pregnancy, measurements consistent with SGA, disorders relating to short gestation and unspecified low birthweight, and total cost of care for up to 280 days before delivery. Maternal comorbidities such as diabetes, hypertension, and infections, along with substance abuse and receipt of teratogenic drugs during pregnancy, were identified using diagnostic codes and medication claims.

2.9. Statistical Analysis. Descriptive statistical analyses were conducted using SAS® (Cary, NC). Frequency analyses were carried out for categorical variables and means and standard deviations were calculated for continuous variables, such as the number of physician visits.

Data were analyzed separately for women who fulfilled the criteria for ITP or cITP prior to pregnancy and those who fulfilled the criteria during pregnancy. For infants with claims of congenital anomalies, data were categorized according to maternal age at conception as follows: 14 years and under, 5-year intervals from 15 years through 49 years, and over 50 years.

3. Results

We identified 585 women with at least one claim of ITP and claims indicating pregnancy during the study period (January 1, 1994, through December 31, 2009). Of those, 139 did not meet the eligibility criteria and were excluded. The remaining 446 women made up the claims-based ITP cohort for this study. Medical records were sought to provide more detailed information on the patients' pregnancy characteristics not captured in the claims data, and charts for 311 of 446 women (69.7%) were obtained. Figure 1 provides a schematic view of the claims-based pregnancy outcomes observed in this cohort of 446 women with claims for ITP and the results of chart-based review. Among the 311 women with charts, outcome data were unavailable for 42 of them. Of the remaining, 260 charts had a confirmed live birth and 9 (3.3%) indicated a fetal loss with no further details.

Among the 446 pregnancies in women with a claims-based diagnosis of ITP, the mean age at pregnancy was 30.3 (SD: ±5.3) years. The claims-based diagnosis was available in 432 cases before or during the pregnancy (Table 1). Approximately half of the women reside in the South/Southeast regions of the United States and, of those with ethnicity reported in the enrollment data, approximately 70% are Caucasian. Of the 446 women, 84 (18.8%) were identified as having cITP before or during pregnancy.

Of all 446 pregnancies with claims-based diagnosis of ITP, 346 (77.6%) indicated a live birth (Table 2). When stratified by timing of ITP diagnosis, live births were more frequent among women diagnosed with ITP during pregnancy (290 of 357 or 81.2%) than in pregnant women diagnosed with ITP before pregnancy (56 of 89 or 62.9%). Of those who were diagnosed with ITP during pregnancy, 14/357 (3.9%) were fetal losses compared with 10/89 (11.2%) of those diagnosed with ITP prior to pregnancy. The magnitude and trend of this difference (7.3%) were not found among women with cITP (9/66 or 13.6% of those diagnosed during pregnancy resulting in fetal loss compared to 2/18 or 10.2% among those diagnosed prior to pregnancy).

The prevalence of low birthweight was higher among women with a diagnosis of ITP before pregnancy (10 of 56 or 17.9%) compared to women with a diagnosis of ITP during pregnancy (28 of 290 or 9.7%). The prevalence of low birthweight in women with cITP was similar in both groups, but the sample size was too small to reach a conclusion.

Table 3 presents the prevalence of major congenital anomalies (MCAs) among the 346 infants of mothers with claims for ITP. There were 27 infants ($n = 27/346$; 7.8%) who had a claim for at least one major malformation and charts were available for 17 of them. The most frequent claims were for ostium secundum type atrial septal defects [$n = 10/346$ (2.9%)], hypospadias [$n = 8/151$ (5.3%)], patent ductus arteriosus [$n = 6/346$ (1.7%)], and ventricular septal defect [$n = 4/346$ (1.2%)]. A total of 4 infants (1.2%) had claims for 3 or more major malformations. Of all infants of mothers with claims for ITP that were assumed to have no MCA and whose charts were obtained ($n = 336$), 10 (3.0%) had at least one chart-confirmed major malformation (Table 4). The most frequent of these confirmed MCAs were hypospadias

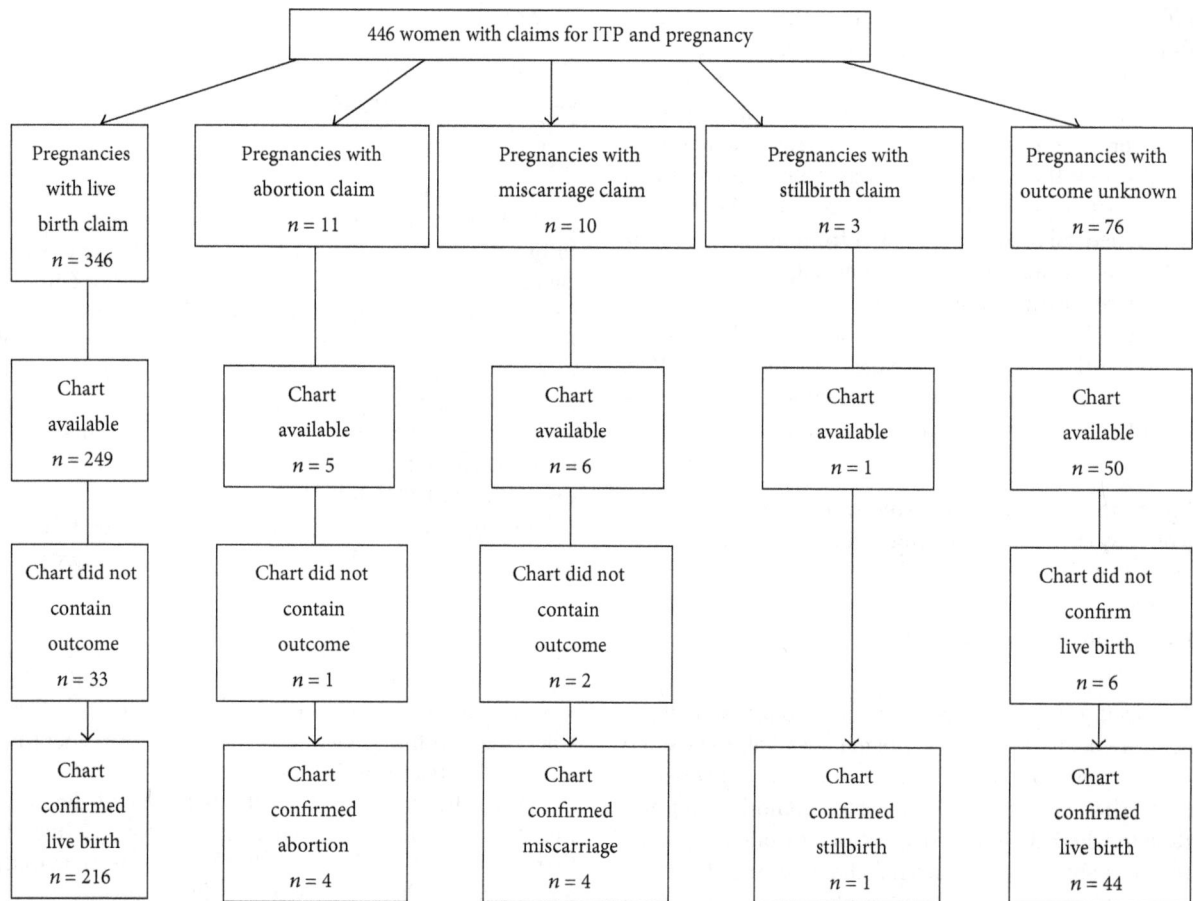

FIGURE 1: Chart review results of claims for pregnancy outcomes.

$[n = 4/336 \ (1.2\%)]$, ventricular septal defect [VSD, $n = 3/336 \ (0.9\%)]$, and patent ductus arteriosus [PDA, $n = 2 \ (0.6\%)]$. Two infants (0.6%) had 3 or more confirmed major malformations.

Among the subgroup of 68 infants of women with claims for cITP, 7/68 (10.3%) had a claim for at least one major malformation. The most frequent claims were for hypospadias $[n = 4/30 \ (13.3\%)]$, ostium secundum type atrial septal defects $[n = 2/68 \ (2.9\%)]$, and patent ductus arteriosus $[n = 2/68 \ (2.9\%)]$. Two of these 68 infants (2.9%) had claims for 3 or more major malformations. Of all infants of mothers with claims for cITP that were assumed to have no MCA and whose charts were obtained ($n = 66$), 4 (6.1%) had at least one chart-confirmed major anomaly (Table 4). The most frequent of these major congenital anomalies was hypospadias $[n = 3/66 \ (4.5\%)]$. One infant (1.5%) had claims for 3 or more confirmed major malformations. There was no statistically significant difference between the prevalences of malformations in the infants of mothers with ITP compared to those with cITP, regardless of whether the data was claims-based or chart-based (Table 4).

4. Discussion

The risks associated with ITP in pregnancy remain controversial [4]. Although severe maternal or neonatal bleeding is rare when pregnant women with ITP are managed by an expert team, a recent questionnaire of women with ITP revealed that 14/50 women were advised to avoid becoming pregnant [18]. Our study is unique because of the availability of data on congenital anomalies in infants born to mothers with ITP and cITP. In addition, the sample size of the population we evaluated is larger than previously published.

The findings of this study are consistent with other published reports. In one prior publication, preterm birth was present in 16/58 (27.6%) infants born to mothers with ITP diagnosed prior to pregnancy and in 15/75 (20%) infants born to mothers with ITP diagnosed during pregnancy, with an overall prevalence of 23.3% [15]. Premature birth affects 5–10% of newborns in most developed countries and approximately 12% of live births in the United States. Therefore, a prevalence of prematurity of 23.3% among pregnancies complicated by ITP represents approximately a 2- to 4-fold increased frequency. In a study by Debouverie et al. [14]

TABLE 1: Demographic characteristics of women with ITP and cITP.

	ITP (446)		cITP (84)	
	N	%	N	%
Age at pregnancy				
15–19	14	3.1	4	4.8
20–29	180	40.4	32	38.1
30–39	237	53.1	46	54.8
40+	15	3.4	2	2.8
Race				
African American	18	4.0	3	3.6
Asian	9	2.0	2	2.4
Caucasian	162	36.3	35	41.7
Hispanic	24	5.4	2	2.4
Unknown	213	47.8	36	42.9
Other race	20	4.5	6	4.6
Region				
Midwest	138	30.9	29	34.5
Northeast	55	12.3	10	11.9
South/Southeast	206	46.2	37	44.1
West	47	10.5	8	9.5
Other diseases				
Diabetes mellitus or gestational diabetes	38	8.5	6	7.1
Hypertension or pregnancy-related hypertension	50	11.2	7	8.3

TABLE 2: Pregnancy outcomes among women with ITP and cITP.

Outcomes	All pregnancies among women with ITP		ITP prior to pregnancy		ITP during pregnancy	
	N	%	N	%	N	%
	446	100	89	100	357	100
Live birth	346	77.6	56	62.9	290	81.2
Spontaneous or elective termination or stillbirth	24	5.4	10	11.2	14	3.9
Outcome unknown	76	17.0	23	25.8	53	14.9
Premature delivery[1]	38	8.5	10	11.2	28	7.8
Low birthweight[1]	6	1.4	1	1.1	5	1.4
Outcomes	All pregnancies among women with cITP		cITP prior to pregnancy		cITP during pregnancy	
	N	%	N	%	N	%
	84	100	18	100	66	100
Live birth	57	67.9	11	61.1	46	69.7
Spontaneous or elective termination or stillbirth	11	13.1	2	10.2	9	13.6
Outcome unknown	16	19.0	5	27.8	11	16.7
Premature delivery[1]	8	9.5	2	11.1	6	9.1
Low birthweight[1]	1	1.2	1	5.6	0	0.0

[1] Premature delivery defined as delivery at less than 37 weeks of gestational age; low birthweight defined as birthweight less than 2500.

of 50 women with cITP who had platelet counts below 150 $\times 10^9$/L for at least one year, there were no fetal deaths in 62 pregnancies but 9 (14%) were premature, 6 (9%) were small for gestational age, and 2 (3%) demonstrated evidence of hemorrhage. In a group of women treated for severe thrombocytopenia (platelet count $< 10 \times 10^9$/L) during pregnancy, the average gestational age at delivery was 36 weeks [13]. There was one intrauterine death and the remaining 25 infants were born without complications [13]. Won et al. [11] studied pregnancies among 30 women with ITP or cITP.

TABLE 3: Claims-based congenital anomalies among newborns of women with ITP or cITP.

Congenital anomaly	Pregnancies with ITP		Pregnancies with cITP	
	N	%	N	%
	346	100.0	68	100.0
Any anomaly	27	7.8	7	10.3
Ostium secundum type atrial septal defect	10	2.9	2	2.9
Hypospadias	8	5.3*	4	13.3**
Patent ductus arteriosus	6	1.7	2	2.9
Ventricular septal defect	4	1.2	1	1.5
3 or more anomaly codes	4	1.2	2	2.9
Unspecified congenital cataract	1	0.3	—	—
Bulbus cordis anomalies and anomalies of cardiac septal closure and common truncus	1	0.3	1	1.5
Congenital stenosis of pulmonary valve	1	0.3	—	—
Congenital stenosis of aortic valve	1	0.3	1	1.5
Hypoplastic left heart syndrome	1	0.3	—	—
Congenital anomalies of pulmonary artery	1	0.3	—	—
Congenital tracheoesophageal fistula, esophageal atresia, and stenosis	1	0.3	—	—
Esophageal atresia	1	0.3	—	—
Congenital hypertrophic pyloric stenosis	1	0.3	—	—
Congenital dislocation of hip, bilateral	1	0.3	—	—
Congenital dislocation of one hip with subluxation of the other hip	1	0.3	—	—
Other congenital anomalies of abdominal wall	1	0.3	—	—
Ostium secundum type atrial septal defect + hypoplastic left heart syndrome + patent ductus arteriosus + congenital anomalies of pulmonary artery + esophageal atresia	1	0.3	—	—
Ostium secundum type atrial septal defect + patent ductus arteriosus	2	0.6	—	—
Ostium secundum type atrial septal defect + patent ductus arteriosus + other congenital anomalies of abdominal wall	1	0.3	—	—
Ostium secundum type atrial septal defect + congenital stenosis of aortic valve + patent ductus arteriosus	1	0.3	1	1.5
Ostium secundum type atrial septal defect + ventricular septal defect + patent ductus arteriosus	1	0.3	1	1.5

*Denominator: 151 male infants.
**Denominator: 30 male infants.

TABLE 4: Prevalence of congenital anomalies by ITP and cITP and by source.

Diagnosis	Claims-based	Chart-based
ITP	27/346 = 7.8%	10/336 = 3.0%
cITP	7/68 = 10.3%	4/66 = 6.1%

$P > 0.05$ comparing ITP to cITP.

There were 29 live births from 31 pregnancies, with a mean gestational age of 36.5 weeks (range, 7–43 weeks). There was one missed abortion at 7 weeks and one termination because of intrauterine death at 16 weeks of gestation [11]. A third newborn died because of premature delivery and respiratory failure at 27 weeks. This child was born to a mother who had complications of a bleeding gastric ulcer due to severe thrombocytopenia (platelet count $< 20 \times 10^9$/L) and who died from acute pulmonary edema following a caesarean section. The remaining 28 newborns had no complications.

The duration of ITP may be important for determining the risk of complications. Thrombocytopenia attributed to aplastic anemia or myelodysplasia was associated with a 53.8% rate of premature birth compared to incidental thrombocytopenia in pregnancy (11.3%) and ITP (16.7%) [12]. Namavar Jahromi et al. [15] contrasted the characteristics of infants born to 57 mothers with ITP diagnosed before pregnancy to 75 women diagnosed with ITP during pregnancy. In the group of mothers with ITP diagnosed prior to pregnancy, there were 2 intrauterine fetal deaths at 224 and 247 days of pregnancy and a higher frequency of infants requiring admission to the neonatal intensive care unit (20/57 or 34.48% versus 12/75 or 16%; $p = 0.01$). Maternal age and platelet count, gestational age at delivery, 5-minute Apgar scores <7, rate of caesarean deliveries, mean neonatal birthweight, and the mean neonatal platelet count did not differ between the two groups. There were three neonates (3/84; 2.3%) with platelet counts < $50 \times 10^9/L$ that were all born to mothers with ITP diagnosed prior to pregnancy, but there were no severe bleeding complications and no intracranial hemorrhage in the infants. However, maternal ITP refractory to splenectomy has been correlated with a higher risk of intracranial hemorrhage in the infants [19].

Webert et al. [10] conducted a retrospective study of women with ITP in pregnancy, most of whom (83/92) had ITP prior to pregnancy. There were 119 pregnancies and two fetal deaths: one stillbirth at 39 weeks of gestation and a stillbirth at 27 weeks of gestation that had extensive hemorrhage throughout the brain, born to a mother with a 4-year history of severe ITP (postsplenectomy) and platelets counts < $50 \times 10^9/L$. There were no reports of fetal malformations and the authors estimated that the fetal loss rate was approximately 1-2%.

No case of hydrocephalus was found in the present study. Hydrocephalus can occur as a rare complication of intracranial hemorrhage in fetuses born to mothers with ITP [20]. Kim and Choi [21] described a neonate with severe thrombocytopenia (platelet count $1 \times 10^9/L$), multiple bruises on the face and scalp, widespread petechiae, cleft palate, and moderate to severe hydrocephalus without evidence of intraventricular hemorrhage. Computerized tomography confirmed severe hydrocephalus without significant compression of the brain parenchyma, diffuse ischemia, and encephalomalacia of both cerebral hemispheres.

Ostium secundum, a type of atrial septal defect (ASD), is found in less than 1% of newborns in the general population [22]. In our study, this congenital heart defect occurred approximately three times more frequently among infants born to mothers with ITP. In infants born to mothers with cITP, the incidence of ostium secundum was 2/68 (2.9%) and there were two additional infants with ostium secundum plus other cardiac malformations (Table 3). Ventricular septal defect and patent ductus arteriosus were also noted in other babies born to mothers with cITP (Table 3). However, the numbers in the group of cITP pregnancies were small and the significance of this finding is unclear.

This study provides a claims-based and chart-based evaluation of pregnancy outcomes among women with ITP and cITP in the United States. The wide range inclusion criteria and large source population (more than 1.2 million pregnancies) allowed us to obtain results that reflect pregnancy outcomes broadly among women with ITP and cITP. However, the database has some limitations and valuable information may be missing or misdiagnosed. We aimed to minimize

these limitations by performing medical record abstraction. This effort resulted in further data, including additional maternal characteristics and birth outcomes. However, there were a small number of pregnancy cases in women with ITP and cITP with no linkage to births. In addition, data from women with different medical or pharmacy coverage and from those without medical coverage could not be assessed by this study. Anomalies documented in live newborns and those requiring billable medical intervention were assessed in this study. However, minor or major anomalies that may have occurred in stillborn infants and in fetuses of elective or spontaneous abortions were not available for analysis. In addition, clinical validation of the diagnoses of ITP and cITP by a specialist was not feasible in this study. While referral to a maternal-fetal specialist is likely for these patients, the documentation from specialists was generally not included in the primary obstetrical records. Finally, the dataset did not include maternal medical conditions other than ITP, nor medical treatments performed during the pregnancy for ITP or other conditions. Therefore, it was not possible to evaluate their potential effects on the pregnancy and birth outcomes.

5. Conclusion

Based on the evaluation of 446 pregnant women with ITP, a diagnosis of ITP or cITP prior to their estimated date of conception may indicate a higher risk for stillbirth or fetal loss, premature delivery, and infants with specific congenital anomalies than an ITP diagnosis during pregnancy. Therefore, the results of this study provide further evidence that the duration of maternal ITP may be an important determinant of the outcomes of pregnancy.

Competing Interests

The authors declare that they have no competing interests.

References

[1] J. N. George, S. H. Woolf, G. E. Raskob et al., "Idiopathic thrombocytopenic purpura: a practice guideline developed by explicit methods for the American Society of Hematology," *Blood*, vol. 88, no. 1, pp. 3–40, 1996.

[2] J. N. George, G. E. Raskob, S. R. Shah et al., "Drug-induced thrombocytopenia: a systematic review of published case reports," *Annals of Internal Medicine*, vol. 129, no. 11, pp. 886–890, 1998.

[3] R. J. Klaassen, S. D. Mathias, G. Buchanan et al., "Pilot study of the effect of romiplostim on child health-related quality of life (HRQoL) and parental burden in immune thrombocytopenia (ITP)," *Pediatric Blood and Cancer*, vol. 58, no. 3, pp. 395–398, 2012.

[4] J. G. Kelton, "Idiopathic thrombocytopenic purpura complicating pregnancy," *Blood Reviews*, vol. 16, no. 1, pp. 43–46, 2002.

[5] K. K. Gill and J. G. Kelton, "Management of idiopathic thrombocytopenic purpura in pregnancy," *Seminars in Hematology*, vol. 37, no. 3, pp. 275–289, 2000.

[6] A. Fujita, R. Sakai, S. Matsuura et al., "A retrospective analysis of obstetric patients with idiopathic thrombocytopenic purpura: a

single center study," *International Journal of Hematology*, vol. 92, no. 3, pp. 463–467, 2010.

[7] V. Suri, N. Aggarwal, S. Saxena, P. Malhotra, and S. Varma, "Maternal and perinatal outcome in idiopathic thrombocytopenic purpura (ITP) with pregnancy," *Acta Obstetricia et Gynecologica Scandinavica*, vol. 85, no. 12, pp. 1430–1435, 2006.

[8] F. E. Al-Jama, J. Rahman, S. A. Al-Suleiman, and M. S. Rahman, "Outcome of pregnancy in women with idiopathic thrombocytopenic purpura," *The Australian and New Zealand Journal of Obstetrics and Gynaecology*, vol. 38, no. 4, pp. 410–413, 1998.

[9] A. Belkin, A. Levy, and E. Sheiner, "Perinatal outcomes and complications of pregnancy in women with immune thrombocytopenic purpura," *The Journal of Maternal-Fetal & Neonatal Medicine*, vol. 22, no. 11, pp. 1081–1085, 2009.

[10] K. E. Webert, R. Mittal, C. Sigouin, N. M. Heddle, and J. G. Kelton, "A retrospective 11-year analysis of obstetric patients with idiopathic thrombocytopenic purpura," *Blood*, vol. 102, no. 13, pp. 4306–4311, 2003.

[11] Y.-W. Won, W. Moon, Y.-S. Yun et al., "Clinical aspects of pregnancy and delivery in patients with chronic idiopathic thrombocytopenic purpura (ITP)," *Korean Journal of Internal Medicine*, vol. 20, no. 2, pp. 129–134, 2005.

[12] S. Chao, C. M. Zeng, and J. Liu, "Thrombocytopenia in pregnancy and neonatal outcomes," *Zhongguo Dang Dai Er Ke Za Zhi*, vol. 13, pp. 790–793, 2011.

[13] D.-P. Wang, M.-Y. Liang, and S.-M. Wang, "Clinical analysis of pregnancy complicated with severe thrombocytopenia," *Zhonghua Fu Chan Ke Za Zhi*, vol. 45, no. 6, pp. 401–405, 2010.

[14] O. Debouverie, P. Roblot, F. Roy-Péaud, C. Boinot, F. Pierre, and O. Pourrat, "Chronic idiopathic thrombocytopenia outcome during pregnancy (62 cases)," *Revue de Medecine Interne*, vol. 33, no. 8, pp. 426–432, 2012.

[15] B. Namavar Jahromi, Z. Shiravani, and L. Salarian, "Perinatal outcome of pregnancies complicated by immune thrombocytopenia," *Iranian Red Crescent Medical Journal*, vol. 14, no. 7, pp. 430–435, 2012.

[16] J. A. Cole, J. G. Modell, B. R. Haight, I. S. Cosmatos, J. M. Stoler, and A. M. Walker, "Bupropion in pregnancy and the prevalence of congenital malformations," *Pharmacoepidemiology and Drug Safety*, vol. 16, no. 5, pp. 474–484, 2007.

[17] J. A. Cole, S. A. Ephross, I. S. Cosmatos, and A. M. Walker, "Paroxetine in the first trimester and the prevalence of congenital malformations," *Pharmacoepidemiology and Drug Safety*, vol. 16, no. 10, pp. 1075–1085, 2007.

[18] A. C. Matzdorff, G. Arnold, A. Salama, H. Ostermann, S. Eberle, and S. Hummler, "Advances in ITP—therapy and quality of life—a patient survey," *PLoS ONE*, vol. 6, no. 11, Article ID e27350, 2011.

[19] S. Koyama, T. Tomimatsu, T. Kanagawa, K. Kumasawa, T. Tsutsui, and T. Kimura, "Reliable predictors of neonatal immune thrombocytopenia in pregnant women with idiopathic thrombocytopenic purpura," *American Journal of Hematology*, vol. 87, no. 1, pp. 15–21, 2012.

[20] P. Tampakoudis, H. Bili, E. Lazaridis, E. Anastasiadou, A. Andreou, and S. Mantalenakis, "Prenatal diagnosis of intracranial hemorrhage secondary to maternal idiopathic thrombocytopenic purpura: a case report," *American Journal of Perinatology*, vol. 12, no. 4, pp. 268–270, 1995.

[21] M. W. Kim and H. M. Choi, "Fetal hydrocephalus in a pregnancy complicated by idiopathic thrombocytopenic purpura," *Journal of Ultrasound in Medicine*, vol. 25, no. 6, pp. 777–780, 2006.

[22] P. Moons, T. Sluysmans, D. De Wolf et al., "Congenital heart disease in 111 225 births in Belgium: birth prevalence, treatment and survival in the 21st century," *Acta Paediatrica*, vol. 98, no. 3, pp. 472–477, 2009.

20

Antenatal Weight Management: Women's Experiences, Behaviours, and Expectations of Weighing in Early Pregnancy

J. A. Swift,[1] J. Pearce,[1] P. H. Jethwa,[1] M. A. Taylor,[1] A. Avery,[1] S. Ellis,[1] S. C. Langley-Evans,[1] and S. McMullen[2]

[1]School of Biosciences, University of Nottingham, Sutton Bonington, Loughborough LE12 5RD, UK
[2]National Childbirth Trust, 30 Euston Square, London NW1 2FB, UK

Correspondence should be addressed to S. C. Langley-Evans; simon.langley-evans@nottingham.ac.uk

Academic Editor: E. R. Lumbers

The current emphasis on obstetric risk management helps to frame gestational weight gain as problematic and encourages intervention by healthcare professionals. However pregnant women have reported confusion, distrust, and negative effects associated with antenatal weight management interactions. The MAGIC study (MAnaging weiGht In pregnanCy) sought to examine women's self-reported experiences of usual-care antenatal weight management in early pregnancy and consider these alongside weight monitoring behaviours and future expectations. 193 women (18 yrs+) were recruited from routine antenatal clinics at the Nottingham University Hospital NHS Trust. Self-reported gestation was 10–27 weeks, with 41.5% ($n = 80$) between 12 and 14 and 43.0% ($n = 83$) between 20 and 22 weeks. At recruitment 50.3% of participants ($n = 97$) could be classified as overweight or obese. 69.4% of highest weight women (≥ 30 kg/m^2) did not report receiving advice about weight, although they were significantly more likely compared to women with BMI < 30 kg/m^2. The majority of women (regardless of BMI) did not express any barriers to being weighed and 40.8% reported weighing themselves at home. Women across the BMI categories expressed a desire for more engagement from healthcare professionals on the issue of bodyweight. Women are clearly not being served appropriately in the current situation which simultaneously problematizes and fails to offer constructive dialogue.

1. Introduction

The antenatal period is often considered to be an important opportunity for health promotion and guidance, offering the so-called "teachable moments" [1]. Usual antenatal care associated with normal pregnancy puts women into greater contact with health professionals [2], and it is thought that responsibility for their developing baby can be an important motivator for behaviour change [1]. Pregnancy-related physical changes can also be said to cause a renegotiation of women's identity towards functionality and mothering [3], explaining why women can become more perceptive to health education [4].

In the context of maternal obesity, the UK's National Institute of Health and Care Excellence (NICE) recommends that the main focus of weight loss lies in the periconceptual period and that during pregnancy a woman should receive advice on healthy lifestyles and weight *management* [5]. Weight gain during pregnancy and changes in shape can be considered both expected and healthy [6], and NICE does not recommend weight loss during pregnancy as it may pose a risk by impairing foetal nutrition [5]. However, the UK does not have any formal, evidence-based recommendations for amount of gestational weight gain, although a guidance range of 10–12.5 kg (22–26 lbs) is used by NHS England [7] and has been recommended by the Department of Health in the past [8]. In contrast the USA has specific recommendations for weight gain for different BMI groupings published in the Institute of Medicine's "Weight Gain During Pregnancy: Reexamining the Guidelines" [9]. Women with a BMI of 20–25 kg/m^2 are advised to gain 11–16 kg during pregnancy, whereas women with obesity are recommended to limit weight gain to no more than 9 kg. Since the late 1990s regular weighing has not been encouraged in the UK [10] and the current NICE [5] advises weighing women only at booking (usually ~10 weeks of gestation), while a joint guideline from the Centre for Maternal and Child Enquires and the Royal College of Obstetrics and Gynaecology recommended follow-up weighing in the 3rd trimester only if the women has a BMI that can be classified as obese at booking [11]. Despite recent evidence that pregnant women with BMI 18–29.9 kg/m^2 found regular weighing to be acceptable and useful [12] and the observation that monitoring can be reassuring [13], there remain fears that this practice would draw (negative) attention to the body, fuelling body image problems [14], particularly among those with internalised weight stigma.

There is also a lack of detailed, evidence-based guidance for clinicians on *how* to achieve appropriate weight gain. NICE [5] recommends that practitioners adopt a patient-centred approach, asking women if they would like advice about their weight and if so when they would like to receive it. This assumes that weight and weight gain have already been defined by the practitioner and women as a topic in need of discussion, but no guidance is given as to how—or indeed whether—the practitioner should take responsibility for raising the issue.

This lack of guidance is positioned within a society that has a significant pro-thin bias [15] and substantial anti-fat attitudes [16]. Women may be increasingly concerned about weight gain during pregnancy [17] and aware of the health risks associated with higher weights [18], but this can be opposed by the general acceptance of the inevitability of gestational weight gain (as opposed to weight gain outside of pregnancy) which temporarily exempts women from adherence to ideal [3]. Taken together it is, therefore, not surprising that there is confusion, contradiction, distrust, and negative effects associated with antenatal weight management interactions—both on the part of practitioners and on pregnant women [19]—along with ambivalence among midwives who are considering both women-centeredness and risk management as priorities [20].

The current study—the MAnaging weiGht In pregnanCy (MAGIC) study—sought to examine women's experiences of routine antenatal weight management provision in Nottingham, where the prevalence of obesity in pregnant women is 20% higher compared to England as a whole [21, personal communication]. In addition to giving a perspective on local needs, this observational study extends previous research by recruiting a cohort of women in early pregnancy and collecting follow-up data (until 12 months postpartum) on a wide range of biological, psychological, social, and behavioural factors. This allows an examination of an objective weight measurement (at baseline) as a dynamic variable subject to individual, ongoing appraisal. It also allows consideration of how advice on weight is positioned alongside advice on diet and physical activity, as well as assessments of dietary and physical activity behaviour, through the whole antenatal and postnatal period. The current analysis uses quantitative and qualitative data collected at recruitment (baseline) only and aims to describe the sample's experiences, behaviours, and expectations of antenatal weight management in early pregnancy.

2. Materials and Methods

2.1. Ethical Approval. This study was approved by the NHS Health Research Authority (NRES Committee East Midlands) and Nottingham University Hospitals NHS Trust, Research and Innovation Department (12/EM/0267).

2.2. Sample and Recruitment. Women were recruited from the antenatal clinic at Queens Medical Centre (QMC, Nottingham University Hospitals NHS Trust) while waiting for either their "dating scan" (an ultrasound scan, usually between 10 weeks 0 days and 13 weeks 6 days, to determine gestational age) or their "18–20-week anomaly scan" (ultrasound screening for structural anomalies, normally between 18 weeks 0 days and 20 weeks 6 days), both of which are routine appointments for all women according to NICE antenatal care pathway [2]. Women aged 18 years or over and of any sociodemographic background, bodyweight, and parity were approached by a researcher and provided with information about the study. Once they had read the information and if they agreed to take part, written consent was obtained. No incentive was offered.

2.3. Measures. Participants completed a paper-based questionnaire collecting data on a number of social, physiological, psychological, and behavioural measures. The variables used in the current analysis were as follows. (1) Sociodemographics: participants self-reported their age, ethnicity, gestation and number of embryos of current pregnancy, and number of other children. In addition, participants self-reported their own and partner's (if applicable) occupation, which were coded using the Standard Occupation Classification 2010 and then classified using the National Statistics Socioeconomic Classification (rebased on SOC2010; NS-SEC) [22]. To assess the socioeconomic status of the household, the highest reported NS-SEC score was taken as the Household Reference Point. (2) Anthropometrics: measurements of weight and height were taken by trained researchers on calibrated equipment (Leicester Height Measure, Marsden, UK, and bathroom scales, Salter, UK). Body Mass Index (BMI) was calculated using the standard formula (kg/m^2) and classified using the World Health Organization's criteria (underweight <18 kg/m^2, recommended weight 18–24.9 kg/m^2, overweight 25–29.9 kg/m^2, and obese ≥30 kg/m^2) [23]. Participants were also asked to self-report their prepregnancy weight in stones and pounds or in kilogrammes and describe how this prepregnancy weight was measured with the options "bathroom scales," "measured on scales by a midwife, by GP, and at a hospital appointment," "I have guessed my weight," and "other." (3) Weight monitoring behaviour and advice: participants were asked to report whether they had been weighed and by which healthcare professional during their current pregnancy and whether they had received specific advice about their weight following being weighed. Open questions were asked to women to describe the advice received following being weighed and how they felt about being weighed and any subsequent advice. Participants also responded to the question "which statement best describes what you were doing at the moment?" with the options "trying to lose weight," "trying to keep my weight at the same level," "not trying to do anything about my weight," and "trying to put on weight." (4) Current shape concern and antenatal weight change expectations: shape concern was assessed using 7 items from the shape concern subscale of the Eating Disorders Examination Questionnaire Version EDE-Q [24]. The item "have you felt fat?" was omitted due to its multidimensionality and value-laden terminology. A summative score was calculated using the mean of all 7 items; scores ranged 0–6 with higher scores indicating more shape concern. Cronbach's alpha for the 7 items in the current sample was 0.91, indicating internal consistency [25]. Participants were also asked whether they expected their weight to change and if so in what direction and by how much. (5) Awareness of guidance and sources of information: participants were asked whether they were aware of the Department of Health's guidance around weight gain and if so what this was. Participants reported what they perceived to be the main sources of information around bodyweight, diet, and exercise, and an open question was asked to women to describe what they thought about sources of information available.

2.4. Data Analysis. Quantitative data were analysed using SPSS version 22 (SPSS Inc., Chicago, IL, USA). Data entry was conducted by three members of the research team and all data entry was double-checked by another member of the team. The dataset was inspected for univariate outliers and missing data. Normality of continuous variables was assessed using the Kolmogorov–Smirnov test, and appropriate parametric and nonparametric statistics were then used to describe the sample. Chi-squared and Kruskal-Wallis tests were used to investigate the relationship between weight classification at recruitment and receiving advice and shape concerns, respectively. These were followed by *post hoc* 2 × 2 chi-squared tests and Mann-Whitney U tests as appropriate. The relationship between shape concerns and amount of weight women expected to gain during pregnancy was analysed using Spearman's rank correlation. Qualitative data from open questions were subjected to an inductive, descriptive content analysis [26].

3. Results

3.1. Sociodemographics. The research team approached 786 women in clinic and 360 consented to participate, were weighed and measured, and took the study materials home with them. Questionnaires were returned by 193 women and these women were considered to be recruited onto the study. At recruitment the participants' age was normally distributed with a mean of 32.8 years (SD 5.2 yrs, min 18.9 yrs, and max 47.1 yrs). 86% ($n = 166$) of the sample self-identified with a white ethnicity, 94.6% ($n = 181$) were living in a household with at least the equivalent of one full-time salary, and 79.6% ($n = 121$) were living in a household with a Household Reference Point of 1-2 (data were missing on ethnicity and occupation for 4 and 2 participants, resp.).

Participants' self-reported gestation was between 10 and 27 weeks with 41.5% ($n = 80$) participants in weeks 12–14 and 43.0% ($n = 83$) in weeks 20–22. The majority were expecting

a singleton ($n = 177$, 91.7%). 43.5% ($n = 84$) of the sample were primiparous, 40.9% ($n = 79$) had one child, and 15.5% ($n = 30$) had two or three children.

3.2. Anthropometrics. At recruitment participants' Body Mass Index (BMI) had a non-Gaussian distribution with a median of 25.1 kg/m^2 (IQR 6.5 kg/m^2, min 17.5 kg/m^2, and max 53.5 kg/m^2), and 50.3% ($n = 97$) of the sample could be classified as overweight or obese (Table 1). There were no significant differences in terms of recruitment BMI between participants and those 167 women consented but did not return the study materials (median 25.6 kg/m^2; IQR 7.4 kg/m^2, min 16.4 kg/m^2, and max 47.6 kg/m^2). Self-reported prepregnancy weights were available for 168 women and had a median of 22.8 kg/m^2 (IQR 5.5 kg/m^2, min 15.9 kg/m^2, and max 51.3 kg/m^2). Women were most likely to take measurements using bathroom scales (66.7%, $n = 112$) while 23.2% ($n = 39$) were based on measurements taken by a healthcare professional. Women had, on average, gained 0.26 kg/wk (IQR 0.34 kg/wk, min −1.05 kg/wk, and max 9.83 kg/wk) since conception.

Among the 168 women who had complete data on both variables, 54 self-reported a prepregnancy weight that could be classified as overweight or obese using measurements taken at recruitment (Table 1). However, 26 of the 114 women who self-reported a prepregnancy weight that could be classified as underweight or recommended weight were classified as overweight or obese using measurements taken at recruitment. Further analysis revealed that 20 of these 26 women were recruited at gestation 20–22 weeks (76.9%) and the remainder were recruited between 12 and 19 weeks.

3.3. Weight Monitoring Behaviour and Advice. 95.3% ($n = 184$) of women reported having been weighed by a healthcare professional during their current pregnancy, most commonly a midwife ($n = 181$). 29 of these 184 women (15.8%) reported that they had received specific advice about their weight (Table 2). There was a significant association between receiving advice and weight classification at recruitment ($\chi^2_{(2)} = 9.57$, $p < 0.001$; the one woman with BMI < 18 kg/m^2 was removed from this analysis due to insufficient cell count). Women who could be classified as obese were significantly more likely to receive specific advice about their weight after being weighed, compared to women who could be classified as having a recommended weight ($\chi^2_{(1)} = 9.04$, $p < 0.01$) or overweight ($\chi^2_{(1)} = 4.20$, $p < 0.05$) at recruitment. Content analysis of the advice reported by participants who had received comments about weight from health professionals covered a range of themes, as did women's feelings about being weighed (Table 2).

40.4% ($n = 78$) of participants reported that they had weighed themselves during their current pregnancy, and the majority of these weighed themselves weekly or fortnightly (57.7%, $n = 45$). The majority of women reported that they were not trying to do anything about their weight at the moment ($n = 142$, 73.6%) while 19.2% ($n = 37$) were trying to keep the same weight. Women with a BMI at recruitment that could be classified as overweight or obese were significantly

TABLE 1: Body Mass Index (BMI) classifications of participants calculated using weight measured at recruitment and self-reported prepregnancy weight.

	BMI* calculated using weight measured at recruitment ($n = 193$)	BMI* calculated using self-reported prepregnancy weight ($n = 168$)
BMI $< 18\,\text{kg/m}^2$	2 (1%)	7 (4.2%)
BMI $18\text{–}24.9\,\text{kg/m}^2$	94 (48.7%)	107 (63.7%)
BMI $25\text{–}29.9\,\text{kg/m}^2$	61 (31.6%)	33 (19.6%)
BMI $\geq 30\,\text{kg/m}^2$	36 (18.7%)	21 (12.5%)

*Both BMI calculations used height assessed at recruitment.

TABLE 2: Weight advice received by participants after being weighed, by BMI classification at recruitment.

	Weight advice received ($n = 29$)	Themes of feelings about being weighed and advice received* ($n = 26$)	Themes of weight advice received after being weighed* ($n = 27$)
BMI $< 18\,\text{kg/m}^2$	1 (3.4%)	Embarrassed ($n = 1$)	Advised that BMI required consultant-led care ($n = 1$)
BMI $18\text{–}24.9\,\text{kg/m}^2$	13 (44.8%)	Grateful/happy ($n = 3$) Fine/did not mind ($n = 7$) Embarrassed ($n = 1$)	Advised that BMI is "low" ($n = 3$) Advised that BMI is "healthy" ($n = 3$) Recommended healthy diet ($n = 4$) Emphasised need for weight gain ($n = 2$) Emphasised need for monitoring ($n = 1$)
BMI $25\text{–}29.9\,\text{kg/m}^2$	4 (13.8%)	Very sensible ($n = 1$) Fine ($n = 1$)	Advised not to lose weight but maintain ($n = 1$) Recommended avoidance of "sugary & fatty" foods ($n = 1$)
BMI $\geq 30\,\text{kg/m}^2$	11 (37.9%)	Fine/did not mind ($n = 4$) Grateful/happy ($n = 4$) Shocked but reassured ($n = 1$) Sceptical of advice ($n = 1$)	Advised to maintain weight/avoid weight gain ($n = 3$) Recommended healthy diet ($n = 2$) Recommended exercise ($n = 1$) Recommended commercial weight loss organization ($n = 2$)

*Themes are not mutually exclusive, and some responses could not be coded as they did not provide a description of the specific advice received.

more likely to be trying to keep the same weight, compared to women with a BMI $< 25\,\text{kg/m}^2$ ($\chi^2_{(1)} = 6.65$, $p < 0.05$). The two women who reported trying to lose weight both had a BMI at recruitment that could be classified as obese.

3.4. *Current Shape Concern and Antenatal Weight Change Expectations.* There was a significant association between BMI classification at recruitment and shape concerns ($\chi^2_{(2)} = 19.71$, $p < 0.001$). Women with a BMI at recruitment which could be classified as a recommended weight had significantly lower shape concern scores than women with a BMI which could be classified as overweight ($Z = -3.35$, $p < 0.01$) or obese ($Z = -3.85$, $p < 0.001$). There were no significant differences between women with a BMI which could be classified as overweight and obese (Table 3).

None of the women reported that they expected to lose weight during pregnancy while 1.6% ($n = 3$) expected no change in their weight, and 5.7% ($n = 11$) reported that they had no idea what to expect. 50.3% ($n = 97$) reported that they were expecting to gain weight but were not able quantify it, while 42.5% ($n = 82$) of the sample were able to quantify their expected weight gain (median 10.1 kg, SD 4.58 kg, min 2.27 kg, and max 22.23 kg; excluding one woman with multiple pregnancy who provided that data on this variable did

TABLE 3: Shape concern subscale scores by BMI classification at recruitment.

	Median	Interquartile range	Min	Max
BMI $18\text{–}24.9\,\text{kg/m}^2$	0.86	1.29	0.14	5.71
BMI $\geq 25\text{–}29.9\,\text{kg/m}^2$	1.71	1.86	0.14	5.00
BMI $\geq 30\,\text{kg/m}^2$	2.14	2.29	0.14	4.71

not significantly alter the distribution). There was no significant association between those women who expected no weight change, weight gain (but not quantified), and quantified weight gain and BMI classification at recruitment. There was small, significant, positive correlation between shape concerns and amount of weight women expected to gain during pregnancy ($r_s = 0.34$, $p < 0.01$, and $n = 82$).

3.5. *Awareness of Guidance and Sources of Information.* 39.4% ($n = 76$) of the sample reported that they were aware of guidance around weight change during pregnancy, and 59 women reported that guidance recommended a weight gain of 11.3 kg (IQR 4.2 kg, min 2 kg, and max 19.1 kg). 80.8% of the sample reported that healthcare professionals were main sources of information, 79.3% print and online information, and 37.8% family and friends. Women's responses to the open question about what they thought about sources of information available ($n = 137$) were often lengthy (max 157 words). Women across the BMI categories were more likely to report that sources of information were adequate or good rather than insufficient, and the thematic content analysis revealed three themes: general adequacy, healthcare professionals' role, and lay sources (Table 4).

4. Discussion

This study reports the broad range of women's experiences, behaviours, and expectations of routine antenatal weight management provision in Nottingham. In line with the recommendations of the NICE [5] guidelines and similar to a small UK study by Brown and Avery [27], most women in the sample reported having been weighed in early pregnancy and by a midwife. It is, however, notable that a low proportion of women weighed reported having received advice after these measurements—even less than that observed by McDonald et al. [28]. Presumably practitioners are using the information to refer higher weight women to consultant-led care, and from an ethical perspective women should be aware of why these measurements are being taken and how it will be used to plan their care. However, NICE also recommended that women with a BMI over 30 should be referred to a dietitian or appropriately trained professional to receive personalised advice on healthy eating and physical activity. Although significantly more women of a higher weight received advice, excessive gestational weight gain can occur regardless of prepregnancy BMI classification. It has been suggested that midwives are optimally placed to deliver advice on gestational weight gain [29] and that as they deal with sensitive issues and women's anxieties as a core part of their role, they are very well equipped [12]. Indeed, NICE recommended discussion of how to achieve a healthy lifestyle during antenatal contacts for all pregnant women. However, other researches reveal that midwives fear offending and alienating women by discussing the issue early in the therapeutic relationship [30]. These are valid concerns due to the moralistic nature of weight, reports of stigma in antenatal settings [18, 30–32], and in the current sample women both of higher and lower weights were embarrassed. However, women in this sample who were weighed and received advice were generally not negative about the experience and more similar to the views expressed by women in research by Olander et al. [33]. The language employed by women in this sample could not be said to be overwhelmingly positive either—rather the tone was one of confirmation of something uncontroversial.

Taken together the majority of women in the sample (regardless of BMI) did not express any barriers to being weighed and as 40.8% reported weighing themselves at home on scales, there is some justification for providing women with an opportunity to take accurate measurements using reliable equipment under supervision. This phenomenon of self-monitoring has been reported elsewhere; for example, women who disengaged from an antenatal weight service cited confusion and disappointment about not being weighed regularly [34, 35] and reported self-monitoring in half of the sample of women which included those who exhibited both

recommended and excess gestational weight gain. What is less clear are women's motivations for regular weighing. It is perhaps being used as a means to motivate behaviour as suggested by Daley et al. [12] but—due to the lack of agreed targets—it might also reflect women's scientific curiosity and fascination as to their new-found functionality [3]. This would explain the relatively low levels of shape concern seen in the sample, even among higher weight women. Tiggemann [36] describes that while body image might be a relatively stable construct, the importance vested in it is dynamic.

Considering the lack of dialogue between women in this sample and their practitioners, it is perhaps unsurprising that the majority are unable to recall the guideline expectations for weight gain used by NHS England and the Department of Health or what to expect during their own pregnancy beyond a sense that they will "gain weight." Those women who did have an expected weight gain that could be quantified varied widely but were, on average, consistent with 10–12.5 kg.

When asked about the advice generally available on weight, diet, and exercise, participants used more positive than negative comments. However, a deeper examination revealed several narratives. In line with previous work [18, 27, 32, 33, 35, 37], women did not feel that their weight or indeed diet and exercise were priorities for midwives and other healthcare professionals. In the current study practitioners detached from the subject by employing terminology such as "BMI" and actions such as "keep an eye on [your weight]." Women also reported that there were not ready opportunities to ask questions about "nonroutine" or "nonemergency" topics. This perhaps also accounts for the equal reliance on Internet sources as "main sources of information," despite the awareness of their limitations. Olander et al. [33], Arden et al. [31], and Brown and Avery [27] have also described how gaps in knowledge on weight can be filled using self-study.

For those who had accessed advice, there was frustration that it was too general, not personalised, and diet-focused. Women are not, therefore, perceiving the advice to be "practical and tailored" as recommended by NICE [5]. Similarly, Heslehurst et al. [38] described how dietary information was provided *ad hoc* and not linked to weight management, while Brown and Avery [27] report that many participants stated advice was brief and lacking in detail. Interestingly women of a higher weight reported that the advice they received was too idealistic and not supported by advice on process.

In contrast to those who want to be better informed, there are women who actively avoided information about weight, diet, and exercise. The issue of bodyweight was sometimes deemed to be not salient (at all or due to time at which it is received) and previously authors have reported women preferring to wait until after birth [34, 39]. Worryingly advice from practitioners was in some cases dismissed as unreliable and Arden et al. [31] also describe how women can lack trust in "official" advice. Others reported a wish to avoid potential negative emotions which once again speaks to the value-laden nature of bodyweight.

4.1. Strengths and Limitations. As with previous work in the UK (e.g., [31]), the current sample is not wholly representative of the population. It had twice the proportion of women from

TABLE 4: Participants' feelings about sources of information during pregnancy on weight, diet, and exercise, by BMI classification at recruitment.

Themes*	BMI < 18 kg/m² (n = 1)	BMI 18–24.9 kg/m² (n = 69)	BMI ≥ 25–29.9 kg/m² (n = 43)	BMI ≥ 30 kg/m² (n = 24)
General adequacy				
Generally fine/good/plenty		14 (20.3%)	11 (25.6%)	4 (16.7%)
Generally not sufficient		8 (11.6%)	4 (9.3%)	2 (8.3%)
Not salient in very early pregnancy	1		3 (7.0%)	
Not salient until postpartum				3 (12.5%)
Emphasis on diet, not weight			5 (11.6%)	
Too general/no guidelines		13 (18.8%)	4 (9.3%)	2 (8.3%)
Individualised advice preferred		6 (8.70%)		
To idealistic			1 (2.3%)	1 (4.2%)
No information on *how* to change			4 (9.3%)	1 (4.2%)
No information on *why* to change			2 (4.7%)	1 (4.2%)
Healthcare professionals role				
Do not appear concerned		3 (4.3%)	3 (7.0%)	1 (4.2%)
Information can be confusing/unreliable/conflicting			3 (7.0%)	3 (12.5%)
Have to ask/seek information		7 (10.1%)	6 (14.0%)	3 (12.5%)
More active engagement preferred		3 (4.3%)	1 (2.3%)	
Subject too personal for HCP		2 (2.90%)	2 (4.7%)	
Do not seek/avoid information		9 (13.0%)		4 (16.7%)
Lay sources				
Happy with information available via the Internet/apps/magazines/books		5 (7.2%)		
Information can be confusing/unreliable/conflicting	1	8 (11.6%)	1 (2.3%)	3 (12.5%)
NHS web resources good/reliable		8 (11.6%)	2 (4.7%)	
Better signposting required		1 (1.4%)		

*Themes are not mutually exclusive.

a household with an NS-SEC score of 1 or 2 compared to the census data for the East Midlands (<65 yrs) [40], and the average age of mothers (32.8 yrs) was also higher than the 30.0 years reported in the Office for National Statistics data [41]. However, the majority of women were recruited at 12–14 weeks of gestation and 20–22 weeks of gestation which reflects the function of the clinics recruited from (namely, the 10–12-week dating scan and 18–20-week anomaly scan), and higher weight women were represented at a level similar to that from national statistics (i.e., 50% overweight or obese at the start of pregnancy [41]). It is interesting to observe that higher weight women were not systematically deterred from participation due to the objective weight and height measurements taken by the researchers, but when taking into account participants' low body shape concerns it may be that women (across the BMI categories) with body image and weight concerns may be underrepresented. This limits the generalisability of the findings and it would be inappropriate to conclude that weighing is generally acceptable across the socioeconomic spectrum and in various ethnic identities. However, the findings do reveal an unmet need for engagement on the issue of bodyweight among some women across the BMI categories.

The uses of BMI categories to identify obesity, indicate risk, and decide upon care are controversial but are widely used in research and clinical practice. Measurements can be taken throughout pregnancy, from prepregnancy [42, 43] to the 3rd trimester [44]. The mismatch between BMI figures in Table 1, calculated using both the self-reported prepregnancy and measured recruitment weights, is possibly due to misreporting and/or gestational weight gain, and it is not possible with the current study design to separate out these potential influences.

5. Conclusion

The positioning of prepregnancy bodyweight and gestational weight gain as *problematic* in the national consciousness has for many years been encapsulated in guidelines such Department of Health, National Institute of Health and Care Excellence, and the Royal College of Obstetrics and Gynaecology. Indeed, the focus has intensified of late, most recently with comments from the Chief Medical Officer [45] who described obesity as the "biggest threat to women's health" and the subsequent media coverage. It is, therefore, unsurprising that the current study revealed a desire for engagement on the issue of bodyweight among some women across the BMI categories. However, the lack of specific guidelines, the lack of available support around process, and the reluctance of some practitioners to engage in this complex and value-laden topic are all barriers.

Women are clearly not being served appropriately in the current situation which simultaneously problematizes and fails to offer solutions. Given the weight of medical opinion that bodyweight should be an issue to be addressed during pregnancy, future work needs to move away from the current obstetric risk management framework to an empowerment approach [6] and build the capacity of practitioners to

deliver individualised weight-related advice without prejudice. Arguably the antenatal period offers a unique opportunity to counter the current negative reductionist dialogue around weight gain with one that emphasises the body's capabilities. Specific behavioural guidelines and positive framed advice could be developed and applied in a flexible, nonjudgmental manner to offer reassurance and empowerment.

Competing Interests

The authors declare that they have no competing interests.

Acknowledgments

First and foremost, the authors would like to thank the women who participated in this study. They would also like to thank Louise Dyason, Charlotte Whitmore, Kimberley Burton, and Aisling McAleer (3rd-year Masters of Dietetics students at the University of Nottingham) who recruited participants alongside members of the research team and entered data, as part of their undergraduate project work. The authors are also extremely grateful to Professor Helen Budge and Dr. George Bugg (Nottingham University Hospitals NHS Trust) for their advice and support regarding data collection. This study was funded by the School of Biosciences, University of Nottingham, and the Revere Charitable Trust.

References

[1] S. Phelan, "Pregnancy: a 'teachable moment' for weight control and obesity prevention," *American Journal of Obstetrics and Gynecology*, vol. 202, no. 2, pp. 135.e1–135.e8, 2010.

[2] National Institute of Health and Care Excellence, "Schedule of appointments in routine antenatal care," Antenatal Care Pathway, http://pathways.nice.org.uk/pathways/antenatal-care#path=view%3A/pathways/antenatalcare/schedule-of-appointments-in-routine-antenatal-care.xml&content=view-index.

[3] E. L. Hodgkinson, D. M. Smith, and A. Wittkowski, "Women's experiences of their pregnancy and postpartum body image: a systematic review and meta-synthesis," *BMC Pregnancy and Childbirth*, vol. 14, no. 1, article 330, 2014.

[4] A. Hui, L. Back, S. Ludwig et al., "Lifestyle intervention on diet and exercise reduced excessive gestational weight gain in pregnant women under a randomised controlled trial," *An International Journal of Obstetrics and Gynaecology*, vol. 119, no. 1, pp. 70–77, 2012.

[5] National Institute for Health and Care Excellence, *Weight Management before During and after Pregnancy*, vol. 27 of *NICE Public Health Guidance*, National Institute for Health and Care Excellence, London, UK, 2010.

[6] M. Ahluwalia, "Supporting the individual needs of obese pregnant women: effects of risk-management processes," *British Journal of Midwifery*, vol. 23, no. 10, pp. 702–708, 2015.

[7] National Health Service Choices, "Your pregnancy and baby guide," 2014, http://www.nhs.uk/conditions/pregnancy-and-baby/pages/pregnancy-and-baby-care.aspx.

[8] Department of Health, *The Pregnancy Book*, Department of Health, London, UK, 2009.

[9] Institute of Medicine, "Weight Gain During Pregnancy: Reexamining the Guidelines," 2009, http://www.nationalacademies

.org/hmd/Reports/2009/Weight-Gain-During-Pregnancy-Re-examining-the-Guidelines.aspx.

[10] V. Allen-Walker, J. Woodside, V. Holmes et al., "Routine weighing of women during pregnancy—is it time to change current practice?" *An International Journal of Obstetrics and Gynaecology*, vol. 123, no. 6, pp. 871–874, 2015.

[11] J. Modder and K. J. Fitzsimons, *Management of Women with Obesity in Pregnancy*, Centre for Maternal and Child Enquiries and Royal Collage of Obstetricians and Gynaecologists, London, UK, 2010.

[12] A. J. Daley, K. Jolly, S. A. Jebb et al., "Feasibility and acceptability of regular weighing, setting weight gain limits and providing feedback by community midwives to prevent excess weight gain during pregnancy: randomised controlled trial and qualitative study," *BMC Obesity*, vol. 2, article 35, 2015.

[13] F. Campbell, J. Messina, M. Johnson, L. Guillaume, J. Madan, and E. Goyder, *Systematic Review of Dietary and/or Physical Activity Interventions for Weight Management in Pregnancy*, ScHARR Public Health Collaborating Centre, Sheffield, UK, 2009.

[14] A. Brown, J. Rance, and L. Warren, "Body image concerns during pregnancy are associated with a shorter breast feeding duration," *Midwifery*, vol. 31, no. 1, pp. 80–89, 2015.

[15] D. Čuržik, Z. Topolovec, and S. Šijanović, "Maternal overnutrition and pregnancy," *Acta Medica Croatica*, vol. 56, no. 1, pp. 31–34, 2002.

[16] R. M. Puhl, J. D. Latner, K. O'Brien, J. Luedicke, S. Danielsdottir, and M. Forhan, "A multinational examination of weight bias: predictors of anti-fat attitudes across four countries," *International Journal of Obesity*, vol. 39, no. 7, pp. 1166–1173, 2015.

[17] H. Skouteris, "Body image issues in obstetrics and gynecology," in *Body Image: A Handbook of Science, Practice, and Prevention*, T. Cash and L. Smolak, Eds., pp. 342–349, Guilford Press, New York, NY, USA, 2nd edition, 2011.

[18] P. J. Furness, K. McSeveny, M. A. Arden, C. Garland, A. M. Dearden, and H. Soltani, "Maternal obesity support services: a qualitative study of the perspectives of women and midwives," *BMC Pregnancy and Childbirth*, vol. 11, article 69, 2011.

[19] M. Johnson, F. Campbell, J. Messina, L. Preston, H. Buckley Woods, and E. Goyder, "Weight management during pregnancy: a systematic review of qualitative evidence," *Midwifery*, vol. 29, no. 12, pp. 1287–1296, 2013.

[20] C. E. Foster and J. Hirst, "Midwives' attitudes towards giving weight-related advice to obese pregnant women," *British Journal of Midwifery*, vol. 22, no. 4, pp. 254–262, 2014.

[21] N. Heslehurst, J. Rankin, J. R. Wilkinson, and C. D. Summerbell, "A nationally representative study of maternal obesity in England, UK: trends in incidence and demographic inequalities in 619 323 births, 1989–2007," *International Journal of Obesity*, vol. 34, no. 3, pp. 420–428, 2010.

[22] Office for National Statistics, "Standard occupational classification 2010," 2010, http://www.ons.gov.uk/ons/guide-method/classifications/current-standard-classifications/soc2010/index.html.

[23] World Health Organization, *Physical Status: The Use and Interprestation of Anthropometry*, vol. 854 of *Report of a WHO Expert Committee. Technical Report Series*, World Health Organization, Geneva, Switzerland, 1995.

[24] C. G. Fairburn and S. J. Beglin, "Assessment of eating disorders: interview or self-report questionnaire?" *International Journal of Eating Disorders*, vol. 16, no. 4, pp. 363–370, 1994.

[25] A. N. Oppenheim, *Questionnaire Design, Interviewing and Attitude Measurement*, Continuum, London, UK, 2nd edition, 2000.

[26] S. A. Fade and J. A. Swift, "Qualitative research in nutrition and dietetics: data analysis issues," *Journal of Human Nutrition and Dietetics*, vol. 24, no. 2, pp. 106–114, 2011.

[27] A. Brown and A. Avery, "Healthy weight management during pregnancy: what advice and information is being provided," *Journal of Human Nutrition and Dietetics*, vol. 25, no. 4, pp. 378–387, 2012.

[28] S. D. McDonald, E. Pullenayegum, V. H. Taylor et al., "Despite 2009 guidelines, few women report being counseled correctly about weight gain during pregnancy," *American Journal of Obstetrics and Gynecology*, vol. 205, no. 4, pp. 333–e6, 2011.

[29] J. Baker, "Developing a care pathway for obese women in pregnancy and beyond," *British Journal of Midwifery*, vol. 19, no. 10, pp. 632–643, 2011.

[30] N. Heslehurst, S. Russell, H. Brandon, C. Johnston, C. Summerbell, and J. Rankin, "Women's perspectives are required to inform the development of maternal obesity services: a qualitative study of obese pregnant women's experiences," *Health Expectations*, vol. 18, no. 5, pp. 969–981, 2015.

[31] M. A. Arden, A. M. S. Duxbury, and H. Soltani, "Responses to gestational weight management guidance: a thematic analysis of comments made by women in online parenting forums," *BMC Pregnancy and Childbirth*, vol. 14, article 216, 2014.

[32] C. M. Furber and L. McGowan, "A qualitative study of the experiences of women who are obese and pregnant in the UK," *Midwifery*, vol. 27, no. 4, pp. 437–444, 2011.

[33] E. K. Olander, L. Atkinson, J. K. Edmunds, and D. P. French, "The views of pre- and post-natal women and health professionals regarding gestational weight gain: An Exploratory Study," *Sexual and Reproductive Healthcare*, vol. 2, no. 1, pp. 43–48, 2011.

[34] L. Atkinson, E. K. Olander, and D. P. French, "Why don't many obese pregnant and post-natal women engage with a weight management service?" *Journal of Reproductive and Infant Psychology*, vol. 31, no. 3, pp. 245–256, 2013.

[35] C. H. Chuang, M. R. Stengel, S. W. Hwang, D. Velott, K. H. Kjerulff, and J. L. Kraschnewski, "Behaviours of overweight and obese women during pregnancy who achieve and exceed recommended gestational weight gain," *Obesity Research and Clinical Practice*, vol. 8, no. 6, pp. e577–e583, 2014.

[36] M. Tiggemann, "Body image across the adult life span: stability and change," *Body Image*, vol. 1, no. 1, pp. 29–41, 2004.

[37] E. A. Duthie, E. M. Drew, and K. E. Flynn, "Patient-provider communication about gestational weight gain among nulliparous women: a qualitative study of the views of obstetricians and first-time pregnant women," *BMC Pregnancy and Childbirth*, vol. 13, article 231, 2013.

[38] N. Heslehurst, R. Lang, J. Rankin, J. R. Wilkinson, and C. D. Summerbell, "Obesity in pregnancy: a study of the impact of maternal obesity on NHS maternity services," *BJOG*, vol. 114, no. 3, pp. 334–342, 2007.

[39] E. K. Olander and L. Atkinson, "Obese women's reasons for not attending a weight management service during pregnancy," *Acta Obstetricia et Gynecologica Scandinavica*, vol. 92, no. 10, pp. 1227–1230, 2013.

[40] Office for National Statistics, *Regional Statistics East Midlands 2011*, 2011, http://www.ons.gov.uk/ons/regional-statistics/region.html?region=East+Midlands.

[41] Health and Social Care Information Centre Statistics, "Obesity, Physical Activity and Diet: England 2014," 2014, http://www.hscic.gov.uk/catalogue/PUB13648/Obes-phys-acti-diet-eng-2014-rep.pdf.

[42] L. M. Bodnar, A. M. Siega-Riz, H. N. Simhan, J. C. Diesel, and B. Abrams, "The impact of exposure misclassification on associations between prepregnancy BMI and adverse pregnancy outcomes," *Obesity*, vol. 18, no. 11, pp. 2184–2190, 2010.

[43] E. Han, B. Abrams, S. Sridhar, F. Xu, and M. Hedderson, "Validity of self-reported pre-pregnancy weight and body mass index classification in an integrated health care delivery system," *Paediatric and Perinatal Epidemiology*, vol. 30, no. 4, pp. 314–319, 2016.

[44] Royal Cornwall Hospitals NHS Trust, "Increased Body Mass Index (BMI) in Pregnancy, Labour, and Post Delivery," 2016, http://www.rcht.nhs.uk/DocumentsLibrary/RoyalCornwall-HospitalsTrust/Clinical/MidwiferyAndObstetrics/Increased-BodyMassIndexBMIInPregnancyLabourAndPostDelivery-ClinicalGuidelineForTheManagementOfAWomanWith.pdf.

[45] Department of Health, "Annual Report of the Chief Medical Officer, 2014—The Health of the 51%: Women," 2015, https://www.gov.uk/government/publications/chief-medical-officer-annual-report-2014-womens-health.

21

Magnesium Supplementation and Blood Pressure in Pregnancy: A Double-Blind Randomized Multicenter Study

Maria Bullarbo [ID],[1,2] **Helena Mattson,**[3] **Anna-Karin Broman,**[4]
Natalia Ödman,[3] **and Thorkild F. Nielsen**[1]

[1]*Department of Obstetrics and Gynecology, Sahlgrenska Academy, University of Gothenburg, Gothenburg, Sweden*
[2]*Department of Gynecology, Närhälsan, Mölndal, Sweden*
[3]*Women's Clinic, Södra Älvsborgs Hospital, Borås, Sweden*
[4]*Women's Clinic, Norra Älvsborgs Hospital, Trollhättan, Sweden*

Correspondence should be addressed to Maria Bullarbo; maria.bullarbo@vgregion.se

Academic Editor: Fabio Facchinetti

Objective. To investigate the effect of magnesium (Mg) supplementation in healthy pregnant women for prevention of blood pressure increase. Secondary outcomes were comparison of biomarkers for hypertensive disorders and labour and fetal outcomes between the groups. *Methods.* Two hundred nulliparous healthy pregnant women were double-blind randomized to receive Mg daily or placebo. *Results.* There were no differences in blood pressure increase. However, among the Mg-treated women, there was a significant negative correlation between increase in blood levels of magnesium and increase in systolic blood pressure ($p = 0.042$). Magnesium supplementation seems to be safe for both mother and infant. *Conclusion.* Magnesium supplementation in healthy first-time pregnant women is not to be recommended for prevention of blood pressure increase. Supplementation in risk pregnancies needs to be further investigated. The study is listed on the ISRCTN registry with study ID 13890849.

1. Introduction

High blood pressure during pregnancy is a risk factor for developing preeclampsia (PE) and eclampsia (E) and affects approximately 6–8% of all pregnant women [1]. A systolic/diastolic blood pressure (SBP/DBP) of 140/90 mm Hg is defined as gestational hypertension (HT). The etiology of HT is multifactorial, but nulliparity, obesity, stress, heredity, high maternal age, multiple pregnancy, diabetes, thrombophilia, kidney disease, chronic HT, and nutritional deficiency are all risk factors [2]. When HT is accompanied by proteinuria of at least 0.3g/day, it is defined as PE. PE can be complicated by elevated liver enzymes, low platelets, or changes in the coagulation system, which are life-threatening conditions. PE can further lead to general convulsions, called eclampsia (E), for which the only known curative treatment is termination of the pregnancy. The mechanisms underlying the development of HT and PE are still largely unknown and seem to be multifactorial, involving both placental pathology and immunological or genetic disorders [3, 4]. If HT is complicated by PE, oxidative stress occurs, followed by the release of inflammatory mediators such as IL-6 [5–7]. Blood levels of both the renal marker cystatin C and the inflammatory marker CRP have also been shown to be elevated in women with hypertensive disorders [8–10]. Some studies have supported a link between HT and/or PE and deficiencies in calcium, vitamins C, D, and E [11–14], and folic acid [12, 15], but the evidence is not conclusive. However, a daily low dose of antiplatelet agents, such as aspirin, of at least 100 mg in risk pregnancies has in recent years been shown to prevent PE and intrauterine growth restriction (IUGR) [16–18]. It is important to note that most studies have focused on prevention of PE and not of gestational HT. There are very few, if any, human studies on the prevention of gestational HT, and, in fact, an animal study demonstrated contradictory results, showing that low-dosage aspirin treatment led to increased risk of HT [19]. It is risky to draw conclusions about effects in humans based on an animal study, but the results do indicate a need for further research on possible preventive agents against gestational HT.

Several studies suggest that the risk of gestational HT is related to changes in magnesium (Mg) homeostasis. Associations have also been reported between mortality in cardiovascular disease and Mg intake in nonpregnant populations [20]. Mg is one of the five most common minerals in the human body and is present in more than 300 human enzymes. Mg plays a major role in the normal functioning of muscles, carbohydrate metabolism, and the skeletal structure [21, 22]. In a Cochrane meta-analysis of Mg supplementation in pregnant women, Makrides et al concluded that it had not been proven to be efficient in preventing gestational HT, but many of the studies were classified as low quality [23] and more studies were therefore recommended. Of interest is the fact that one study showed a correlation between low plasma levels of Mg in pregnant women and PE [24]. The same study also showed that 16% of all pregnant women had low plasma levels of Mg. After the publication of the Cochrane review by Makrides, our research group demonstrated a positive correlation between the urinary secretion of Mg and calcium in early pregnancy and BP increase in late pregnancy [25]. In a follow-up double-blind randomized placebo-controlled study of 60 pregnant women, 300 mg Mg or placebo was administered daily as a supplement from gestational week 25 until labour. Women included were classified to belong to a risk group for developing BP increase due to high urinary secretion of calcium/Mg. The DBP increase during late pregnancy was significantly lower in the study group receiving Mg compared to the placebo group [26]. The same study showed that the expression of Mg-sensitive genes was also related to SBP and DBP and to Mg excretion in the urine. The results suggested that Mg is involved in the regulation of BP during pregnancy [27]. The same conclusion was reached by Rylander in a review of Mg and BP in pregnancy [28]. A retrospective study comparing women with and without PE also showed that an increase in DBP of ≥15 mm Hg was a risk indicator for developing PE, indicating that preventing gestational HT might also prevent the development of PE [29]. As early as 1998, it was shown that lowered red cell Mg concentrations were correlated to severe HT in pregnancy, suggesting that Mg deficiency could be a contributory factor in the development of hypertensive disorders of pregnancy [30]. The association of a low dietary Mg intake and an increased risk of PE has also been confirmed in a meta-analysis studying the effects of various dietary factors on the risk of pregnancy-induced high BP [31]. Spätling et al. concluded in a review on Mg and pregnancy that the need for Mg intake increases during pregnancy, with a daily recommended dose of supplemented Mg of 240–480 mg [32].

2. Objective

The primary aim of the study was to investigate whether a daily supplementation with 400 mg Mg during pregnancy compared to a placebo group in a double-blind setting could prevent an increase of diastolic BP of at least 15 mm Hg. Secondary outcomes were comparison of biomarkers for hypertensive disorders and labour and fetal outcomes between the groups.

3. Methods

The study was a placebo-controlled double-blind interventional multicenter study. A total of 199 nulliparous women in gestational weeks 12–14 were recruited at 3 antenatal care units (ACU) in west Sweden (in the cities of Borås, Alingsås, and Trollhättan). Inclusion criteria were nulliparity, no regular medication, normotension, singleton pregnancy, and maternity age >18 years and <40 years. Exclusion criteria were age <18 or >40 years, multiple pregnancies, trombophilia, previous labour, diabetes, chronic HT, kidney disease, heart disease, regular medication, history of cardiac arrhythmia, or heredity of sudden cardiac arrest. Abdominal ultrasound examination was performed for dating and verification of singleton and viable pregnancy. After oral and written consent, participants were randomized in a computerized double-blind procedure to receive either Mg (400 mg Magnesium Extra, Diasporal®) or placebo. The code was not broken until all participants had given birth. Blood samples were collected at gestational weeks 12–14 and 35 for analysis of IL-6, CRP, urate, cystatin C, Mg, Ca, albumin, creatinine, and glomerular filtration rate (GFR). BP was measured at the ACU at 2-3 weeks' intervals throughout the pregnancy, with the women seated with arm and backrest support, down to Korotkoff V with a manual sphygmomanometer. BP data registered at the ACU and labour ward were collected from medical records. Records were obtained on gestational length at birth, labour outcomes including excessive bleeding >1000 ml, instrumental delivery, and duration of active labour, and fetal outcomes including Apgar score at five minutes, pH in the arterial umbilical cord, birth weight, and need of care at a neonatal intensive care unit (NICU). Possible additional multivitamin intake containing extra Mg obtained from medical records was also registered.

4. Statistical Analyses

A sample size of 178 women was estimated to achieve 80% power at 5% significance level, assuming that 25% of Mg-treated women experience an increase of <15 mm Hg in DBP during pregnancy compared to 45% in the placebo group. This hypothesis was based on results from the first interventional pilot study of 60 women. Due to expected dropout in the study due to miscarriage or nausea, 200 women were calculated to participate in the study, of whom 100 women received Mg and 100 women received placebo. A p value < 0.05 was interpreted as statistically significant. For differences between the groups, the Mann–Whitney U test and Fisher's exact test were used. Spearman's test was used to analyze correlations between different variables. Mean (SD)/median (min; max) were used for descriptive purposes.

TABLE 1: Baseline data (PP).

Variable	Magnesium ($n = 83$)	Placebo ($n = 93$)	p value
Maternal age	27.0 (3.4)	26.9 (3.5)	0.92
	27.0 (20.0; 36.0)	27.0 (18.0; 36.0)	
	$n = 83$	$n = 93$	
BMI (body mass index)	24.7 (4.7)	24.1 (3.8)	0.62
	24.0 (18.0; 43.0)	24.0 (18.0; 35.0)	
	$n = 83$	$n = 93$	
Smoking habit	14 (16.9%)	17 (18.3%)	0.96
DBP at week 12	67.5 (7.9)	67.0 (6.1)	0.61
	70.0 (50.0; 85.0)	70.0 (55.0; 85.0)	
	$n = 83$	$n = 93$	
SBP at week 12	114.6 (10.8)	112.7 (10.1)	0.19
	115.0 (90.0; 135.0)	110.0 (90.0; 135.0)	
	$n = 83$	$n = 93$	
Gestational length at inclusion	12.7 (1.5)	12.8 (1.7)	0.94
	12.6 (9.4; 16.9)	12.6 (8.9; 17.7)	
	$n = 83$	$n = 93$	
Extra Mg (mg/day in multivitamin tablets)	31.7 (47.5)	33.9 (48.3)	0.70
	0.0 (0.0; 150.0)	0.0 (0.0; 150.0)	
	$n = 81$	$n = 92$	
Mg intake (n)			
0 (no)	53 (65.4%)	58 (63.0%)	
1 (yes)	28 (34.6%)	34 (37.0%)	0.87

For categorical variables, n (%) is presented.
For continuous variables, mean (SD)/median (min; max)/n is presented.
For comparison between groups, Fisher's exact test (lowest 1-sided p value multiplied by 2) was used for dichotomous variables and the Mann–Whitney U test was used for continuous variables.

5. Results

For all outcomes regarding BP, labour, and infants' analyses, statistics on both intention to treat (ITT) and per protocol (PP) were calculated. As there were no statistically significant differences in any outcomes between ITT and PP groups, results for mainly the PP groups are described. The study had a dropout rate of 11% (7 women in the placebo group and 16 in the Mg group). Main reasons were nausea and difficulty in intake of the randomized supplementation. One exclusion occurred in the Mg group before randomization because of accidental damage of the randomized supplement, and therefore a total of 199 women were randomized (99 to the Mg group and 100 to the placebo). Baseline data were equal between the two study groups (Table 1). As there was no difference between the groups of women taking additional supplements of Mg, no regression analysis was performed.

The main outcome was BP increase, illustrated in Tables 2(a) and 2(b) (Table 2(b) only including women taking no extra Mg) and in Figures 1(a) and 1(b). For the primary outcome, there was no difference between the groups regarding increase in DBP or SBP. The number of women diagnosed with gestational HT and PE was equally distributed between the Mg and placebo groups (17 versus 20 and 3 versus 4, resp.). As regards secondary outcomes (Table 3), there were no differences in fetal or labour outcomes except for gestational length at birth ($p = 0.03$ for PP and 0.048 for ITT). Mean gestational length at birth was 40,2 (Mg) versus 39,9 weeks (placebo). Blood parameters were equal between the groups at gestational week 12, at week 35, and in change over time from week 12 to week 35 (Δ DBP and Δ SBP, Table 4). Scatter plots with Spearman's correlation showed no correlations between blood parameters or change in blood parameters and SBP or DBP (no table shown). However, when analyzing only the Mg group regarding correlations between Δ Mg levels from week 12 to week 35 and Δ SDP and DBP, there was a negative correlation regading SBP ($p = 0,042$) but not regarding DBP ($p = 0,13$), shown in Figures 2(a) and 2(b). It was not possible to analyze Mg-deficient women as they were too few (only 2 in the Mg group and 5 in the placebo group).

Of 199 women included in the study, 35% in the Mg group and 37% in the placebo group were supplemented with additional multivitamin tablets containing Mg. The doses of extra Mg varied between 30 and 150 mg/day.

TABLE 2

(a) Primary outcome. Increase from gestational week 12 to labour in diastolic (DBP) and systolic (SBP) blood pressure

Variable	Magnesium (n = 83)	Placebo (n = 93)	p value
Increase in DBP ≥15 or SBP ≥30 mm Hg			
0 (no)	46 (56.1%)	56 (60.2%)	
1 (yes)	36 (43.9%)	37 (39.8%)	0.69
Increase in DBP of ≥15 mm Hg (maximum increase)			
0 (no)	47 (57.3%)	57 (61.3%)	
1 (yes)	35 (42.7%)	36 (38.7%)	0.70
Maximum increase in DBP	12.4 (8.3)	10.6 (9.4)	0.17
	10.0 (-5.0; 35.0)	10.0 (-10.0; 30.0)	
	n = 83	n = 93	
Increase in SBP of ≥30 mm Hg (maximum increase)			
0 (no)	77 (93.9%)	84 (90.3%)	
1 (yes)	5 (6.1%)	9 (9.7%)	0.56
Maximum increase in SBP	12.6 (10.7)	12.9 (11.7)	0.96
	10.0 (-10.0; 55.0)	10.0 (-5.0; 60.0)	
	n = 83	n = 93	
Gestational HT			
0 (no)	62 (75.6%)	78 (83.9%)	
1 (yes)	20 (24.4%)	15 (16.1%)	0.24

For categorical variables, n (%) is presented.
For continuous variables, mean (SD)/median (min; max)/n is presented.
For comparison between groups, Fisher's exact test (lowest 1-sided p value multiplied by 2) was used for dichotomous variables and the Mann–Whitney U test was used for continuous variables.

(b) Primary outcome. Increase from gestational week 12 to labour in diastolic blood pressure (DBP) and systolic blood pressure (SBP). Women taking extra Mg were excluded

Variable	Magnesium (n = 53)	Placebo (n = 58)	p value
Increase in DBP ≥15 or SBP ≥30 mm Hg			
0	27 (50.9%)	32 (55.2%)	
1	26 (49.1%)	26 (44.8%)	0.80
Increase in DBP of ≥15 mm Hg (maximum increase)			
0	28 (52.8%)	33 (56.9%)	
1	25 (47.2%)	25 (43.1%)	0.81
Maximum increase in DBP	12.8 (8.0)	11.6 (8.4)	0.34
	10.0 (-5.0; 30.0)	10.0 (0.0; 30.0)	
	n = 53	n = 58	
Increase in SBP of ≥30 mm Hg (maximum increase)			
0	50 (94.3%)	52 (89.7%)	
1	3 (5.7%)	6 (10.3%)	0.58
Maximum increase in SBP	12.5 (9.0)	12.4 (11.2)	0.70
	10.0 (0.0; 35.0)	10.0 (-5.0; 50.0)	
	n = 53	n = 58	

TABLE 2: Continued.

Variable	Magnesium (n = 53)	Placebo (n = 58)	p value
Gestational HT			
0	42 (79.2%)	48 (82.8%)	
1	11 (20.8%)	10 (17.2%)	0.82

For categorical variables, n (%) is presented.
For continuous variables, mean (SD)/median (min; max)/n is presented.
For comparison between groups, Fisher's exact test (lowest 1-sided p value multiplied by 2) was used for dichotomous variables and the Mann–Whitney U test was used for continuous variables.
2018-04-26 analys.sas.

6. Discussion

Healthy first-time pregnant women with no risk factors for developing gestational HT seem to have no need of extra daily supplementation of Mg to protect against BP increase. Therefore, a general recommendation of oral Mg supplementation during pregnancy remains controversial, despite an increased need for Mg during pregnancy. However, these results are somewhat unexpected, as our research group in earlier studies found correlations between supplementation with Mg and prevention of DBP increase. It must be emphasised, however, that the earlier promising results were achieved among pregnant nulliparous women with high urinary excretion of Mg and calcium in early pregnancy, indirectly indicating Mg deficiency. Participants in our earlier study were accordingly classified to belong to a risk group for developing BP increase during pregnancy.

Excretion of Mg is increased during stress reactions, including merely the state of being pregnant. The major question in this study is whether the participants were deficient in Mg or not. If not, they would be unlikely to benefit from supplementation with Mg, as the results indicate in this study. It is established that Mg deficiency is difficult to measure, as only 1% of all Mg is measurable in the blood, and blood levels decrease only when the deficiency is very serious. Hence, normomagnesemia does not exclude Mg deficiency [33]. Interpreting the results of biomarkers was difficult, as only two-thirds of the 199 participants gave a blood test in the third trimester. Despite this fact, it was unexpected to find no difference between the groups in plasma levels of Mg in the third trimester of pregnancy, despite differences in Mg intake.

The main shortcoming of the study was the fact that the participants were allowed to take multivitamin tablets containing Mg, which in general is recommended for pregnant women. Also, given current knowledge regarding increased need for Mg during pregnancy, performing a placebo-controlled study is hard to justify from an ethical point of view. However, they were not allowed to take extra Mg on their own as a supplement without reporting that to the study group, which no one did, nor was any registration of such use seen in the medical records. Furthermore, the possibility cannot be excluded that, after being informed about the study, an additional unknown number of participants took over-the-counter Mg. Consequently, there could be a treatment bias. Notably, however, Makrides, who authored the Cochrane meta-analysis on Mg supplementation during pregnancy, classified the Sibai study as high quality, despite the fact that it allowed extra Mg intake [34]. Another possible explanation to equal plasma levels of Mg between the study groups is that the bioavailability of Mg supplementation could be changed during pregnancy, and plasma Mg level is in fact a poor indicator of the total body magnesium content and availability. To our knowledge, studies on the bioavailability of multivitamin tablets during pregnancy have not been performed, and hence the possible impact on the results of such intake is unknown. Unfortunately, approximately 1/3 declined to leave blood samples in pregnancy week 35, most likely because the women had to pay an extra visit to the laboratory at a nearby hospital. To conclude, results from our study on Mg supplementation should be interpreted with caution.

Among secondary outcomes, there were statistical differences regarding gestational length and modes of delivery. These results should also be interpreted with caution given the small number of cases in our study, especially as our results are not confirmed by earlier studies summarized in the Cochrane review by Makrides [23]. There were no differences in fetal outcomes, indicating that Mg supplementation seems to be safe for the fetus. However, it would have been a strength to have also measured umbilical levels of Mg, as more studies are needed on possible effects in infants.

The strength of this study is that it is a randomized double-blind placebo-controlled trial that was completely blinded for the study group as well, since the randomization was performed by the manufacturing company and kept secret until onset of data collection. According to baseline data, the study groups were equivalent, with no statistical differences between groups (Table 1). The study protocol was followed correctly, the primary and secondary aims are clearly defined, and power calculation was performed. The number of dropouts was in line with power calculations (11%). The causes of dropout were registered and mainly linked to side effects. The study group was completely independent from the manufacturing company and had no conflicts of interest. Another important strength of the study is that Mg citrate was used for supplementation, with proven good bioavailability [35].

Finally, it must be underlined that research on the prevention of HT disorders during pregnancy is mainly focused on risk pregnancies. For instance, aspirin is only

TABLE 3: Labour and fetal outcomes. Missing results are due to labour at other hospitals and no access to medical records (PP).

Variable	Magnesium ($n = 83$)	Placebo ($n = 93$)	p value
Gestational length at birth	40.2 (2.0)	39.9 (1.5)	**0.03**
	40.7 (29.3; 42.4)	40.1 (35.0; 42.4)	
	$n = 80$	$n = 89$	
Premature labour (<37+0 weeks)	5 (6.3%)	3 (3.4%)	0.60
Duration of labour (active labour in hours)	7.27 (3.81)	7.07 (3.60)	0.85
	7.00 (1.00; 18.00)	7.00 (1.00; 17.00)	
	$n = 63$	$n = 74$	
Mode of delivery			
Emergency Cesarean Section	14 (17.9%)	7 (8.1%)	0.10
Elective Cesarean Section	1 (1.3%)	5 (5.8%)	0.26
Normal vaginal delivery	59 (75.6%)	62 (72.1%)	0.76
Vacuum extraction	4 (5.1%)	12 (14.0%)	0.10
Blood loss, mL	499.7 (351.5)	518 (347)	0.48
	400.0 (50.0; 2200.0)	425 (150; 2000)	
	$n = 78$	$n = 86$	
Birth weight (g)	3482 (597)	3511 (454)	0.99
	3570 (1335; 4594)	3575 (2540; 4860)	
	$n = 79$	$n = 86$	
Apgar score at 5 minutes	9.73 (0.80)	9.73 (0.64)	0.72
	10.00 (5.00; 10.00)	10.00 (7.00; 10.00)	
	$n = 78$	$n = 86$	
Umbilical arterial pH	7.25 (0.08)	7.25 (0.09)	0.92
	7.27 (7.08; 7.45)	7.26 (7.03; 7.43)	
	$n = 72$	$n = 80$	
NICU care			
0 (no)	62 (80.5%)	76 (88.4%)	
1 (yes)	15 (19.5%)	10 (11.6%)	0.24

For categorical variables, n (%) is presented.
For continuous variables, mean (SD)/median (min; max)/n is presented.
For comparison between groups, Fisher's exact test (lowest 1-sided p value multiplied by 2) was used for dichotomous variables and Chi-square test was used for nonordered categorical variables and the Mann–Whitney U test was used for continuous variables.

recommended to pregnant women at risk of developing PE or intrauterine growth restriction (IUGR). Results from our studies on Mg supplementation suggest that pregnant women with risk factors for developing hypertension disorders could benefit from extra Mg intake but are less likely to benefit if they have no risk factors. It is consequently reasonable to suggest that pregnant women at risk to a greater extent have Mg deficiency.

proven to be effective in preventing BP increase among healthy nulliparous women. Interestingly, however, Mg-treated women who had an increase in plasma levels of Mg in fact had a prevention of SBP inrease. It is possible and even likely that women at risk of developing gestational HT or being Mg-deficient could benefit from Mg supplementation. Further studies are needed.

7. Conclusion

Mg supplementation during pregnancy seems to be safe for mother and infant and is inexpensive but is yet not

Disclosure

The authors alone are responsible for the content and writing of the article.

TABLE 4: Blood levels of Mg, CRP, calcium, albumin, uric acid, cystatin C, IL-6, creatinine, and glomerular filtration rate (GFR) at gestational weeks 12 and 35 and change in levels (Δ) from week 12 to week 35 (PP).

Variable	Magnesium ($n = 83$)	Placebo ($n = 93$)	p value
Mg 12 Reference interval 0,71–0,94 mmol/L	0.78 (0.06)/0.78 (0.66; 0.92) $n = 82$	0.77 (0.04)/0.78 (0.68; 0.87) $n = 90$	0.30
Mg 35	0.75 (0.06)/0.76 (0.63; 0.90) $n = 56$	0.73 (0.05)/0.73 (0.62; 0.86) $n = 69$	0.08
Δ Mg 12–35	-0.04 (0.05)/-0.05 (-0.16; 0.08) $n = 56$	-0.04 (0.06)/-0.04 (-0.21; 0.06) $n = 67$	0.72
CRP 12	5.45 (4.80)/4.00 (2.00; 26.00) $n = 82$	4.70 (3.88)/3.00 (2.00; 23.00) $n = 90$	0.26
CRP 35	5.98 (5.14)/4.00 (2.00; 28.00) $n = 55$	5.38 (4.14)/4.00 (2.00; 25.00) $n = 69$	0.74
Δ CRP 12–35	0.62 (5.52)/0.00 (-11.00; 25.00) $n = 55$	0.82 (4.50)/0.00 (-21.00; 20.00) $n = 67$	0.27
Calcium 12	2.32 (0.08)/2.31 (2.12; 2.54) $n = 81$	2.31 (0.08)/2.31 (2.08; 2.58) $n = 90$	0.52
Calcium 35	2.29 (0.10)/2.30 (2.08; 2.51) $n = 55$	2.28 (0.08)/2.27 (2.11; 2.46) $n = 69$	0.32
Δ calcium 12–35	-0.02 (0.11)/0.01 (-0.26; 0.24) $n = 54$	-0.03 (0.12)/-0.04 (-0.26; 0.25) $n = 68$	0.44
Albumin 12	37.6 (2.7)/38.0 (30.0; 44.0) $n = 80$	37.4 (2.5)/37.0 (31.0; 43.0) $n = 89$	0.42
Albumin 35	30.8 (2.2)/31.0 (25.0; 36.0) $n = 55$	30.8 (2.3)/31.0 (26.0; 37.0) $n = 69$	0.73
Δ albumin 12-35	-7.00 (2.85)/-7.00 (-13.00; 1.00) $n = 54$	-6.69 (3.03)/-6.00 (-13.00; 2.00) $n = 67$	0.49
Uric acid 12	199.6 (40.2)/200.0 (103.0; 320.0) $n = 80$	198.4 (39.9)/ 198.0 (99.0; 286.0) $n = 91$	0.96
Uric acid 35	266.7 (66.8)/265.0 (140.0; 460.0) $n = 56$	276.5 (63.0)/271.0 (153.0; 490.0) $n = 67$	0.36
Δ Uric acid 12–35	70.7 (54.5)/71.0 (-34.0; 219.0) $n = 55$	78.5 (49.8)/73.5 (-40.0; 232.0) $n = 66$	0.35
Cystatin C 12	0.596 (0.10)/0.59 (0.36; 0.85) $n = 77$	0.580 (0.10)/0.56 (0.40; 0.89) $n = 81$	0.19
Cystatin C 35	0.99 (0.19)/0.97 (0.62; 1.51) $n = 51$	1.05 (0.31)/1.02 (0.64; 2.61) $n = 59$	0.34
Δ C 12–35	0.41 (0.18)/0.40 (0.16; 1.03) $n = 47$	0.47 (0.29)/0.42 (0.01; 1.74) $n = 51$	0.31
IL-6 12	6.72 (8.48)/3.60 (0.70; 50.00) $n = 79$	7.76 (11.30)/4.65 (0.50; 96.00) $n = 88$	0.33
IL-6 35	11.7 (10.0)/8.3 (1.9; 55.0) $n = 51$	12.7 (10.6)/9.7 (2.9; 73.0) $n = 67$	0.32
Δ IL-6 12–35	5.97 (8.92)/4.05 (-7.00; 36.10) $n = 48$	4.72 (14.67)/4.50 (-79.00; 52.00) $n = 63$	0.80
Creatinine 12	50.8 (6.7)/51.0 (39.0; 76.0) $n = 82$	50.3 (8.0)/49.0 (34.0; 82.0) $n = 91$	0.58

TABLE 4: Continued.

Creatinine 35	50.6 (7.4)/52.0 (35.0; 69.0)	49.9 (9.1)/48.0 (36.0; 95.0)	0.33
	$n = 56$	$n = 69$	
Variable	Magnesium ($n = 83$)	Placebo ($n = 93$)	p value
Δ creatinine 12–35	-0.59 (6.77)/-1.000 (-22.0;24.0) $n = 56$	-1.03 (6.55)/-1.00 (-15.00; 24.00) $n = 68$	0.55
GFR 12	177.2 (46.7)/171.5 (101.0; 345.0) $n = 78$	182.1 (43.7)/185.5 (94.0; 299.0) $n = 80$	0.24
GFR 35	86.3 (21.7)/84.0 (44.0; 138.0) $n = 52$	82.1 (24.8)/78.0 (20.0; 151.0) $n = 59$	0.26
Δ GFR 12–35	-95.6 (45.4)/-84.0 (-229.0; -27.0) $n = 49$	-97.9 (35.1)/-97.5 (-168.0; -15.0) $n = 50$	0.29

For continuous variables, mean (SD)/median (min; max)/n is presented.
For comparison between groups, the Mann–Whitney U test was used for continuous variables.

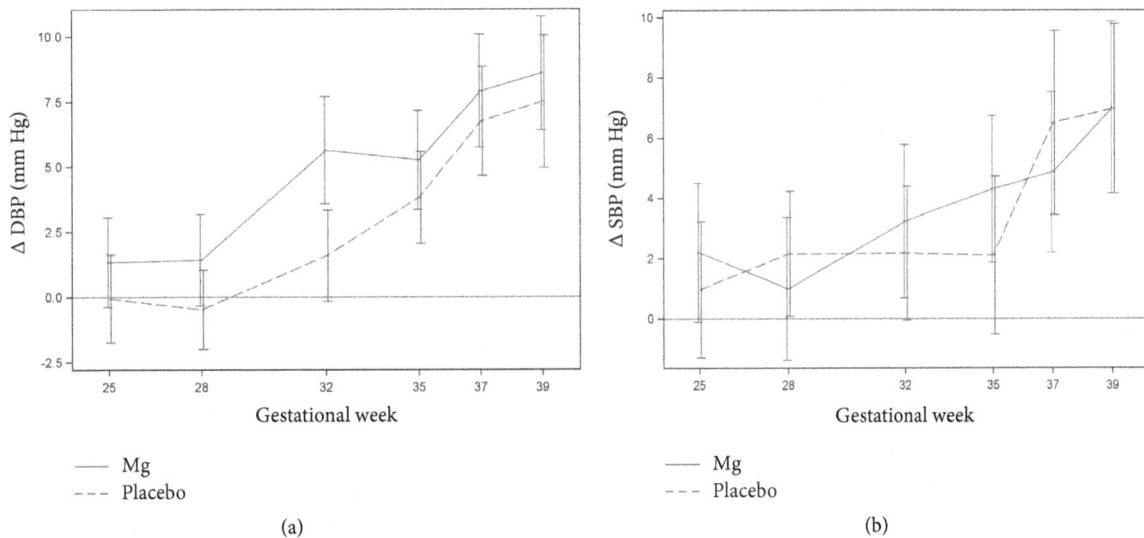

FIGURE 1: (a) Change (Δ) in DBP during pregnancy (PP). (b) Change (Δ) in SBP during pregnancy (PP).

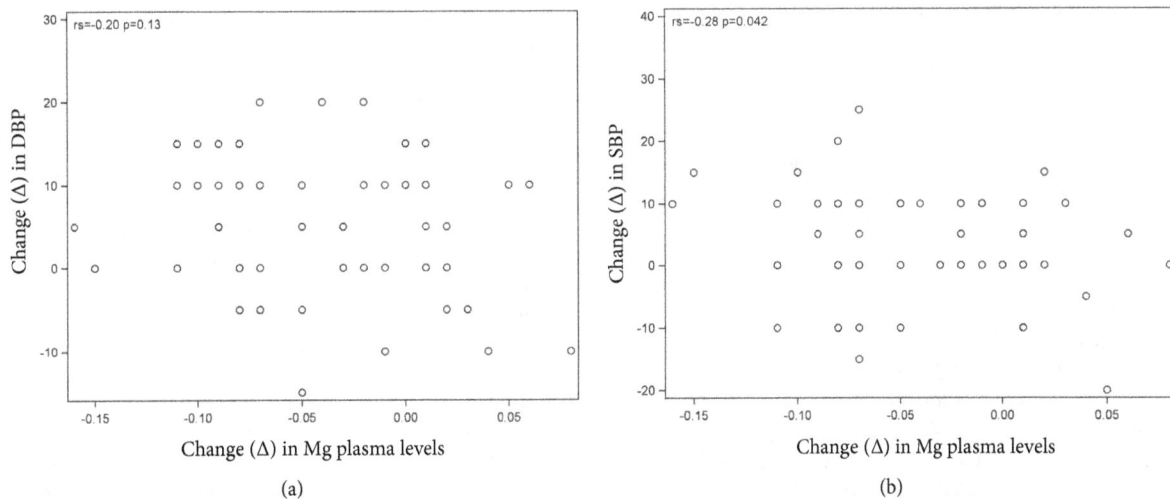

FIGURE 2: (a) Mg group. Spearman's correlation between change in DBP from week 12 to week 35 and change in Mg plasma levels from week 12 to week 35. (b) Mg group. Spearman's correlation between change in SBP from week 12 to week 35 and change in Mg plasma levels from week 12 to week 35.

Conflicts of Interest

The authors report no conflicts of interest.

Authors' Contributions

Maria Bullarbo and Thorkild F. Nielsen contributed to study design, planning, and data analysis; Maria Bullarbo, Helena Mattson, Anna-Karin Broman, and Natalia Ödman contributed to study conduct; Maria Bullarbo and Thorkild F. Nielsen contributed to manuscript writing.

Acknowledgments

The study was supported by grants from the Research and Development Foundation at Region Halland and Södra Älvsborg. Thanks are due to Protina GmbH, Ismaning/Munich, Germany, for the distribution of study agents and randomization procedure. Special thanks are due to Nils-Gunnar and Anders Pehrsson for statistical help.

References

[1] E. J. Roccella, "Report of the national high blood pressure education program working group on high blood pressure in pregnancy," *American Journal of Obstetrics & Gynecology*, vol. 183, no. 1, pp. S1–S22, 2000.

[2] C. Antza, R. Cifkova, and V. Kotsis, "Hypertensive complications of pregnancy: a clinical overview," *Metabolism*, 2017.

[3] J. M. Roberts and C. A. Hubel, "The two stage model of preeclampsia: variations on the theme," *Placenta*, vol. 30, Suppl A, pp. S32–S37, 2009.

[4] B. C. Young, R. J. Levine, and S. A. Karumanchi, "Pathogenesis of preeclampsia," *Annual Review of Pathology: Mechanisms of Disease*, vol. 5, pp. 173–192, 2010.

[5] C. V. Redman and I. L. Sargent, "Pre-eclampsia, the placenta and the maternal systemic inflammatory response - a review," *Placenta*, vol. 24, pp. S21–S27, 2003.

[6] U. D. Anderson, M. G. Olsson, K. H. Kristensen, B. Åkerström, and S. R. Hansson, "Review: biochemical markers to predict preeclampsia," *Placenta*, vol. 33, pp. S42–S47, 2012.

[7] J. P. Xiao, Y. X. Yin, Y. F. Gao et al., "The increased maternal serum levels of IL-6 are associated with the severity and onset of preeclampsia," *Cytokine*, vol. 60, no. 3, pp. 856–860, 2012.

[8] K. Kristensen, D. Wide-Swensson, C. Schmidt et al., "Cystatin C, β-2-microglobulin and β-trace protein in pre-eclampsia," *Acta Obstetricia et Gynecologica Scandinavica*, vol. 86, no. 8, pp. 921–926, 2007.

[9] K. Kristensen, I. Larsson, and S. R. Hansson, "Increased cystatin C expression in the pre-eclamptic placenta.," *Molecular Human Reproduction*, vol. 13, no. 3, pp. 189–195, 2007.

[10] D. Cemgil Arikan, M. Aral, A. Coskun, and A. Ozer, "Plasma IL-4, IL-8, IL-12, interferon-γ and CRP levels in pregnant women with preeclampsia, and their relation with severity of

disease and fetal birth weight," *The Journal of Maternal-Fetal and Neonatal Medicine*, vol. 25, no. 9, pp. 1569–1573, 2012.

[11] L. C. Chappell, P. T. Seed, A. L. Briley et al., "Effect of antioxidants on the occurrence of pre-eclampsia in women at increased risk: a randomised trial," *The Lancet*, vol. 354, no. 9181, pp. 810–816, 1999.

[12] L. M. Bodnar, G. Tang, R. B. Ness, G. Harger, and J. M. Roberts, "Periconceptional multivitamin use reduces the risk of preeclampsia," *American Journal of Epidemiology*, vol. 164, no. 5, pp. 470–477, 2006.

[13] L. M. Bodnar, J. M. Catov, H. N. Simhan, M. F. Holick, R. W. Powers, and J. M. Roberts, "Maternal vitamin D deficiency increases the risk of preeclampsia," *The Journal of Clinical Endocrinology & Metabolism*, vol. 92, no. 9, pp. 3517–3522, 2007.

[14] J. M. Purswani, P. Gala, P. Dwarkanath, H. M. Larkin, A. Kurpad, and S. Mehta, "The role of vitamin D in pre-eclampsia: A systematic review," *BMC Pregnancy and Childbirth*, vol. 17, p. 231, 2017.

[15] S. W. Wen, X.-K. Chen, M. Rodger et al., "Folic acid supplementation in early second trimester and the risk of preeclampsia," *American Journal of Obstetrics & Gynecology*, vol. 198, no. 1, pp. 45.e1–45.e7, 2008.

[16] D. L. Rolnik, D. Wright, L. C. Poon et al., "Aspirin versus Placebo in Pregnancies at High Risk for Preterm Preeclampsia," *The New England Journal of Medicine*, vol. 377, no. 7, pp. 613–622, 2017.

[17] M. C. Tolcher, D. M. Chu, L. M. Hollier et al., "Impact of USP-STF recommendations for aspirin for prevention of recurrent preeclampsia," *American Journal of Obstetrics & Gynecology*, vol. 217, no. 3, pp. 365.e1–365.e8, 2017.

[18] S. Roberge, K. Nicolaides, S. Demers, J. Hyett, N. Chaillet, and E. Bujold, "The role of aspirin dose on the prevention of preeclampsia and fetal growth restriction: systematic review and meta-analysis," *American Journal of Obstetrics & Gynecology*, vol. 216, no. 2, pp. 110–120.e6, 2017.

[19] O. Osikoya, P. A. Jaini, A. Nguyen, M. Valdes, and S. Goulopoulou, "Effects of low-dose aspirin on maternal blood pressure and vascular function in an experimental model of gestational hypertension," *Pharmacological Research*, vol. 120, pp. 267–278, 2017.

[20] W. Zhang, H. Iso, T. Ohira, C. Date, and A. Tamakoshi, "Associations of dietary magnesium intake with mortality from cardiovascular disease: The JACC study," *Atherosclerosis*, vol. 221, no. 2, pp. 587–595, 2012.

[21] PJ. Porr, M. Nechifor, and J. Durlach, "Advances in magnesium research," *John Libbey Eurotext*, pp. 1–206, 2006.

[22] L. Kass, J. Weekes, and L. Carpenter, "Effect of magnesium supplementation on blood pressure: A meta-analysis," *European Journal of Clinical Nutrition*, vol. 66, no. 4, pp. 411–418, 2012.

[23] M. Makrides, D. D. Crosby, E. Bain, and C. A. Crowther, "Magnesium supplementation in pregnancy," *Cochrane Database of Systematic Reviews*, vol. 4, Article ID CD000937, 2014.

[24] N. O. Enaruna, A. Ande, and E. E. Okpere, "Clinical significance of low serum magnesium in pregnant women attending the University of Benin Teaching Hospital," *Nigerian Journal of Clinical Practice*, vol. 16, no. 4, pp. 448-53, 2013.

[25] T. F. Nielsen and R. Rylander, "Urinary calcium and magnesium excretion relates to increase in blood pressure during pregnancy," *Archives of Gynecology and Obstetrics*, vol. 283, no. 3, pp. 443–447, 2011.

[26] M. Bullarbo, N. Ödman, A. Nestler et al., "Magnesium supplementation to prevent high blood pressure in pregnancy: A

randomised placebo control trial," *Archives of Gynecology and Obstetrics*, vol. 288, no. 6, pp. 1269–1274, 2013.

[27] A. Nestler, R. Rylander, M. Kolisek et al., "Blood pressure in pregnancy and magnesium sensitive genes," *Pregnancy Hypertension: An International Journal of Women's Cardiovascular Health*, vol. 4, no. 1, pp. 41–45, 2014.

[28] R. Rylander, "Magnesium in pregnancy blood pressure and pre-eclampsia - A review," *Pregnancy Hypertension: An International Journal of Women's Cardiovascular Health*, vol. 4, no. 2, pp. 146–149, 2014.

[29] M. Bullarbo and R. Rylander, "Diastolic blood pressure increase is a risk indicator for pre-eclampsia," *Archives of Gynecology and Obstetrics*, vol. 291, no. 4, pp. 819–823, 2015.

[30] S. M. Khedun, D. Ngotho, J. Moodley, and T. Naicker, "Plasma and red cell magnesium levels in black African women with hypertensive disorders of pregnancy," *Hypertension in Pregnancy*, vol. 17, no. 2, pp. 125–134, 1998.

[31] D. Schoenaker, S. S. Soedamah-Muthu, and G. D. Mishra, "The association between dietary factors and gestational hypertension and pre-eclampsia: A systematic review and meta-analysis of observational studies," *BMC Medicine*, vol. 12, pp. 157–174, 2014.

[32] L. Spätling, H. G. Classen, K. Kisters et al., "Supplementation of magnesium in pregnancy," *Journal of Pregnancy and Child Health*, vol. 04, no. 01, 2017.

[33] Y. Ismail, A. A. Ismail, and A. A. A. Ismail, "The underestimated problem of using serum magnesium measurements to exclude magnesium deficiency in adults; A health warning is needed for "normal" results," *Clinical Chemistry and Laboratory Medicine*, vol. 48, no. 3, pp. 323–327, 2010.

[34] B. M. Sibai, M. A. Villar, and E. Bray, "Magnesium supplementation during pregnancy: A double-blind randomized controlled clinical trial," *American Journal of Obstetrics & Gynecology*, vol. 161, no. 1, pp. 115–119, 1989.

[35] R. Rylander, "Bioavailability of magnesium salts - A review," *Journal of Pharmacy and Nutrition Sciences*, vol. 4, no. 1, pp. 57–59, 2014.

22

Predictors of Gestational Weight Gain among White and Latina Women and Associations with Birth Weight

Milagros C. Rosal,[1] Monica L. Wang,[2,3] Tiffany A. Moore Simas,[1] Jamie S. Bodenlos,[4] Sybil L. Crawford,[1] Katherine Leung,[1] and Heather Z. Sankey[5]

[1]Department of Medicine, Division of Preventive and Behavioral Medicine, University of Massachusetts Medical School, 55 Lake Avenue North, Worcester, MA 01655, USA
[2]Boston University School of Public Health, 801 Massachusetts Avenue, Boston, MA 02215, USA
[3]Harvard School of Public Health, 677 Huntington Avenue, Boston, MA 02215, USA
[4]Department of Psychology, Hobart and William Smith Colleges, 217 Gulick Hall, Geneva, NY 14456, USA
[5]Department of Obstetrics and Gynecology, Baystate Medical Center, 759 Chestnut Street, Springfield, MA 01199, USA

Correspondence should be addressed to Milagros C. Rosal; milagros.rosal@umassmed.edu

Academic Editor: Debbie Smith

This study examined racial/ethnic differences in gestational weight gain (GWG) predictors and association of first-trimester GWG to overall GWG among 271 White women and 300 Latina women. Rates of within-guideline GWG were higher among Latinas than among Whites (28.7% versus 24.4%, $p < 0.016$). Adjusted odds of above-guideline GWG were higher among prepregnancy overweight (OR = 3.4, CI = 1.8–6.5) and obese (OR = 4.5, CI = 2.3–9.0) women than among healthy weight women and among women with above-guideline first-trimester GWG than among those with within-guideline first-trimester GWG (OR = 4.9, CI = 2.8–8.8). GWG was positively associated with neonate birth size ($p < 0.001$). Interventions targeting prepregnancy overweight or obese women and those with excessive first-trimester GWG are needed.

1. Introduction

Significant evidence ties gestational weight gain (GWG) to short- and long-term maternal and infant outcomes. To optimize maternal and child health, the Institute of Medicine (IOM) provides guidelines for GWG based on prepregnancy body mass index (BMI) [1]. Greater GWG is recommended for women with prepregnancy BMIs in the underweight (28–40 pounds (lbs), 12.7–18.1 kg) or healthy weight (25–35 lbs, 11.3–15.9 kg) range, with less GWG recommended for prepregnancy overweight (15–25 lbs, 6.8–11.3 kg) and obese (11–20 lbs, 5.0–9.1 kg) women. However, only 22 to 40% of women attain GWG within the recommended ranges [2–8], and women of lower socioeconomic status and racial/ethnic minority women have lower adherence to GWG guidelines [5, 9–11]. Among Latina women and depending on national origin, estimates of excessive GWG range from 36 to 51%, whereas estimates of insufficient GWG range from 17 to 30% [7, 9, 10, 12, 13].

Socioeconomic and racial/ethnic disparities in achieving recommended GWG are further compounded by higher pregnancy rates and greater odds of adverse birth-related outcomes among socioeconomically disadvantaged and racial/ethnic minority populations than their more affluent and White counterparts. The pregnancy rate of Latina women in the US is estimated to be two-thirds higher than that of non-Latino Whites [14]. Within the Latina population, nearly half of Caribbean Latina women experience GWG above IOM guidelines [9], and Puerto Rican Latinas are among women with the highest rates of low birth weight neonates [15] and preterm births [16], both predictors of infant mortality [17]. However, little is known about why adherence to guidelines is low among this population. Identifying and understanding factors driving racial/ethnic differences in

GWG are a priority to target maternal and child health disparities in this growing and at-risk population.

Given the numerous adverse health consequences of excessive and insufficient GWG for the mother and the offspring [1, 4, 18–21], understanding the risk factors for low adherence to IOM-recommended GWG and intervening in at-risk groups are of utmost importance. In targeting interventions, timing of GWG may be important. However, little is known about the influence of early GWG (e.g., first trimester) on overall GWG and other maternal and infant outcomes. A prospective study of a predominantly White female sample indicated that maternal weight change in the first trimester was a stronger predictor of birth weight than weight change in the second or third trimester [22]. However, research on early GWG among Latina women is lacking. The timing and extent of GWG may also be an important determinant of birth weight as well as other maternal and prenatal outcomes; thus, early identification of women who are at risk of excessive or inadequate GWG may be critical to guide the timing and content for intervention delivery to maximize maternal and prenatal health and reduce health disparities.

To address gaps in the literature, this study aimed to examine differences in predictors of gestational weight gain (GWG), assess the association of first-trimester GWG to overall GWG between non-Latina White and Latina women, and examine GWG status with birth outcomes. We hypothesized that women who were overweight or obese before pregnancy would have higher odds of GWG outside of IOM recommendations and that first-trimester GWG status (below, within, or above guideline) would positively correlate with overall GWG.

2. Methods

2.1. Participants and Setting. The study's targeted population included non-Latina White and Latina women who received prenatal care from private providers and hospital clinics (i.e., a resident clinic and a midwifery clinic). The study was conducted at Baystate Medical Center, a large tertiary care facility in western Massachusetts with an average of 4,300 deliveries each year, approximately 57% of them to Latina women (primarily of Puerto Rican origin).

2.2. Procedures. Identification of participants included two screening steps. First, electronic medical record database searches were performed for a retrospective cohort of women who had live deliveries (preterm or full-term) at the medical center from September 1, 2005, to August 31, 2006. Women with multifetal pregnancies, unknown ethnicity, and primary language other than English or Spanish were excluded. A total of 3,966 (of 4,300) patient records met these criteria. Based on estimates of adherence to IOM guidelines in other samples, a sample size of at least 400 women was required for adequate power analysis for the current study. Thus, the second screening step consisted of randomly selecting one quarter ($n = 1,016$) of eligible patient records, stratified by ethnicity (non-Latina White and Latina) and site of prenatal care (hospital clinics and private providers), for

additional participant eligibility screening via paper medical chart review. A total of 445 records were excluded. Reasons for exclusion included missing data on prepregnancy weight ($n = 226$) or height ($n = 4$), missing dates of prenatal measurements ($n = 138$), no documentation of prenatal visits in the first trimester of pregnancy ($n = 296$), maternal history of gastric bypass ($n = 2$), or maternal diagnosis of pregestational diabetes ($n = 31$). Of excluded records, 60% were excluded for one criterion and 40% were excluded for two or more criteria.

A scannable medical record abstraction form was developed by the research team. The form included fields for recording participant demographics (date of birth, race/ethnicity, primary language, marital status, insurance type, parity, and employment status), psychiatric history (i.e., documented psychiatric diagnosis or use of psychiatric medication), height, and dates and measured weights at each prenatal visit. Three research assistants were trained in the process of data abstraction from paper medical records until 100% interrater reliability was achieved. Data from completed and cross-checked abstraction forms were scanned and were uploaded into a SAS database.

Data abstraction was performed from 2007 to 2008. During this time frame, revisions of IOM's GWG guidelines were anticipated and were available following data cleaning procedures and at the time of analyses. Thus, the investigative team decided *a priori* to utilize 2009 guidelines [1] in categorizing GWG measures (described below) with the goal of providing an estimate of likely nonadherence to new recommendations and associated outcomes. Additionally, the 2009 guidelines did not differ greatly from former guidelines yet offered the benefit of a recommended range of gain for obese women in contrast to the previously stated "at least 15 pounds (6.8 kg)" without an upper bound [17]. All study protocols and procedures were approved by the Baystate Medical Center Institutional Review Board and the University of Massachusetts Medical School Institutional Review Board.

2.3. GWG Measures. Height and prepregnancy weight were obtained from prenatal forms in participants' medical records. Customarily, height is measured by obstetric provider office staff and prepregnancy weight is self-reported by pregnant women at their first prenatal appointment. Prepregnancy BMI was calculated as weight (kg)/height squared (in meters) and categorized as follows: underweight (BMI < 18.5 kg/m^2); healthy weight ($18.5 \text{ kg/m}^2 \leq \text{BMI} < 25 \text{ kg/m}^2$); overweight ($25 \text{ kg/m}^2 \leq \text{BMI} < 30 \text{ kg/m}^2$); and obese ($30 \text{ kg/m}^2 \leq \text{BMI}$) [17, 23].

Gestational weight measures were routinely obtained by clinical staff as part of standard obstetric care appointments, as is customary. At each visit, women are weighed and their weight is recorded in prenatal health records, along with gestational age. Each participant's GWG status was determined based on prepregnancy BMI, gestational age, and weight gain at the time of the weight measure. For each prepregnancy weight status category, IOM-recommended trajectories of weight gain were defined (1) in terms of minimum and maximum total weight gain at week 13 (end of first trimester) and (2) for subsequent weeks in terms of minimum and maximum weight gain per week. Thus, for each week of gestational age, a minimum and maximum recommended weight gain were calculated.

First-trimester GWG status was determined using the last weight measure recorded during the first trimester. GWG status in the first trimester was assessed by comparing first-trimester GWG (calculated by subtracting pregravid weight from weight at the last first-trimester prenatal visit) to the IOM-recommended GWG range for gestational age at the last first-trimester prenatal visit. Similarly, GWG status at delivery was determined using weight measured from the last recorded prenatal appointment and was assessed by comparing total GWG (calculated by subtracting pregravid weight from weight at the last prenatal visit prior to delivery) to the IOM-recommended GWG range for gestational age at the last prenatal visit (the average period between the last prenatal visit and delivery is estimated at 6.6 days) [24]. GWG status was categorized as follows: inadequate or "below" if weight gain for gestational age was below the lowest value of the recommended range; appropriate or "within" if weight gain for gestational age was between the recommended range lowest and highest values; and excessive or "above" if weight gain for gestational age was above the highest value of the recommended range.

2.4. Outcome Measures. Gestational age at delivery was calculated based on best dates for estimated date of confinement (EDC). EDC is determined as per clinician evaluation considering concordance of the last menstrual period and first-trimester ultrasound [25] and documented on the medical record based on clinical care standards. Pregnancies delivered at < 37 weeks were categorized as preterm and those delivered at ≥ 37 weeks were full term. Neonate birth weight recorded by nursing staff at the time of delivery was abstracted from the inpatient record. Neonates were categorized as small for gestational age (SGA) and large for gestational age (LGA) if birth weight was <10th and ≥90th percentile, respectively, of 1999-2000 US national reference data for singleton gestations, accounting for gestational age and gender [26, 27]. Regardless of gestational age, low birth weight (LBW) was defined as < 2,500 grams [28] and high birth weight (HBW) or macrosomia as ≥ 4,000 grams [26].

2.5. Statistical Analysis. Descriptive statistics of the study sample stratified by ethnicity were conducted using Chi-square tests or Fisher Exact tests for categorical variables and t-tests for continuous variables. Estimated means and standard errors for total GWG were computed for each ethnic group and by prepregnancy weight status category within ethnic group, adjusting for gestational age at the last prenatal visit. Unadjusted associations of GWG status (below, within, or above IOM-recommended range) with participant characteristics were estimated using contingency tables and Chi-square tests. Adjusted associations of GWG status with participant characteristics were estimated using multinomial logistic regression models (within GWG guidelines as the outcome reference category) to allow for the possibility of

associations that violated the proportional odds assumption (e.g., a positive association with both above and below GWG guidelines).

Potential effect modification by ethnicity was examined by stratifying contingency tables of GWG status with participant characteristics by ethnicity and by including interaction terms of ethnicity with other predictors in logistic regression models. Model fit was assessed using the Hosmer-Lemeshow goodness-of-fit Chi-square statistic [29]. Infant outcomes were compared by GWG status for the entire group and by ethnicity using contingency tables, Chi-square tests, and logistic regression. Supplemental analyses included conducting backward elimination in the logistic regression analyses to assess whether results were similar after omitting irrelevant or redundant predictors and performing sensitivity analysis comparing results based on the 1990 IOM GWG guidelines versus the 2009 IOM GWG guidelines.

3. Results

The final analytic sample included 571 participants (47% White and 53% Latina). The majority of participants were single (64%) and unemployed (53%) and had public health insurance (64%) (Table 1). Less than half (46%) of women had prepregnancy BMIs within the healthy weight range, a quarter were obese, and more than half (58%) exceeded GWG recommendations at the time of delivery. Compared to White women, Latina women were younger and more likely to be single and unemployed, have public insurance, and have higher parity (p values < 0.05). White women had higher prevalence of documented tobacco and alcohol use, were more likely to have a documented psychiatric history, and were more likely to deliver LGA neonates than Latina women (p values < 0.05). No other differences by ethnicity were observed. A comparison by prenatal care site revealed that women receiving care in hospital clinics were more likely to be younger, unmarried, unemployed, and nulliparous, have public insurance, have a psychiatric history, and have lower levels of education than those receiving care in private clinics (p values < 0.01).

Average GWG adjusted for gestational age at delivery was 36.3 lbs (SE = 0.92) (16.5 kg (SE = 0.42)) for White women and 32.4 lbs (SE = 0.88) (14.7 kg (SE = 0.36)) for Latina women (p < 0.0001). Average GWG by prepregnancy weight status category were as follows: 37.9 lbs (SE = 2.3) (17.48 kg (SE = 1.0)) for underweight participants; 36.7 lbs (SE = 0.9) (16.6 kg (SE = 0.4)) for healthy weight participants; 35.3 lbs (SE = 1.2) (35.3 kg (SE = 0.5)) for overweight participants; and 28.0 lbs (SE = 1.2) (12.7 kg (SE = 0.5)) for obese participants. Across prepregnancy weight status categories, adherence to IOM GWG recommendations was poor among both ethnic groups, with only 27% gaining within recommended ranges. Ethnic differences in GWG status at time of delivery for the overall sample were observed, with Latina women less likely to gain in excess than White women (p = 0.016) (Figure 1). Latina women were more likely to gain within the IOM-recommended range than White women across all prepregnancy weight status categories, with the exception of the underweight category (among underweight participants,

TABLE 1: Sample characteristics of overall study sample and by ethnicity ($N = 571$).

Sample characteristics	All women (n = 571)		White non-Latina (n = 271)		Latina (n = 300)		p value
	N	%	N	%	N	%	
	Mean	SD	Mean	SD	Mean	SD	
Demographic factors							
Age category, N (%)							
Age 15–19	127	22.24	39	14.39	88	29.33	<0.001
Age 20–24	155	27.15	64	23.62	91	30.33	
Age 25–29	133	23.29	67	24.72	66	22.00	
Age 30–34	100	17.51	62	22.88	38	12.67	
Age ≥ 35	56	9.81	39	14.39	17	5.67	
Mean (SD)	25.35	6.40	27.09	6.52	23.79	5.88	<0.001
Marital status, N (%)							
Divorced	8	1.41	6	2.21	2	0.67	<0.001
Married	199	35.04	129	47.60	70	23.57	
Single	361	63.56	136	50.18	225	75.76	
Employment at onset of pregnancy N (%)							
Employed	266	46.83	153	56.67	113	37.92	<0.001
Not employed	302	53.17	117	43.33	185	62.08	
Parity, N (%)							
0	233	42.75	114	44.53	119	41.18	0.003
1	160	29.36	86	33.59	74	25.61	
2	89	16.33	39	15.23	50	17.30	
3 or more	63	11.56	17	6.64	46	15.92	
Behavioral factors							
Alcohol use, N (%)							
No	449	78.91	193	71.22	256	85.91	<0.001
Yes, past	112	19.68	74	27.31	38	12.75	
Yes, this pregnancy	8	1.41	4	1.48	4	1.34	
Tobacco use, N (%)							
No	392	68.89	172	63.47	220	73.83	0.016
Yes, past	67	11.78	34	12.55	33	11.07	
Yes, this pregnancy	110	19.33	65	23.99	45	15.10	
Prepregnancy weight categories (body mass index range), N (%)							
Underweight (BMI ≤ 18.4)	33	5.78	16	5.90	17	5.67	
Normal weight (BMI 18.5–24.9)	260	45.53	133	49.08	127	42.33	0.315
Overweight (BMI 25.0–29.9)	138	24.17	64	23.62	74	24.67	
Obese (BMI ≥ 30.0)	140	24.52	58	21.40	82	27.33	
Prenatal care factors							
Week gestation at the 1st prenatal visit	10.57	3.07	10.53	2.72	10.61	3.36	0.760
Gestational age at the last visit	35.76	5.39	35.68	5.84	35.83	4.96	0.740
Number of prenatal visits	9.78	3.24	9.84	3.36	9.72	3.14	0.656
Gestational age at delivery	38.97	5.87	38.87	6.91	39.06	4.76	0.705
Prenatal care site, N (%)							
Private	272	47.64	137	50.55	135	45.00	0.185
Hospital clinic	299	52.36	134	49.45	165	55.00	

TABLE 1: Continued.

Sample characteristics	All women (n = 571)		White non-Latina (n = 271)		Latina (n = 300)		p value
	N	%	N	%	N	%	
	Mean	SD	Mean	SD	Mean	SD	
Insurance type, N (%)							
Commercial/private	201	35.39	139	51.29	62	20.88	<0.001
No insurance/unknown	4	0.70	4	1.48	0	0.00	
Public	363	63.91	128	47.23	235	79.12	
GWG status with respect to IOM guidelines							
GWG status at the last prenatal visit, N (%)							
Within guidelines	152	26.62	66	24.35	86	28.67	0.016
Below guidelines	90	15.76	33	12.18	57	19.00	
Above guidelines	329	57.62	172	63.47	157	52.33	
GWG status in the 1st trimester, N (%)							
Within guidelines	148	26.43	69	26.24	79	26.60	0.537
Above guidelines	256	45.71	126	47.91	130	43.77	
Below guidelines	156	27.86	68	25.86	88	29.63	
Psychiatric factors							
Psychiatric history, N (%)							
None	445	78.21	203	75.19	242	80.94	0.003
Anxiety	15	2.64	11	4.07	4	1.34	
Depression	86	15.11	38	14.07	48	16.05	
Other	23	4.04	18	6.67	5	1.67	
Psychiatric medications, N (%)							
No	539	94.40	251	92.62	288	96.00	0.080
Yes	32	5.60	20	7.38	12	4.00	
Pregnancy outcomes							
Length of pregnancy, N (%)							
Term delivery	504	88.73	244	90.71	260	86.96	0.158
Preterm delivery	64	11.27	25	9.29	39	13.04	
Birth weight parameters							
SGA	56	10.04	20	7.60	36	12.20	0.012
Normal GA	454	81.36	212	80.61	242	82.03	
LGA	48	8.60	31	11.79	17	5.76	
LBW (<2500 gr)	53	9.45	23	8.68	30	10.14	0.390
Normal BW	456	81.28	213	80.38	243	82.09	
HBW (>4000 gr)	52	9.27	29	10.94	23	7.77	

p values are from Chi-square and t-tests for ethnic differences.

White women were more likely to have GWG within recommended ranges than Latinas) (Figure 2).

Table 2 presents unadjusted associations between demographics, behavioral factors and psychiatric history, and GWG status. GWG status was significantly associated with ethnicity, employment status at pregnancy onset, prepregnancy BMI, and first-trimester GWG (p values < 0.05). In logistic regression models, no effect modification by ethnicity

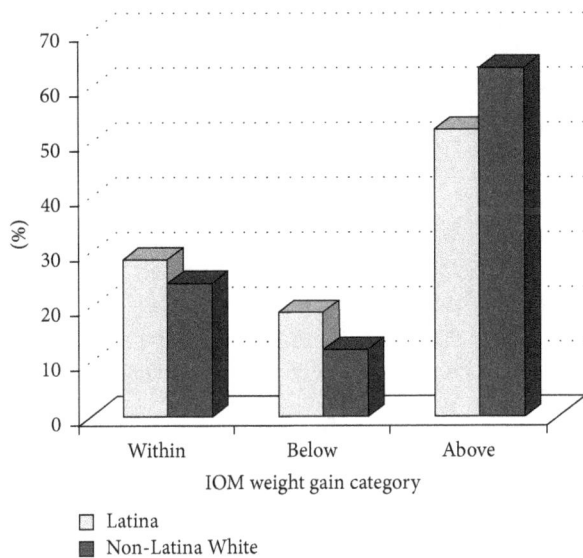

FIGURE 1: Gestational weight gain status among White non-Latina and Latina women.

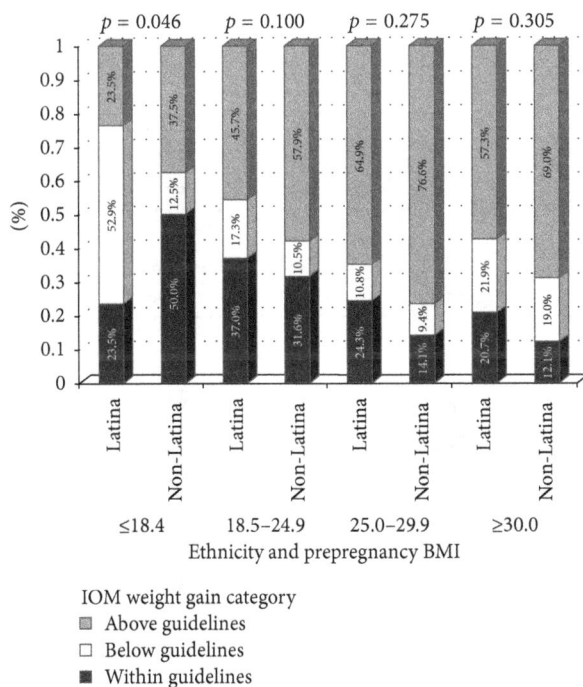

FIGURE 2: Gestational weight gain status by prepregnancy BMI for White non-Latina and Latina women.

was indicated (p values for interaction terms > 0.05); thus, results are presented for the entire sample. Multivariable logistic regression models estimating participant characteristics associated with GWG status at time of delivery (Table 3) indicated that odds of above-guideline GWG at time of delivery were greater among prepregnancy overweight and obese women compared to healthy weight women (OR = 3.4, CI = 1.8–6.5; OR = 4.5, CI = 2.3–9.0, resp.) and among those with first-trimester GWG above guidelines compared

to those with GWG within guidelines (OR = 4.9, CI = 2.8–8.8). Odds of below-guideline GWG at time of delivery were greater among prepregnancy underweight and obese women compared to healthy weight (OR = 5.3, CI = 1.4–20.2; OR = 3.5, CI = 1.4–8.7, resp.) and among women with first-trimester GWG below guidelines compared to within-guideline GWG (OR = 3.0, CI = 1.3–6.8). Odds of below-guideline GWG were lower among women receiving care at hospital clinics compared to those receiving care from a private provider and among past smokers compared to never smokers (OR = 0.3, CI = 0.1–0.9; OR = 0.3, CI = 0.1–1.0, resp.).

A very small number of adverse events were observed within each ethnic group. Thus, Table 4 presents estimates of associations between GWG status and length of pregnancy (preterm versus full-term) and birth weight parameters for the overall sample. GWG status was unrelated to pregnancy length but was associated with birth size (a higher percentage of SGA in pregnancies with below-guideline GWG and a higher percentage of LGA in pregnancies with above-guideline GWG; p values < 0.05). Observed ethnic differences in birth size (Table 1) by which White women were more likely to have LGA neonates and Latina women were more likely to have SGA neonates were not impacted when adjusted for GWG status (data not shown). Supplemental analyses from running more parsimonious models and from sensitivity tests did not yield results that were substantially different from those presented (data not shown).

4. Discussion

Findings from this retrospective cohort study provide insights for identifying women at risk for nonadherence to IOM-recommended GWG and for developing targeted interventions. Above-guideline GWG was greater in this cohort (58%) than in previous studies of multiethnic samples (35%–57% in prior studies) [2–4, 7], suggesting that rates of above-guideline GWG may continue to increase, especially among White women. As noted in other populations [2, 7, 30], prepregnancy weight status predicted GWG in this study. Targeting weight prior to pregnancy is desirable but may be unfeasible for numerous reasons, such as lack of pregnancy intentionality. Targeting weight change during pregnancy may be a more feasible window, as a majority of women seek prenatal care during the first-trimester and are motivated to modify health behaviors [31]. To our knowledge, this is the first study to examine first-trimester GWG status as a predictor of GWG status at time of delivery in a multiethnic sample of women, with first-trimester GWG status predicting overall GWG status among non-Latina White and Latina women. Along with other research [22], study findings indicate that the first trimester of pregnancy may be a critical and feasible window to promote healthy GWG and associated maternal and neonatal outcomes; thus, the identification of women who are at elevated risk for below or above GWG guidelines (e.g., prepregnancy underweight and overweight/obese women) and subsequent delivery of targeted interventions for these subgroups during early prenatal care should be emphasized.

TABLE 2: Univariate associations of demographic, behavioral, and psychological factors and gestational weight gain status based on 2009 IOM recommendations ($N = 571$).

Category	GWG below guidelines		GWG within guidelines		GWG above guidelines		p value
	N	%	N	%	N	%	
Age category							
Age 15–19	26	20.47	26	20.47	75	59.06	0.179
Age 20–24	26	16.77	43	27.74	86	55.48	
Age 25–29	20	15.04	34	25.56	79	59.40	
Age 30–34	14	14.00	35	35.00	51	51.00	
Age ≥ 35	4	7.14	14	25.00	38	67.86	
Ethnicity							
Latina	57	19.00	86	28.67	157	52.33	0.016
White	33	12.18	66	24.35	172	63.47	
Marital status							
Divorced	1	12.50	2	25.00	5	62.50	0.931
Married	29	14.57	57	28.64	113	56.78	
Single	60	16.62	93	25.76	208	57.62	
Employment at onset of pregnancy							
Employed	33	12.41	82	30.83	151	56.77	0.044
Not employed	55	18.21	70	23.18	177	58.61	
Insurance type							
Commercial/private	21	10.45	64	31.84	116	57.71	0.064
No insurance/unknown	1	14.29	2	28.57	4	57.14	
Public	68	18.73	86	23.69	209	57.58	
Obstetric provider							
Private	42	15.44	76	27.94	154	56.62	0.793
Hospital clinic	48	16.05	76	25.42	175	58.53	
Parity							
0	35	15.02	57	24.46	141	60.52	0.913
1	26	16.25	42	26.25	92	57.50	
2	13	14.61	28	31.46	48	53.93	
3 or more	11	17.46	17	26.98	35	55.56	
Prepregnancy BMI							
BMI ≤ 18.4	11	33.33	12	36.36	10	30.30	<0.001
BMI 18.5–24.9	36	13.85	89	34.23	135	51.92	
BMI 25.0–29.9	14	10.14	27	19.57	97	70.29	
BMI ≥ 30.0	29	20.71	24	17.14	87	62.14	
Tobacco use							
No	65	16.58	112	28.57	215	54.85	0.236
Yes, past	8	11.94	18	26.87	41	61.19	
Yes, this pregnancy	17	15.45	21	19.09	72	65.45	
Alcohol use							
No	68	15.14	123	27.39	258	57.46	0.302
Yes, past	21	18.75	23	20.54	68	60.71	
Yes, this pregnancy	1	12.50	4	50.00	3	37.50	
GWG during the 1st trimester							
Above	8	3.13	43	16.80	205	80.08	0.001
Below	61	39.10	53	33.97	42	26.92	
Within	15	10.14	55	37.16	78	52.70	

TABLE 2: Continued.

Category	GWG below guidelines		GWG within guidelines		GWG above guidelines		p value
	N	%	N	%	N	%	
Psychiatric diagnosis							
None	71	15.96	123	27.64	251	56.40	0.955
Depression	13	15.12	21	24.42	52	60.47	
Anxiety	3	20.00	3	20.00	9	60.00	
Other	3	13.04	5	21.74	15	65.22	
Psychiatric medications							
No	86	15.96	143	26.53	310	57.51	0.871
Yes	4	12.50	9	28.13	19	59.38	
Psychiatric history or medications							
No	70	16.55	117	27.66	236	55.79	0.325
Yes	20	13.51	35	23.65	93	62.84	

p value is from a Chi-square test.

For both non-Latina White and Latina women in our study sample, maternal smoking status (previous smoker prior to pregnancy) was associated with lower odds of below-recommended GWG which is consistent with previous research indicating that smoking during pregnancy is related to lower GWG and smoking cessation associated with greater GWG [2, 3, 32, 33]. Between 29% and 70% of women reportedly quit smoking upon becoming pregnant [34]; thus, health care provider attention to smoking history and smoking patterns during pregnancy, with particular focus given to previous or current smokers during early prenatal care, is important to optimize GWG throughout pregnancy.

A larger proportion of SGA infants were born to Latina women than non-Latina White women, with the prevalence of SGA (12.2%) and preterm delivery (13.0%) among Latina women in our sample slightly higher than national estimates for Latina women (9%-10%) [35]. In contrast, a greater proportion of LGA infants were born to White women. We did not find an association between GWG status at time of delivery and pregnancy length as previously found [36]. In addition, we did not find ethnic differences in low or high birth weight, which is in contrast to prior data indicating that Puerto Rican Latinas have some of the highest rates of low birth weight neonates [15] and preterm births [16] in the US. Multiple factors not assessed in this retrospective cohort study (e.g., prior preterm births, gestational diabetes mellitus) may contribute to and account for differences in birth outcomes observed in this study compared to previous studies. In addition, conventional measures of GWG may introduce bias when studying GWG-preterm birth associations [37]. Additional studies with larger, ethnically diverse samples are needed to elucidate predictors driving racial/ethnic disparities in birth weight outcomes.

Study strengths include the sample's ethnic and socioeconomic diversity (i.e., White/Latina women, public/commercial insurance, and hospital clinics/private provider) and

inclusion of women who delivered pre- and full-term (previous studies have been limited to women who delivered full-term) [2, 7]. Although no data were available on place of birth, most Latinos in the region where the study was conducted are of Puerto Rican descent, a largely understudied population with considerable health disparities, including infant mortality [38].

Study limitations include the retrospective study design and the use of existing medical record data (with data gathered within the context of clinical activities rather than by trained research staff). However, all providers completed similar maternal and prenatal medical forms, which were routinely filed in the hospital medical record database prior to delivery. Participants' self-reported prepregnancy weight (as opposed to prepregnancy weight measured in a clinical or research setting) was used to determine GWG status. However, the IOM guidelines are based on studies that similarly use self-reported prepregnancy weight [39], and self-reported prepregnancy weight has been found to be highly correlated with clinically measured weight [40–42]. Information available on smoking patterns during pregnancy (i.e., number of cigarettes, quit date) was restricted. Furthermore, smoking status data was collected in the context of the first prenatal appointment and may be subject to social desirability bias and may only reflect smoking status at the first prenatal visit. However, the prevalence of smoking in our sample (19%) is consistent with smoking rates among White [2, 3, 32, 33] and Latina pregnant women [43] in previous studies. Presence of gestational diabetes, shown to be associated with birth weight [44, 45], was not controlled for. Women without a first-trimester prenatal visit and with missing prepregnancy BMI data were excluded from analysis; as systematic biases might exist between women who were or were not missing these data, findings may not be representative of the larger population from which the study sample was drawn. Study findings may not be generalizable to other (non-Puerto Rican) Latino subgroups. Lastly, the study

TABLE 3: Multivariate analysis of predictors of gestational weight gain status in overall study sample ($N = 571$).

Variable	Adjusted OR for GWG below guidelines		Adjusted OR for GWG above guidelines	
	Odds ratio (95% CI)	p value	Odds ratio (95% CI)	p value
GWG during the 1st trimester				
Within guidelines	Reference	<0.0001		<0.0001
Above guidelines	0.29 (0.08–1.01)		4.92 (2.75–8.81)	
Below guidelines	3.01 (1.33–6.81)		0.39 (0.21–0.74)	
Prepregnancy BMI				
18.5–24.9	Reference	0.0072	Reference	<0.0001
≤18.4	5.26 (1.37–20.17)		0.19 (0.06–0.58)	
25.0–29.9	0.83 (0.27–2.58)		3.44 (1.82–6.50)	
≥30.0	3.47 (1.38–8.70)		4.55 (2.29–9.04)	
Ethnicity				
White	Reference	0.9446	Reference	0.0069
Latina	0.97 (0.43–2.17)		0.46 (0.26–0.81)	
Tobacco use				
No	Reference	0.0402	Reference	0.2008
Yes, past	0.26 (0.07–0.99)		1.09 (0.49–2.42)	
Yes, this pregnancy	1.77 (0.64–4.84)		2.01 (0.93–4.31)	
Alcohol use				
No	Reference	0.5637	Reference	0.1978
Yes, past	1.69 (0.64–4.49)		1.15 (0.57–2.30)	
Yes, this pregnancy	0.85 (0.05–13.18)		0.15 (0.02–1.29)	
Age group				
25–29	Reference	0.2141	Reference	0.1470
15–19	3.07 (0.87–10.91)		1.50 (0.61–3.67)	
20–24	1.35 (0.45–4.04)		0.83 (0.40–1.74)	
30–34	0.60 (0.20–1.76)		0.52 (0.25–1.08)	
≥35	0.50 (0.10–2.44)		1.18 (0.49–2.86)	
Insurance				
Commercial/private	Reference	0.3929	Reference	0.1126
Public	1.58 (0.55–4.57)		1.75 (0.88–3.50)	
Employment at onset				
Employed	Reference	0.2533	Reference	0.2683
Not employed	1.63 (0.71–3.76)		1.39 (0.77–2.50)	
Parity				
0	Reference	0.9476	Reference	0.5305
1	0.93 (0.38–2.29)		0.94 (0.51–1.74)	
2	1.24 (0.42–3.61)		0.73 (0.34–1.61)	
3 or more	1.28 (0.35–4.59)		0.52 (0.20–1.30)	
Obstetric provider				
Private	Reference	0.0255	Reference	0.3441
Hospital clinic	0.35 (0.14–0.89)		0.75 (0.41–1.37)	
Psychiatric medications				
No	Reference	0.6482	Reference	0.2837
Yes	0.67 (0.12–3.72)		0.51 (0.15–1.73)	
Psychiatric diagnosis				
None	Reference	0.6362	Reference	0.5163
Anxiety	2.08 (0.25–17.06)		1.26 (0.25–6.50)	
Depression	1.14 (0.37–3.52)		1.27 (0.60–2.67)	
Other	3.16 (0.42–23.92)		3.57 (0.66–19.31)	

was not adequately powered to examine ethnic differences in pregnancy outcomes by GWG status; thus, results of GWG associated with outcomes of interest by ethnicity are exploratory.

Understanding factors that contribute to inadequate and excessive GWG is critical to the development of interventions that seek to optimize recommended GWG. Additional researches on racial/ethnic differences in the influence of

TABLE 4: Prevalence of selected pregnancy outcomes by gestational weight status in overall study sample ($N = 571$).

| Outcomes | Gestational weight gain status | | |
	Below	Within	Above
Length of pregnancy ($p = 0.966$)[1]			
Term delivery	80 (88.9)	134 (88.2)	290 (89.0)
Preterm delivery	10 (11.1)	18 (11.8)	36 (11.0)
Birth weight ($p = 0.001$)[1]			
SGA	18 (20.7)	15 (10.1)	23 (7.1)
Normal GA	66 (75.9)	124 (83.2)	264 (82.0)
LGA	3 (3.4)	10 (6.7)	35 (10.9)
Birth weight ($p = 0.061$)[1]			
LBW (<2500)	10 (11.5)	18 (12.1)	25 (7.7)
Normal BW	73 (83.9)	122 (81.9)	261 (80.3)
HBW (>4000)	4 (4.6)	9 (6.0)	39 (12.0)

[1] p value for association between GWG status and selected pregnancy outcomes in the entire sample.
GA: gestational age; SGA: small for gestational age; LGA: large for gestational age; BW: birth weight; LBW: low birth weight; HBW: high birth weight.

early GWG on GWG and other maternal and neonatal outcomes are needed to guide the development of interventions tailored for socioeconomically and ethnically diverse populations.

Additional Points

Implications for Practice and/or Policy. Study findings highlight the importance of identifying and targeting populations at high risk for excessive GWG, particularly in early pregnancy. Emphasizing early prenatal care and facilitating adherence to GWG recommendations in the first trimester are particularly relevant among prepregnancy underweight and overweight/obese women. Within the clinical setting, identifying populations at risk for both above- and below-guideline GWG during early prenatal care is critical for optimizing GWG. Timely targeted interventions are needed for health care providers and practitioners to deliver throughout pregnancy with the ultimate goal of improving maternal and neonatal short- and long-term outcomes.

Competing Interests

The authors have no competing financial interests to declare.

Acknowledgments

This study was funded by the Division of General Obstetrics & Gynecology Research Fund, Baystate Medical Center, Springfield, MA, USA.

References

[1] Institute of Medicine, *Weight Gain During Pregnancy: Reexamining the Guidelines*, National Academic Press, Washington, DC, USA, 2009.

[2] C. S. Wells, R. Schwalberg, G. Noonan, and V. Gabor, "Factors influencing inadequate and excessive weight gain in pregnancy: Colorado, 2000–2002," *Maternal and Child Health Journal*, vol. 10, no. 1, pp. 55–62, 2006.

[3] C. M. Olson and M. S. Strawderman, "Modifiable behavioral factors in a biopsychosocial model predict inadequate and excessive gestational weight gain," *Journal of the American Dietetic Association*, vol. 103, no. 1, pp. 48–54, 2003.

[4] N. E. Stotland, Y. W. Cheng, L. M. Hopkins, and A. B. Caughey, "Gestational weight gain and adverse neonatal outcome among term infants," *Obstetrics and Gynecology*, vol. 108, no. 3, pp. 635–643, 2006.

[5] B. E. Gould Rothberg, U. Magriples, T. S. Kershaw, S. S. Rising, and J. R. Ickovics, "Gestational weight gain and subsequent postpartum weight loss among young, low-income, ethnic minority women," *American Journal of Obstetrics and Gynecology*, vol. 204, no. 1, pp. 52.e1–52.e11, 2011.

[6] C. M. Olson, M. S. Strawderman, P. S. Hinton, and T. A. Pearson, "Gestational weight gain and postpartum behaviors associated with weight change from early pregnancy to 1 y postpartum," *International Journal of Obesity and Related Metabolic Disorder*, vol. 27, no. 1, pp. 117–127, 2003.

[7] P. Brawarsky, N. E. Stotland, R. A. Jackson et al., "Pre-pregnancy and pregnancy-related factors and the risk of excessive or inadequate gestational weight gain," *International Journal of Gynecology and Obstetrics*, vol. 91, no. 2, pp. 125–131, 2005.

[8] S. Y. Chu, S. Y. Kim, and C. L. Bish, "Prepregnancy obesity prevalence in the United States, 2004-2005," *Maternal and Child Health Journal*, vol. 13, no. 5, pp. 614–620, 2009.

[9] L. Chasan-Taber, M. D. Schmidt, P. Pekow, B. Sternfeld, C. G. Solomon, and G. Markenson, "Predictors of excessive and inadequate gestational weight gain in Hispanic women," *Obesity*, vol. 16, no. 7, pp. 1657–1666, 2008.

[10] H. Sangi-Haghpeykar, K. Lam, and S. P. Raine, "Gestational weight gain among hispanic women," *Maternal and Child Health Journal*, vol. 18, no. 1, pp. 153–160, 2014.

[11] I. E. Headen, E. M. Davis, M. S. Mujahid, and B. Abrams, "Racial-ethnic differences in pregnancy-related weight," *Advances in Nutrition*, vol. 3, no. 1, pp. 83–94, 2012.

[12] L. O. Walker, M. M. Hoke, and A. Brown, "Risk factors for excessive or inadequate gestational weight gain among Hispanic women in a U.S.-Mexico border state," *Journal of Obstetric, Gynecologic, and Neonatal Nursing*, vol. 38, no. 4, pp. 418–429, 2009.

[13] A. M. Siega-Riz and C. J. Hobel, "Predictors of poor maternal weight gain from baseline anthropometric, psychosocial, and demographic information in a hispanic population," *Journal of the American Dietetic Association*, vol. 97, no. 11, pp. 1264–1268, 1997.

[14] S. J. Ventura, J. C. Abma, W. D. Mosher, and S. K. Henshaw, "Estimated pregnancy rates by outcome for the United States, 1990-2004," *National Vital Statistics Report*, vol. 56, no. 15, pp. 1–28, 2008.

[15] T. J. Rosenberg, T. P. Raggio, and M. A. Chiasson, "A further examination of the 'epidemiologic paradox': birth outcomes among Latinas," *Journal of the National Medical Association*, vol. 97, no. 4, pp. 550–556, 2005.

[16] C. R. Stein, D. A. Savitz, T. Janevic et al., "Maternal ethnic ancestry and adverse perinatal outcomes in New York City," *American Journal of Obstetrics and Gynecology*, vol. 201, no. 6, pp. 584.e1–584.e9, 2009.

[17] Institute of Medicine, Subcommittee on Nutritional Status, and Weight Gain during Pregnancy, *Nutrition During Pregnancy*, No. 27, National Academy Press, Washington, DC, USA, 1990.

[18] E. Oken, E. M. Taveras, K. P. Kleinman, J. W. Rich-Edwards, and M. W. Gillman, "Gestational weight gain and child adiposity at age 3 years," *American Journal of Obstetrics and Gynecology*, vol. 196, no. 4, pp. 322.e1–322.e8, 2007.

[19] S. Y. Chu, W. M. Callaghan, C. L. Bish, and D. D'Angelo, "Gestational weight gain by body mass index among US women delivering live births, 2004-2005: fueling future obesity," *American Journal of Obstetrics and Gynecology*, vol. 200, no. 3, pp. 271.e1–271.e7, 2009.

[20] Y. Linné, L. Dye, B. Barkeling, and S. Rössner, "Long-term weight development in women: a 15-year follow-up of the effects of pregnancy," *Obesity Research*, vol. 12, no. 7, pp. 1166–1178, 2004.

[21] A. R. Amorim, S. Rössner, M. Neovius, P. M. Lourenço, and Y. Linné, "Does excess pregnancy weight gain constitute a major risk for increasing long-term BMI?" *Obesity*, vol. 15, no. 5, pp. 1278–1286, 2007.

[22] J. E. Brown, M. A. Murtaugh, D. R. Jacobs Jr., and H. C. Margellos, "Variation in newborn size according to pregnancy weight change by trimester," *American Journal of Clinical Nutrition*, vol. 76, no. 1, pp. 205–209, 2002.

[23] K. M. Rasmussen and A. L. Yaktine, Eds., *Weight Gain during Pregnancy: Re-Examining the Guidelines*, National Academy Press, Washington, DC, USA, 2009.

[24] T. A. Moore Simas, D. K. Doyle Curiale, J. Hardy, S. Jackson, Y. Zhang, and X. Liao, "Efforts needed to provide institute of medicine-recommended guidelines for gestational weight gain," *Obstetrics & Gynecology*, vol. 115, no. 4, pp. 777–783, 2010.

[25] American College of Obstetricians and Gynecologists, "ACOG practice Bulletin No. 101: ultrasonography in pregnancy," *Obstetrics and Gynecology*, vol. 113, no. 2, part 1, pp. 451–461, 2009.

[26] American College of Obstetricians and Gynecologists (ACOG), "Intrauterine growth restriction," ACOG Practice Bulletin 12, American College of Obstetricians and Gynecologists (ACOG), Washington, DC, USA, 2000.

[27] C. E. Margerison Zilko, D. Rehkopf, and B. Abrams, "Association of maternal gestational weight gain with short- and long-term maternal and child health outcomes," *American Journal of Obstetrics and Gynecology*, vol. 202, no. 6, pp. 574.e1–574.e8, 2010.

[28] World Health Organization (WHO), *International Statistical Classification of Diseases and Related Health Problems, Tenth Revision*, World Health Organization, Geneva, Switzerland, 1992.

[29] D. W. Hosmer and S. Lemeshow, *Applied Logistic Regression*, John Wiley & Sons, New York, NY, USA, 2nd edition, 2000.

[30] N. E. Stotland, J. S. Haas, P. Brawarsky, R. A. Jackson, E. Fuentes-Afflick, and G. J. Escobar, "Body mass index, provider advice, and target gestational weight gain," *Obstetrics & Gynecology*, vol. 105, no. 3, pp. 633–638, 2005.

[31] J. A. Martin, B. E. Hamilton, P. D. Sutton et al., "Births: final data for 2007," *National Vital Statistics Reports*, vol. 58, no. 24, pp. 1–85, 2010.

[32] J. P. Furuno, L. Gallicchio, and M. Sexton, "Cigarette smoking and low maternal weight gain in medicaid-eligible pregnant women," *Journal of Women's Health*, vol. 13, no. 7, pp. 770–777, 2004.

[33] A. S. Olafsdottir, G. V. Skuladottir, I. Thorsdottir, A. Hauksson, and L. Steingrimsdottir, "Combined effects of maternal smoking status and dietary intake related to weight gain and birth size parameters," *British Journal of Obstetrics and Gynaecology*, vol. 113, no. 11, pp. 1296–1302, 2006.

[34] A report of the Surgeon General, "Tobacco smoke causes disease: The biology and behavioral basis for smoking attributable disease," http://www.mchb.hrsa.gov/whusa11/hstat/hsrmh/pages/228sdp.html.

[35] Centers for Disease Control and Prevention and National Vital Statistics System, "*Annual natality files*," http://www.cdc.gov/nchs/births.htm.

[36] M. Viswanathan, A. M. Siega-Riz, M. K. Moos et al., "Outcomes of maternal weight gain," Evidence Report/Technology Assessment (Full Report) 168, 2008.

[37] J. A. Hutcheon, L. M. Bodnar, K. S. Joseph, B. Abrams, H. N. Simhan, and R. W. Platt, "The bias in current measures of gestational weight gain," *Paediatric and Perinatal Epidemiology*, vol. 26, no. 2, pp. 109–116, 2012.

[38] MassCHIP, *Race/Hispanic Ethnicity Report: Birth and Perinatal Indicators*, Massachusetts Department of Public Health, Boston, Mass, USA, 2010.

[39] A. M. Siega-Riz, L. S. Adair, and C. J. Hob, "Institute of medicine maternal weight gain recommendations and pregnancy outcome in a predominantly hispanic population," *Obstetrics and Gynecology*, vol. 84, no. 4, pp. 565–573, 1994.

[40] S. Avishai-Eliner, K. L. Brunson, C. A. Sandman, and T. Z. Baram, "Stressed-out, or in (utero)?" *Trends in Neurosciences*, vol. 25, no. 10, pp. 518–524, 2002.

[41] C. Stevens-Simon, K. J. Roghmann, and E. R. McAnarney, "Relationship of self-reported prepregnant weight and weight gain during pregnancy to maternal body habitus and age," *Journal of the American Dietetic Association*, vol. 92, no. 1, pp. 85–87, 1992.

[42] C. Stevens-Simon, E. R. McAnarney, and M. P. Coulter, "How accurately do pregnant adolescents estimate their weight prior to pregnancy?" *Journal of Adolescent Health Care*, vol. 7, no. 4, pp. 250–254, 1986.

[43] A. E. Haskins, E. R. Bertone-Johnson, P. Pekow, E. Carbone, R. T. Fortner, and L. Chasan-Taber, "Smoking during pregnancy and risk of abnormal glucose tolerance: a prospective cohort study," *BMC Pregnancy and Childbirth*, vol. 10, p. 55, 2010.

[44] G. Seghieri, R. Anichini, A. De Bellis, L. Alviggi, F. Franconi, and M. C. Breschi, "Relationship between gestational diabetes mellitus and low maternal birth weight," *Diabetes Care*, vol. 25, no. 10, pp. 1761–1765, 2002.

[45] B. Krstevska, S. Mishevska, E. Janevska et al., "Gestational Diabetes Mellitus—the impact of maternal body mass index and glycaemic control on baby's birth weight," *Prilozi*, vol. 30, no. 2, pp. 115–124, 2009.

23

Prevalence, Infectivity, and Associated Risk Factors of Hepatitis B Virus among Pregnant Women in Yirgalem Hospital, Ethiopia: Implication of Screening to Control Mother-to-Child Transmission

Anteneh Amsalu [iD],[1] **Getachew Ferede** [iD],[1] **Setegn Eshetie** [iD],[1]
Agete Tadewos,[2] **and Demissie Assegu**[2]

[1]*Department of Medical Microbiology, University of Gondar, Gondar, Ethiopia*
[2]*Department of Medical Laboratory Sciences, Hawassa University, Hawassa, Ethiopia*

Correspondence should be addressed to Anteneh Amsalu; ant.amsalu@gmail.com

Academic Editor: Olav Lapaire

Background. Hepatitis B surface antigen (HBsAg) and hepatitis B e antigen (HBeAg) positive mother has up to 90% likelihood of mother-to-child transmission (MTCT) of hepatitis B virus (HBV) to newborns in the absence of any prophylaxis or antiviral therapy utilization. However, routine antenatal screening and intervention strategies are not yet practiced in Ethiopia. Therefore, this study was conducted to determine the prevalence, infectivity, and associated risk factors of HBV among pregnant women. *Methods.* A cross-sectional study was conducted from October 2015 to August 2016 in Yirgalem Hospital. A total of 475 pregnant women were recruited, and data on sociodemography and potential risk factors were collected using a structured questionnaire. In addition, blood samples were tested for HBsAg, and HBsAg positive samples were retested for HBeAg using commercially available strip test. The status of HIV was collected from the records. *Results.* The seroprevalence of HBsAg was 34 (7.2%), of whom 13 (38.8%) were positive for HBeAg. The prevalence of HIV infection was 10.1% (48/475). Ten out of 34 HBV positive cases (29.4%) were coinfected with HIV. The overall HBV/HIV coinfection rate was 2.1% (10/475). Women with history of multiple sexual partners and being HIV positive were significantly associated with HBsAg positivity. Among the study participants, 35.4% were aware of MTCT of HBV and only 12 (2.5%) have taken HBV vaccine. *Conclusions.* High prevalence of HBsAg and HBeAg as well as low awareness and practices of HBV prevention methods suggests that perinatal transmission of HBV might be the prevailing mode of HBV transmission in the study area. Thus, screening of all pregnant women, particularly those who had history of multiple sexual partners and HIV coinfection, and provision of health education about HBV prevention methods are inevitable.

1. Introduction

Hepatitis B virus (HBV) is thought to be the main etiological agent for chronic liver disease (CLD) worldwide. Over 2 billion people today have been infected with HBV and 350 million of them are chronically infected, with annual death of more than 1 million of HBV-related CLD [1–3]. Mother-to-child transmission (MTCT) is responsible for approximately one-half of chronic hepatitis B (CHB) infection worldwide [4]. In endemic areas, where carrier rates are greater than 5%, perinatal transmission is common, especially when HBV-infected mothers are also HBeAg positive [5, 6]. Without

any prophylaxis or antiviral therapy, women who are acutely infected with HBV or are chronic carriers of HBV are likely to transmit the virus to their offspring at the time of delivery [7].

The risk of MTCT among infants born to HBV-infected mothers ranges from 10 to 40% in HBeAg negative mothers and to as high as 90% in HBeAg-positive mothers with HBV deoxyribonucleic acid (DNA) level (>200,000IU/ml, equivalent to 6 log copies/ml). The majority (> 95%) of perinatally acquired infection results in CHB infection, due to induction of an immune tolerant state of variable duration [8, 9] and has a 15 to 25 percent risk of dying in adulthood from cirrhosis or liver cancer [10]. The risk of developing

CHB infection is inversely proportional to the age at time of exposure and immune status [6, 9]. In addition, concurrent viral (hepatitis A, C, or D viruses or HIV) infection, high maternal HBV viral load and activity of viral replication (determined by detection of HBeAg) in the third trimester of pregnancy, increases the risk of perinatal transmission [6, 11].

Regardless of whether they have been previously tested or vaccinated, screening of all pregnant women for HBV infection at the first prenatal visit is important in view of the morbidity and mortality of pregnant women, its effect on the pregnancy outcome, and the risk of vertical transmission from mother to child [12]. In Ethiopia, the HBsAg prevalence rate among pregnant women varies between 3% and 7.8% [13–17]. Despite its prevalence, there is a paucity of data regarding on HBeAg status among pregnant women which helps to understand the frequency of highly infective HBV carriers in the given region which in turn helps to design and implement preventive and control measures and awareness of transmission route of HBV infection. Hence, the present study was designed to determine seroprevalence, infectivity, and associated risk factor of HBV among pregnant women attending the Yirgalem Hospital.

2. Materials and Methods

2.1. Ethical Consideration. This study was reviewed and approved by the Institutional Review Board (IRB) of Hawassa University College of Medicine and Health Sciences. Then support letter was obtained from the Yirgalem Hospital administration. The purpose and importance of the study were explained to each study participant. To ensure confidentiality of participant's information, anonymous typing was applied for every study participant. Study participants were interviewed alone to keep the privacy and all participants did not pay for the test. The test results were given to the clinicians who are working on ANC clinic of the hospital and all women who tested positive for HBsAg were counseled on their status, the route of disease transmission, the need for immunization to their neonate at birth, and close-contact screening against hepatitis. Then, they were referred to internal medicine for further diagnosis and management.

2.2. Study Design, Area, and Period. A cross-sectional study was conducted among pregnant women attending Yirgalem Hospital ANC clinic from October 2015 to August 2016. The hospital was located 70 km far from Hawassa, the capital city of Southern Nations and Nationalities People's Region (SNNPR), and 345 km from Addis Ababa, the capital city of Ethiopia. It is the largest hospital in the region and provides medical education and training in addition to medical care. The hospital ANC clinic gives services for more than 15 pregnant women per a day and has 30 bed rooms to serve pregnant women. At the time of their first visit of the ANC clinic, pregnant women have been screened for HIV, syphilis, anemia, and proteinuria. However, women were screened for HBV only when there is any suspicion of risk.

2.3. Population. Sample size was estimated to be 423 using single population proportion formula, assuming 50% HBeAg prevalence (infectivity) in pregnant women, 5% precision, and 95% level of confidence. However, in attempting to enhance the statistical power of detecting the rate difference by exposure status, we investigated a total of 500 pregnant women, prospectively. 475 consecutive pregnant women attending antenatal care (ANC) clinic in Yirgalem Hospital during the study period were enrolled. Pregnant women who are healthcare workers and refused to give consent for the blood test were exempted from the study.

2.4. Data Collection

2.4.1. Sociodemographic Data. A written informed consent was obtained after careful explanation, about the concept of the study to each pregnant woman, before their inclusion in the study. Two midwives were trained for 2 days on study procedures, facts on HBV infections and transmission, counseling, and safety issues. Data on sociodemography and potential risk factors were collected using structured questionnaires. HIV result and ART status were obtained from their medical records.

2.5. Specimen Collection and Handling. About 5 ml of venous blood was collected from all pregnant women in Yirgalem Hospital Laboratory. The blood was allowed to clot and serum was separated by centrifugation at room temperature at 3000 rpm, and HBsAg was performed. About 2 ml serum was stored in the freezer at $-20°C$ and transported to Hawassa University Teaching Laboratory using a cold box for further test.

2.6. Laboratory Testing. All samples were screened for the presence of HBsAg using a commercial test strip (Shanghai Eugene Biotech Co., Ltd, China). The sensitivity and specificity of the HBsAg kit were 100% and 99.34%, respectively. All samples that tested positive were retested for confirmation using the same kit and there were no discordant results. All HBsAg positive samples were retested for HBeAg using a commercial test strip, the INSIGHT HBeAg test (Tulip Diagnostics (P) Ltd, India). The sensitivity and specificity of the HBeAg kit were 99% and 97%, respectively. All tests were carried out according to the manufacturer's instructions as outlined in the package inserts. In addition, HIV result was taken from the medical records, which is a routine test recommended for all pregnant women in Ethiopia and is uniformly performed using the established national rapid testing algorithm: the Kehua Bioengineering (KHB) test kit (Shanghai, China) is used as a screening test, followed by the HIV1/2 STAT-PAK assay if positive. If the STAT-PAK and KHB results are discordant, the Uni-Gold HIV test is used as a tiebreaker to determine the result.

2.7. Quality Assurance. The validity and completeness of the data were checked by the trained supervisor daily. The performance of the rapid HBsAg test kit was evaluated using known positive and negative controls obtained from enzyme linked immunosorbent assay (ELISA) tested blood donors and have consistent result. Sera of positive HBeAg study subjects were retested by the same method and give the same result. Furthermore, formation of colored band to the control (C) line acts as a procedural control and serves to valid the result.

2.8. Data Analysis. Data were coded, entered, and analyzed using SPSS version 20 (IBM Corp., Armonk, NY, USA). We described data using either proportion or mean with standard deviation (SD). Association between participant characteristics and outcome variables (HBsAg positivity) was assessed using $\chi 2$ test (or Fisher's exact test as appropriate) for categorical predictors. All explanatory variables with a p-value ≤ 0.05 in the bivariate analysis were included in the multivariate logistic regression model to identify variables which have been associated independently. Odds ratios (OR) with their 95% confidence intervals (CI) served to investigate the influence of various factors on the occurrence of HBV infection. A p-value of <0.05 was regarded as significant.

3. Results

3.1. Sociodemographic Characteristics. Out of 500 pregnant women approached during the study period, 25 (5.0%) were excluded because 6 refused to participate and 19 were healthcare workers. Thus, a total of 475 pregnant women aged 18–42 years were enrolled into the study. The mean (standard deviation (SD)) age of the study group was 26.5±4.6 years, and HBV infection rate increased as the age increased. Majority, 416 (87.2%), of the women had the educational status of at least elementary and 323 (68.0%) of women were urban in residence. A large proportion of the women, 428 (90.1%), were currently married, but those who were divorced or widowed were 3.8%, and 322 (67.8%) of them were multigravida. More than half of the study participants were housewives in occupation and majority of them, 209 (44.0%), were in the third trimester (Table 1).

3.2. HBeAg Positivity among HBsAg Positive Pregnant Women. The overall seroprevalence of HBsAg was 34 (7.2%) (95% CI 4.9% - 9.3%). Three of them had known their HBsAg status. Among 34 HBsAg positive women, 13 (38.2%) were also positive for HBeAg (Figure 1). The highest prevalence rate of HBsAg was observed in the age group ≥ 30 years (10.5%) followed by the age group 25–29 years (6.4%); however, no statistically significant difference was observed with age groups. Almost all of the participants with HBsAg positivity were married and 70.6% were multigravida. None of the sociodemographic and obstetrical characteristics of pregnant women assessed in this study was significantly associated with HBsAg positivity (Table 1).

3.3. Associated Risk Factors of HBV Infection. Among 475 pregnant women, 43 (9.1%) had a history of multiple sexual partners, of which 16.3% were positive for HBsAg. Statistically significant association was detected between HBV infection and having multiple sexual partners (p= 0.02). Women having history of multiple sexual partners had higher odds of HBsAg positivity (aOR = 2.92, 95% CI = 1.19-7.16)

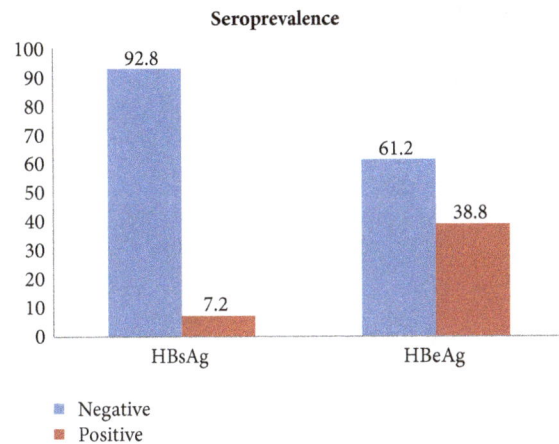

FIGURE 1: Seroprevalence rate of HBsAg among pregnant women and HBeAg positivity in Yirgalem Hospital, October 2015 to August 2016.

as compared to those without history of multiple sexual partners.

In this study, 48 (10.1%) of pregnant women were HIV positive. 36 (75%) of them were on ART. Ten of 48 women were equally infected with the HBV. Eight out of 10 coinfected women started ART and six of them were HBeAg negative while two were HBeAg positive. Overall, 10 (2.1%) pregnant women were coinfected with HIV and HBV. In a bivariate analysis, those pregnant women infected with HIV were 4.4 times (aOR = 4.44, 95% CI = 1.96-10.08) more likely to be HBsAg positive than those who were HIV negative. However, place of birth, a history of previous surgery, history of blood transfusion, a history of tooth extraction or tattoos, family history of liver disease, a previous history of abortion, and being diabetes mellitus (DM) patient were not found to be significantly associated with the HBsAg status (Table 2).

In multivariate analysis of selected variables for independent predictors of HBV in pregnant women, a history of multiple sexual partners (aOR=2.92, 95%CI=1.19-7.16) and HIV positivity (aOR= 4.44, 95%CI=1.96-10.08) remained statistically significant predictors of HBV among pregnant women (Table 2).

3.4. Previous HBV Screening, Vaccination, and Awareness Status of Pregnant Women. Of the total participants who responded to the question whether they were previously screened or vaccinated at the time of interview, seventy-four (15.6%) women have been previously screened for HBV. Of these, 6 (8.1%) participants were currently positive for HBsAg, and six started ART but were negative for HBeAg. During oral interview, out of these six positive participants, three answered that they were positive while the other three had conducted screening and their results were negative. Out of the total participants, only 12 (2.5%) reported that they received one or more doses of hepatitis B vaccine. Of these, only 3(0.6%) pregnant women had received three doses (full dose). About 46.5%, 44.8%, and 35.4% of participants were aware of HBV transmission via sexual contact and blood

TABLE 1: HBsAg in relation to sociodemography in pregnant women attending Yirgalem Hospital, October 2015 to August 2016.

Characteristics	Total women* (N = 475)	Women with* HBsAg (N = 34)	COR(95%CI)	p-value
Age (years)				
< 25	158(33.3)	9(5.7)	1	
25-29	203(42.7)	13(6.4)	1.13(0.47-2.72)	0.78
≥30	114(24.0)	12(10.5)	1.95(0.79-4.79)	0.15
Residence				
Urban	323(68.0)	25(7.7)	1.33(0.61-2.93)	0.47
Rural	152(32.0)	9(5.9)	1	
Education				
Illiterate	59(12.4)	4(6.8)	1.02(0.27-2.77)	0.98
Elementary	165(34.7)	9(5.4)	0.81(0.28-2.35)	0.69
Secondary	161(33.9)	15(9.0)	1.44(0.54-3.85)	0.47
College and above	90(18.9)	6(6.9)	1	
Occupation				
Housewife	246(51.8)	20(8.1)	2.74(0.36-21.17)	0.33
Employed	133(28.0)	12(9.0)	3.07(0.39-24.56)	0.29
Daily labor	12(2.5)	1(8.3)	2.82(0.16-49.00)	0.48
Merchant	52(10.9)	0	0.00	0.99
Student	32(6.7)	1(3.1)	1	
Marital status				
Married	428(90.1)	33(7.7)	1.42(0.18-11.01)	0.74
Single	29(6.1)	0	0.00	0.99
Divorced /Widowed	18(3.8)	1(5.6)	1	
Gestational age				
1st trimester	95(20.0)	9(9.5)	1.88(0.72-4.92)	0.19
2nd trimester	171(36.0)	9(5.3)	1	
3rd trimester	209(44.0)	16(7.7)	1.49(0.64-3.47)	0.35
Gravidity				
Primigravida (1)	153(32.2)	10(6.5)	1	
Multigravida (≥2)	322(67.8)	24(7.5)	1.15(0.54-2.47)	0.72

*Data were shown as N (%); N: number; HBsAg: hepatitis B surface antigen.

and body fluids contact through nonintact skin and mucus membrane and from MTCT, respectively (Table 3).

4. Discussion

Early screening of pregnant women for HBV infection will have paramount importance to investigate the infection and to implement evidence based medical interventions. Since most of the pregnant women are not aware of their HBV infection status, they may serve as an important reservoir to fuel HBV transmission [18]. The seroprevalence of HBsAg in this study was 7.2%, which is in agreement with the studies in Addis Ababa, Central Ethiopia (6%)[19], Deder Hospital, Eastern Ethiopia (6.9%) [20], and Southern Ethiopia (6.1%-7.8%) [16, 17]. Similarly, the current finding was also comparable with the findings of studies in Yaounde, Cameroon (7.7%) [21], in Mali (8.0%) [22], and in Nigeria (6.67%-8.3%) [23, 24]. However, it was higher than previous studies carried out in

other parts of Ethiopia (3%-4.4%) [13–15, 19, 25] and in Dares Salaam, Tanzania (3.9%) [26]. The high HBsAg positivity rate observed in this study might be due to multiple sexual practices and low level of awareness of the different routes of HBV transmission. On the other hand, the prevalence of HBsAg in this study was lower than prevalence rates of 9.7% and 10.2% reported in Cameroon [18, 27], 10.8% in Yemen [28], and 11.8% in northern Uganda[29]. These differences might be attributable to differences in the study population, whereby a selected population exposed to no condom sexual intercourse in a postconflict region with high rates of HIV infection were studied in Uganda [29], cultural practices such as circumcision in Yemen [28], and the obvious natural difference linked with various geographical situations.

The HBeAg status and the HBV viral load are both factors known to be associated with vertical HBV transmission [30]. We have assessed the presence of HBeAg which is a marker of high infectivity, as a proxy measure for the risk of vertical

TABLE 2: Risk factors associated with HBsAg positivity among pregnant women in Yirgalem Hospital, October 2015 to August 2016.

Risk factors	Total women *(N = 475)	HBsAg (N=34) *Positive (%)	COR(95%CI)	aOR(95%CI)	p-value
Place of birth					
No birth	146(30.7)	8(5.5)	1		
Home	93(19.6)	7(7.5)	1.40(0.49-4.01)		
Health institution	236(49.7)	19(8.1)	1.51(0.64-3.55)		
Surgery					
Yes	82(17.3)	7(8.5)	1.27(0.53-3.01)		
No	393(82.7)	27(6.9)	1		
Blood transfusion					
Yes	23(4.8)	1(4.3)	0.58(0.08-4.42)		
No	452(95.2)	33(7.3)	1		
Tattooing					
Yes	91(19.2)	5(5.5)	0.71(0.27-189)		
No	384(80.8)	29(7.6)	1		
Tooth extraction					
Yes	132(27.8)	8(6.1)	0.79(0.35-1.78)		
No	343(72.2)	26(7.6)	1		
Multiple sexual partner					
Yes	43(9.1)	7(16.3)	2.92(1.19-7.16)	2.94(1.17-7.41)	0.02
No	432(90.9)	27(6.2)	1		
Family history of liver disease					
Yes	23(4.8)	1(4.3)	0.58(0.08-4.42)		
No	452(95.2)	33(7.3)	1		
Abortion					
Yes	67(14.1)	5(7.5)	1.05(0.39-2.82)		
No	408(85.9)	29(7.1)	1		
DM					
Yes	28(5.9)	3(10.7)	1.61(0.46-5.63)		
No	447(94.1)	31(6.9)	1		
HIV					
Yes	48(10.1)	10(20.8)	4.42(1.97-9.93)	4.44(1.96-10.08)	0.001
No	427(89.9)	24(5.6)	1		

*Data were shown as N (%); N: number; HBsAg: hepatitis B surface antigen; DM: diabetes mellitus; HIV: human immunodeficiency virus.

TABLE 3: Relation of HBsAg and previous status of participants to HBV, vaccination, andawareness of pregnant women about route of transmission in Yirgalem Hospital, October 2015 to August 2016.

Participant responses	Total women (N = 475)	HBsAg Positive(N=34)
Previously screened for HBV	74(15.6)	6(8.1)
Previous HBV result, positive	3/74(4.1)	3(100)
Have you taken HBV vaccine? Yes	12(2.5)	0
Is HBV transmitted sexually? Yes	221(46.5)	15(6.8)
Is HBV transmitted through contact of blood and body fluid? Yes	213(44.8)	15(7.0)
Is HBV transmitted from mother to child? Yes	168(35.4)	12(7.1)
Other routes of transmission mentioned	154(32.4%)	11(7.1)

HBsAg: hepatitis B surface antigen; HBV: hepatitis B virus.

transmission of HBV. Out of all HBsAg positive patients, 38.2% were positive for HBeAg. This finding was significantly higher as compared to other studies elsewhere [21, 31]. This might be due to difference in diagnostic methods which used ELISA kit [21, 31]. It is known that the risk of vertical transmission and resulting chronic infection from HBsAg (+) mother to her baby is approximately 90% in HBeAg-positive pregnant women [8]. Hence our result suggests that vertical transmission is possibly an important means of HBV transmission in the study area where there is no birth dose vaccination program for newborn of HBsAg carrier mothers.

In the present study, sociodemographic variables like age, marital and educational status, residence, and occupation of participants as well as reproductive variables like gestational age and gravidity were not significantly associated with the risk of HBV infection. This finding is in line with the study conducted in Felege Hiwot Referral Hospital, Ethiopia [15] and Nigeria [32]. However, it contrasted with previous study that showed that pregnant women with no formal education had higher odds of HBV infection [16].

In the current study, pregnant women who had multiple sexual partners were almost three times more likely to have risk of acquiring HBV infection as compared to their counterparts. This is in agreement with the findings in other parts of Ethiopia [15, 20] and in Africa [31, 32]. Although 46.5% of the study participants were aware of sexual route of HBV transmission, women who have awareness had no significant difference as compared to those who have no awareness. This highlights that further health education is needed to protect pregnant women from being infected and to cut off sexual transmission of HBV through change in sexual practice and behavior modification.

In this study, high prevalence of HIV infection (10.1%) among pregnant women attending the ANC was consistent with the previous studies in Gondar (9.6-11.9%) [33–36]. HIV-infected pregnant women were more than 4 times more likely to be coinfected with HBV than HIV-uninfected ones. This is in agreement with the findings of Noubiap et al. [27] who demonstrated that HIV-infected women were 22 times more likely to be coinfected with HBV than HIV-uninfected women during pregnancy. This can be explained by the fact that HBV and HIV share common modes of transmission. Moreover, it has been reported that HIV/HBV coinfection facilitates HBV replication and reactivation, leading to higher HBV-DNA levels and reduced spontaneous clearance of the virus [37]. Although we overlooked salvaging the duration of ART taken and type of ART regimens, lamivudine is the first line ART treatment for HIV positive pregnant women in Ethiopia [38]. It has dual nucleoside reverse transcriptase inhibitor backbone in women with HIV/HBV coinfection; in line with these eight coinfected women who started ART, two women were HBeAg positive, which needs further prospective studies to investigate the effect of lamivudine in reducing HBeAg during coinfection with HIV. The overall HBV/HIV coinfection rate in our study population was 2.1%. This coinfection rate is almost three times the 0.74% rate recently reported among pregnant women in Hawassa [16], greater than the 1.3% rate reported in Northwest Ethiopia [14] and the 1.5% rate in Cameron [27], and significantly lower

than the 4.2% rate reported in Nigeria [24]. The difference in coinfection rate may be due to the relatively small number of HIV positive cases in the previous study.

Since mother-child transmission is the major route of acquisition of HBV worldwide, particularly in endemic countries like Ethiopia, early recognition of HBV carrier pregnant women followed by treatment with safe antiviral agents, if indicated, and vaccination will reduce perinatal HBV infection and its complications [39]. In this study, only 15.6% of pregnant women have been previously screened for HBV. Of them, just 2.5% of pregnant women have been vaccinated against HBV. Moreover, almost two-thirds of the study participants are unaware of perinatal transmission of HBV. Thus, the provision of appropriate and correct information about the common aspects of HBV infection including perinatal transmissions, screening, and prevention by vaccination is warranted to further improve the control of HBV infection in the target group. Though there is an improvement as compared to the previous study in Hawassa [16] which reported that none of the study participants were screened and vaccinated for HBV, this difference in awareness might be because previously screened pregnant women in this study were more likely to have heard about transmission route of HBV compared to those who had no previous experience of HBV testing [40].

Nevertheless, this study has the limitation that other confirmatory methods like ELISA and molecular HBV-DNA test were not performed due to lack of budget and molecular virology laboratory facilities. The generalizability of results to all pregnant women may be limited by selection and information bias due to the institutional based nature of the study and the reliance on participants' report to assess associated factors.

5. Conclusions

High prevalence of HBsAg and HBeAg as well as low awareness and practices of HBV prevention methods suggests that perinatal transmission of HBV might be the prevailing mode of HBV transmission in the study area. Thus, screening of all pregnant women, particularly those who had history of multiple sexual partners and HIV coinfection, and provision of health education about HBV prevention methods are inevitable

Conflicts of Interest

The authors declare that they have no conflicts of interest.

Authors' Contributions

Anteneh Amsalu conceived the idea and developed the proposal. Anteneh Amsalu, Agete Tadewos, and Demissie Assegu reviewed and approved the proposal. Anteneh Amsalu, Getachew Ferede, Setegn Eshetie, Agete Tadewos, and Demissie Assegu contributed to the inception of the research question, design, proposal development, analysis, and preparation of the manuscript. Anteneh Amsalu,

Getachew Ferede, and Setegn Eshetie analyzed the data, were involved in the interpretation of results, and critically reviewed the manuscript. All authors read and approved the final manuscript for publication.

Acknowledgments

The authors express their gratitude to the study participants and data collectors. The authors also thank the Ethiopian Public Health Association (EPHA) for the partial presentation of the manuscript at the 28th Annual Conference and Allied Academies for publishing a poster abstract at the Second World Conference on STDs, STIs, and HIV/AIDS. Finally, special acknowledgment goes to Hawassa University for financial support.

References

[1] T. Shimelis, W. Torben, G. Medhin et al., "Hepatitis B virus infection among people attending the voluntary counselling and testing centre and anti-retroviral therapy clinic of St Paul's General Specialised Hospital, Addis Ababa, Ethiopia," *Sexually Transmitted Infections*, vol. 84, no. 1, pp. 37–41, 2008.

[2] M. Lemoine, S. Eholié, and K. Lacombe, "Reducing the neglected burden of viral hepatitis in Africa: strategies for a global approach," *Journal of Hepatology*, vol. 62, no. 2, pp. 469–476, 2015.

[3] H. B. El-Serag, "Epidemiology of viral hepatitis and hepatocellular carcinoma," *Gastroenterology*, vol. 142, no. 6, pp. 1264–1273, 2012.

[4] B. Navabakhsh, N. Mehrabi, A. Estakhri, M. Mohamadnejad, and H. Poustchi, "Hepatitis B Virus Infection during Pregnancy:Transmission and Prevention," *MEJDD*, vol. 3, no. 2, pp. 92–102, 2011.

[5] Z. Zhang, C. Chen, Z. Li, Y.-H. Wu, and X.-M. Xiao, "Individualized management of pregnant women with high hepatitis B virus DNA levels," *World Journal of Gastroenterology*, vol. 20, no. 34, pp. 12056–12061, 2014.

[6] T. L. Wright, "Introduction to chronic hepatitis B infection," *American Journal of Gastroenterology*, vol. 101, no. 1, pp. S1–S6, 2006.

[7] M.-H. Chang, "Hepatitis B virus infection," *Seminars in Fetal and Neonatal Medicine*, vol. 12, no. 3, pp. 160–167, 2007.

[8] J. R. Lamberth, S. C. Reddy, J.-J. Pan, and K. J. Dasher, "Chronic hepatitis B infection in pregnancy," *World Journal of Hepatology*, vol. 7, no. 9, pp. 1233–1237, 2015.

[9] A. Bertoletti and P. T. Kennedy, "The immune tolerant phase of chronic HBV infection: new perspectives on an old concept," *Cellular & Molecular Immunology*, vol. 12, pp. 258–263, 2015.

[10] N. Camvulam, P. Gotsch, and R. C. Langan, "Caring for Pregnant Women and Newborns with Hepatitis B or C," *American Family Physician*, vol. 82, no. 10, pp. 1225–1229, 2010.

[11] N. P. Nelson, D. J. Jamieson, and T. V. Murphy, "Prevention of perinatal hepatitis B virus transmission," *Journal of the Pediatric Infectious Diseases Society*, vol. 3, no. 1, pp. S7–S12, 2014.

[12] E. E. Mast, H. S. Margolis, A. E. Fiore et al., "A comprehensive immunization strategy to eliminate transmission of hepatitis B virus infection in the United States: recommendations of the Advisory Committee on Immunization Practices (ACIP) part 1: immunization of infants, children, and adolescents," *MMWR Recommendations and Reports*, vol. 54, no. RR16, pp. 1–23, 2005.

[13] D. Tegegne, K. Desta, B. Tegbaru, and T. Tilahun, "Seroprevalence and transmission of Hepatitis B virus among delivering women and their new born in selected health facilities, Addis Ababa, Ethiopia: A cross sectional study," *BMC Research Notes*, vol. 7, no. 1, p. 239, 2014.

[14] Y. Zenebe, W. Mulu, M. Yimer, and B. Abera, "Sero-prevalence and risk factors of hepatitis B virus and human immunodeficiency virus infection among pregnant women in Bahir Dar city, Northwest Ethiopia: a cross sectional study," *BMC Infectious Diseases*, vol. 14, no. 1, p. 118, 2014.

[15] S. Molla, A. Munshea, and E. Nibret, "Seroprevalence of hepatitis B surface antigen and anti HCV antibody and its associated risk factors among pregnant women attending maternity ward of Felege Hiwot Referral Hospital, northwest Ethiopia: A cross-sectional study Hepatitis viruses," *Virology Journal*, vol. 12, no. 1, p. 204, 2015.

[16] Y. Metaferia, W. Dessie, I. Ali, and A. Amsalu, "Seroprevalence and associated risk factors of hepatitis B virus among pregnant women in southern Ethiopia: a hospital-based cross-sectional study," *Epidemiology and Health*, vol. 38, p. e2016027, 2016.

[17] J. M. Ramos, C. Toro, F. Reyes, A. Amor, and F. Gutiérrez, "Seroprevalence of HIV-1, HBV, HTLV-1 and Treponema pallidum among pregnant women in a rural hospital in Southern Ethiopia," *Journal of Clinical Virology*, vol. 51, no. 1, pp. 83–85, 2011.

[18] A. A. B. Frambo, J. Atashili, P. N. Fon, and P. M. Ndumbe, "Prevalence of HBsAg and knowledge about hepatitis B in pregnancy in the Buea Health District, Cameroon: A cross-sectional study," *BMC Research Notes*, vol. 7, no. 1, p. 394, 2014.

[19] Z. Desalegn, L. Wassie, H. B. Beyene, A. Mihret, and Y. A. Ebstie, "Hepatitis B and human immunodeficiency virus co-infection among pregnant women in resource-limited high endemic setting, Addis Ababa, Ethiopia: Implications for prevention and control measures," *European Journal of Medical Research*, vol. 21, no. 1, article no. 16, 2016.

[20] A. Umare, B. Seyoum, T. Gobena, and T. H. Mariyam, "Hepatitis B virus infections and associated factors among pregnant women attending antenatal care clinic at deder hospital, eastern Ethiopia," *PLoS ONE*, vol. 11, no. 11, Article ID e0166936, 2016.

[21] N. J. Fomulu, F. L. I. Morfaw, J. N. Torimiro, P. Nana, M. V. Koh, and T. William, "Prevalence, correlates and pattern of Hepatitis B among antenatal clinic attenders in Yaounde-Cameroon: Is perinatal transmission of HBV neglected in Cameroon?" *BMC Pregnancy and Childbirth*, vol. 13, p. 158, 2013.

[22] B. MacLean, R. F. Hess, E. Bonvillain et al., "Seroprevalence of hepatitis B surface antigen among pregnant women attending the hospital for women & children in Koutiala, Mali," *South African Medical Journal*, vol. 102, no. 1, pp. 47–49, 2012.

[23] G. R. Pennap, E. T. Osanga, and A. Ubam, "Seroprevalence of hepatitis B surface antigen among pregnant women attending antenatal clinic in federal medical center Keffi, Nigeria," *Research Journal of Medical Sciences*, vol. 5, no. 2, pp. 80–82, 2011.

[24] A. C. Eke, U. A. Eke, C. I. Okafor, I. U. Ezebialu, and C. Ogbuagu, "Prevalence, correlates and pattern of hepatitis B surface antigen in a low resource setting," *Virology Journal*, vol. 8, no. 12, 2011.

[25] T Yohanes, Z. Zerdo, and N. Chufamo, "Seroprevalence and Predictors of Hepatitis B Virus Infection among Pregnant Women Attending Routine Antenatal Care in Arba Minch Hospital, South Ethiopia," *Hepatitis Research and Treatment*, vol. 2016, Article ID 9290163, 7 pages, 2016.

[26] S. Rashid, C. Kilewo, and S. Aboud, "Seroprevalence of hepatitis B virus infection among antenatal clinic attendees at a tertiary hospital in Dar es Salaam, Tanzania," *Tanzania Journal of Health Research*, vol. 1, no. 16, pp. 1–8, 2014.

[27] J. J. Noubiap, J. R. Nansseu, S. T. Ndoula, J. J. Bigna, A. M. Jingi, and J. Fokom-Domgue, "Prevalence, infectivity and correlates of hepatitis B virus infection among pregnant women in a rural district of the Far North Region of Cameroon," *BMC Public Health*, vol. 15, p. 454, 2015.

[28] E. A. Murad, S. M. Babiker, G. I. Gasim, D. A. Rayis, and I. Adam, "Epidemiology of hepatitis B and hepatitis C virus infections in pregnant women in Sana'a, Yemen," *BMC Pregnancy and Childbirth*, vol. 13, article 127, 2013.

[29] P. Bayo, E. Ochola, C. Oleo, and A. D. Mwaka, "High prevalence of hepatitis B virus infection among pregnant women attending antenatal care: A cross-sectional study in two hospitals in northern Uganda," *BMJ Open*, vol. 4, no. 11, Article ID 005889, 2014.

[30] A. K. W. Kfutwah, M. C. Tejiokem, and R. Njouom, "A low proportion of HBeAg among HBsAg-positive pregnant women with known HIV status could suggest low perinatal transmission of HBV in Cameroon," *Virology Journal*, vol. 9, article no. 62, 2012.

[31] C. G. Anaedobe, A. Fowotade, C. E. Omoruyi, and R. A. Bakare, "Prevalence, socio-demographic features and risk factors of Hepatitis B virus infection among pregnant women in South-western Nigeria," *Pan African Medical Journal*, vol. 20, article no. 406, 2015.

[32] K. A. Rabiu, O. I. Akinola, A. A. Adewunmi, O. M. Omololu, and T. O. Ojo, "Risk factors for hepatitis B virus infection among pregnant women in Lagos, Nigeria," *Acta Obstetricia et Gynecologica Scandinavica*, vol. 89, no. 8, pp. 1024–1028, 2010.

[33] M. Melku, A. Kebede, and Z. Addis, "Magnitude of HIV and syphilis seroprevalence among pregnant women in gondar, northwest ethiopia: a cross-sectional study," *HIV/AIDS—Research and Palliative Care*, vol. 7, no. 175, 2015.

[34] M. Endris, T. Deressa, Y. Belyhun, and F. Moges, "Seroprevalence of syphilis and human immunodeficiency virus infections among pregnant women who attend the University of Gondar teaching hospital, Northwest Ethiopia: A cross sectional study," *BMC Infectious Diseases*, vol. 15, no. 1, article no. 111, 2015.

[35] M. Tiruneh, "Seroprevalence of multiple sexually transmitted infections among antenatal clinic attendees in Gondar Health Center, northwest Ethiopia," *Ethiopian Medical Journal*, vol. 46, no. 4, pp. 359–366, 2008.

[36] G. Andargie, A. Kassu, F. Moges et al., "Brief communication: low prevalence of HIV infection, and knowledge, attitude and practice on HIV/AIDS among high school students in Gondar, Northwest Ethiopia," *Ethiopian Journal of Health Development*, vol. 21, no. 2, pp. 179–182, 2007.

[37] C. L. Thio, "Hepatitis B and human immunodeficiency virus coinfection," *Hepatology*, vol. 49, no. 5, pp. S138–S145, 2009.

[38] Federal Democratic Republic of Ethiopia Ministry of Health: National guidelines for comprehensive HIV prevention, care and treatment. 2014.

[39] K. Yogeswaran and S. K. Fung, "Chronic hepatitis B in pregnancy: unique challenges and opportunities.," *Clinical and Molecular Hepatology*, vol. 17, no. 1, pp. 1–8, 2011.

[40] O. K. Chan, T. T. Lao, S. S. H. Suen, T. K. Lau, and T. Y. Leung, "Knowledge on hepatitis B infection among pregnant women in a high endemicity area," *Patient Education and Counseling*, vol. 85, no. 3, pp. 516–520, 2011.

24

The Impact of Scientific and Technical Training on Improving Routine Collection of Antenatal Care Data for Maternal and Foetal Risk Assessment

Dewi Anggraini ®,[1,2,3] Mali Abdollahian,[1] Kaye Marion,[1] Supri Nuryani,[4,5] Fadly Ramadhan,[2] Rezky Putri Rahayu,[2] Irfan Rizki Rachman,[2] and Widya Wurianto[2]

[1] School of Science (Mathematical and Geospatial Sciences), College of Science, Engineering, and Health, RMIT University, GPO Box 2476, Melbourne, VIC 3001, Australia
[2] Study Program of Mathematics, Faculty of Mathematics and Natural Sciences, University of Lambung Mangkurat (ULM), Ahmad Yani Street, Km. 36, Banjarbaru, South Kalimantan 70714, Indonesia
[3] Study Program of Statistics, Faculty of Mathematics and Natural Sciences, University of Lambung Mangkurat (ULM), Ahmad Yani Street, Km. 36, Banjarbaru, South Kalimantan 70714, Indonesia
[4] Ulin Public Hospital, 43 Ahmad Yani Street, Km 2.5, Banjarmasin, South Kalimantan 70233, Indonesia
[5] Abdi Persada Midwifery Academy, 365 Sutoyo S. Street, Banjarmasin, South Kalimantan 70115, Indonesia

Correspondence should be addressed to Dewi Anggraini; dewi.anggraini@ulm.ac.id

Academic Editor: Irene Hoesli

Objectives. First, to assess the impact of scientific and technical training on midwives' abilities in collecting and recording the results of routine antenatal care examinations. Second, to explore midwives' views with regard to factors affecting their abilities to successfully complete the data documentation tasks. *Methods.* The study was conducted in South Kalimantan, Indonesia (April 2016-October 2017). Nineteen urban and rural midwives were selected. Access to antenatal care information on 4,946 women (retrospective cohort study) and 381 women (prospective cohort study) was granted. A descriptive and exploratory design was used to describe midwives' abilities and challenges pertaining to timely collection and recording of results concerning antenatal care examinations. *Results.* Scientific and technical training has significantly improved the average amount of recorded antenatal care data (from 17.5% to 62.1%, p-value < 0.0005). Lack of awareness, high workload, and insufficient skills and facilities are the main reasons for the database gaps. *Conclusions.* The training has equipped midwives with scientific knowledge and technical abilities to allow routine collection of antenatal care data. Provision and adequate use of this information during different stages of pregnancy is crucial as an evidence-based guideline to assess maternal and foetal risk factors to ending preventable mortality.

1. Introduction

Antenatal care (ANC) utilisation is highly recommended as a preventative action to improve pregnancy outcomes. Access to this service has been identified as one of the most effective interventions to prevent or manage complications and adverse birth outcomes [1–3]. ANC services provided across Indonesian healthcare centres are expected to comply with a quality integrated ANC standard to improve maternal and child health offerings, including recording and reporting the results of ANC examinations [4, 5]. This investment can provide sufficient information to be analysed and evidence to be used for informed planning, decision making, and monitoring policy progress to end preventable maternal and neonatal mortality [6–8].

Adequate use of ANC information and its systematic analysis during different stages of pregnancy is crucial to monitoring, detecting, and assessing the risks and preventable factors linked to maternal and neonatal mortality. In Indonesia, the access to timely, complete, and reliable data on pregnancy-related outcomes and the causes and the impacts of interventions remain challenging. This hinders planning programs, decision making, and allocating resources appropriately to reduce maternal, foetal, and neonatal mortality [5, 9–11]. Improvement of the ANC data availability, consistency, and quality during pregnancy can help medical practitioners detect the risks of abnormal delivery; consequently, proper interventions be initiated in a timely manner [7, 8, 12–14].

In the Indonesian ANC model, midwives are the key practitioners across provinces (87.8% of medical practitioners) [15, 16]. They are expected to provide a comprehensive and integrated ANC service to pregnant women and document the results of examinations in local health recording and reporting systems, such as pregnancy registers, mothers' medical cards, and maternal and child health (MCH) booklets [5]. They are also expected to detect early signs of potential complications and abnormalities during pregnancy and delivery and provide appropriate interventions or referrals in a timely manner. Nevertheless, their abilities in documenting the results of ANC examinations have been reportedly low, with a 20% rate in hospitals and a 42.5% rate in primary healthcare (PHC) centres [11]. Unrecorded or unavailable local data on maternal, foetal, and neonatal care have been acknowledged as a major cause of hampering evidence-based interventions to track, review, and assess the causes and preventable factors associated with maternal and neonatal mortality [13, 17].

This study has assessed the impact of scientific and technical training on midwives' abilities in collecting and recording the results of routine ANC examinations in local pregnancy registers. Particularly, midwives were recruited who work in urban and rural PHC centres as these are the most locally recommended and cost-effective first level of healthcare in Indonesia. The study also explored midwives' views with regard to factors affecting their abilities to complete the data documentation tasks.

2. Methods

2.1. Research Design. A descriptive and exploratory design using both quantitative and qualitative methods was used. The study was carried out in two phases: quantitative design (phase 1) and qualitative design (phase 2). During the quantitative phase, a review of local pregnancy registers was conducted. The purpose of this phase was to assess and compare midwives' abilities in collecting and recording the results of recommended ANC examinations (Table 1) during service provision. This took place on two occasions: before hands-on scientific and technical training (retrospective cohort study using current manual pregnancy registers) and after the training program (prospective cohort study using electronic pregnancy registers). Meanwhile, during the qualitative phase, i.e., after the training program, electronic questionnaires were distributed to the midwives. This phase was used to gather information from the participating midwives regarding their

views on challenges of documenting the results of ANC examinations in a timely manner.

2.2. Setting. The study was conducted in the province of South Kalimantan, Indonesia, between April 2016 and October 2017. The locality is one of the five provinces recording the highest neonatal mortality rate [11, 18, 19].

2.3. Participants. Nineteen midwives were recommended by the Provincial Health Department and Midwifery Association to participate in this study. They had been rendering antenatal and midwifery services for a minimum of five years at 19 PHC centres comprising 14 public health centres (PKMs) and 5 private midwifery clinics (BPMs). These centres are distributed throughout all administrative areas of the province (2 urban and 11 rural areas).

2.4. The Research Instrument and Data Collection

2.4.1. Phase 1: Quantitative Design

Hands-On Scientific and Technical Training. Scientific and technical training was initiated and conducted amongst Indonesian urban and rural PHC's midwives (21-22 May 2016) to enhance the existing investment program in midwives. The program was intended to reduce maternal and neonatal mortality [9–11, 20]. The training aimed to educate and update midwives with scientific knowledge and technical abilities to allow for routine monitoring, measuring, collecting, and electronically recording of the significant maternal and foetal characteristics during ANC. This initiative was also meant to improve the availability, quantity, quality, and use of ANC information to strengthen routine maternal, foetal, and child health information systems and quality of care [3, 6, 11, 13, 17]. Additionally, the information can be utilised to monitor the progress of policies and programs in ending the preventable deaths due to prematurity, stillbirths, and low birth weight (LBW) [7, 17].

The training was divided into two sessions: scientific and technical. In the scientific domain, the maternal and foetal characteristics that play a vital role in evidence-based intervention decisions to reduce neonatal mortality were discussed. The session also covered scientific reasons for the significance of these characteristics and how their measurements are used to make evidence-based interventions to prevent neonatal mortality. This scientific introduction gave the participating midwives better insights into the importance of complete performance of such measurements and recording of results routinely from the start of pregnancy to delivery time.

An electronic pregnancy register was introduced in the technical part of the training. Each ANC category and its characteristics (Table 1) involved in the electronic register were technically and thoroughly explained and discussed to reach a consensus among the midwives. A demonstration of how to appropriately record and manage the data was also performed. This session provided the representative midwives better knowledge and skills of how to record the

TABLE 1: List of recommended contents of ANC examinations.

ANC category	Recommended/current ANC characteristics	Proposed ANC characteristics
Personal information (PI)	Name, name of partner/husband, date of birth, address, contact number, educational background, occupation, religion, maternal age, date of the first registration/visit, ownership of health insurance, ownership of Maternal and Child Health (MCH) booklet, prepregnancy weight, prepregnancy height, and blood type.	Ethnicity/country of birth and prepregnancy body mass index (BMI).
Obstetric history (OH)	Gravidity, parity, number of deliveries, number of abortions, number of live births, obstetric complication history, chronic diseases and allergies, the last delivery date, the last menstrual period, and the estimated delivery date.	Number of stillbirths, number of premature births, prepregnancy contraception, distance between previous and current pregnancies, the last birth attendance, the last tetanus toxoid (TT) immunisation, and the last mode of delivery.
Delivery plans (DP)	Birth attendance, birth place, birth companion, transportation, and blood donor.	-
Antenatal care utilisation criteria (ANCUC)	Gestational age (GA), the method of antenatal care (ANC) enrolment, date of consultation, and date of the next consultation.	Number of antenatal care (ANC) visits.
Maternal measurements (MM)	Anamnesis, patellar reflex, weight, middle upper arm circumference (MUAC), nutritional status, blood pressure, and fundal height (FH).	Height, body mass index (BMI), body temperature, *blood pressure (column separation between systole and diastole records)*, pulse, breathe, and abdominal palpation (Leopold I, II, III, and IV).
Laboratory tests (LT)	Haemoglobin level, urine protein, syphilis, maternal urine reduction, blood sugar level, thallassemia, hepatitis B surface antigen, prevention of mother to child transmission (human immunodeficiency virus (HIV) test), rapid test (malaria), and tuberculosis.	*Haemoglobin level: before and after having iron tablets*, sputum acid resistant bacteria, and ankylostoma test.
Supplements (S)	Iron tablets and tetanus toxoid (TT) immunisation.	Folic acid, calcium, aspirin, and vitamin C.
Maternal risk detection (MRD)	Maternal complication, referral, and risk detector.	Intervention action.
Foetal measurements: clinical method (CFM)	Number of gestation, foetal weight estimation, foetal heart rate, foetal presentation, and foetal station/descent level (FS).	-
Foetal measurements: ultrasonic method (UFM)	Not available	Gestational age (GA) based on ultrasound scanning, crown-rump length, head circumference, abdominal circumference, biparietal diameter, femur length, humerus length, placenta localisation, foetal presentation, amniotic fluid index, foetal heart rate, and foetal weight estimation.
Foetal risk detection (FRD)	Not available	Foetal complication, intervention action, referral, and risk detector.
Delivery time (DT)	Gestational age (GA) at delivery time, last menstrual period age at delivery time, active phase I and II (date and time), active phase III management, breast feeding initiation, neonatal delivery (date and time), placenta delivery (date and time), new born gender, new born presentation, birth weight, birth length, head circumference, birth place and address, delivery complication, referral, birth attendance, integration programs, bleeding status, mode of delivery, and survival status (mother and new born).	Abdominal circumference, chest circumference, femur length, humerus length, and intervention action towards delivery complications.

Source: [4, 21–28, 30–33, 38–41].

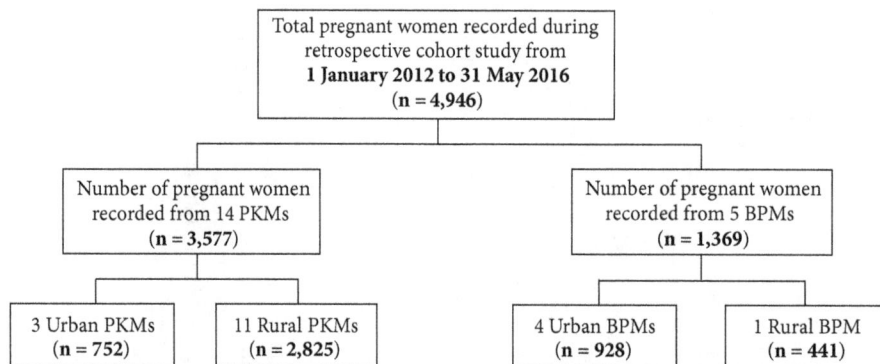

FIGURE 1: Description of retrospective data.

results of standard ANC measurements electronically and appropriately.

Manual Pregnancy Register. During the training, the participating midwives were asked to provide the current manual pregnancy registers (1 January 2012–31 May 2016) available at PHC centres where they were employed. The structure and content of these registers were then closely examined to match and track the recommended ANC characteristics suggested in Table 1. These records were then entered into the developed electronic pregnancy register for quantitative analyses by local graduates and research students who had experiences in the area of data entry. To improve the quality of the data processing task, the team in charge of data entry was trained to understand the content of the manual and electronic registers. This was followed by face-to-face and online communication between the principal investigator, the data collection team, and the midwives to minimise data entry error. The access to manually recorded ANC information on 4,946 women who enrolled, received care, and gave birth in the centres was granted (Figure 1).

Electronic Pregnancy Register. A bilingual electronic pregnancy register was created using a standard platform (Microsoft Excel) containing 12 categories of recommended ANC examinations listed in Table 1. This creation was based on current national application in conjunction with additional characteristics that have not been included but which are recommended nationally [4, 21–23] and internationally [7, 24–38].

The ANC categories are listed in the first column of Table 1. The objective of this tabulation is to stratify maternal and foetal measurements that are routinely undertaken during ANC service. The second column represents the recommended national and international characteristics under each ANC category. In the third column, unrecorded characteristics of the recommended ANC examinations are given. In the developed electronic register, new columns to record these characteristics were created. We proposed that these characteristics should be included in the current ANC data recording and reporting systems in Indonesia.

At the end of the training sessions, the representative midwives agreed to participate in our prospective cohort study (1 June 2016–30 June 2017). By following the national standard operational procedures of ANC, the midwives were expected to longitudinally monitor and measure the recommended ANC examinations (Table 1) and record the results into the developed electronic pregnancy register in a timely manner. Online communication between the principal investigator and the midwives was conducted to improve the quality of the data processing task and minimise data entry error. Therefore, the access to electronically recorded ANC information on 381 women who enrolled, received care, and gave birth in the centres was granted (Figure 2).

2.4.2. Phase 2: Qualitative Design

Electronic Questionnaires. After the training, an electronic feedback questionnaire was distributed to the participating midwives through email and social media platforms. The questionnaire covered questions on the current manual systems of recording and reporting ANC examination results, accessibility to the existing health information systems, and feedback on the training program. The questionnaire responses were used to assess the performance of the current ANC documentation systems, the potential challenges to complete the tasks, and the impact of the training program. The questionnaire responses were electronically collected between August and October 2016. A discussion forum was also conducted through a social media platform, both as personal communication among the midwives to clarify unclear specific responses and as a group to clarify common related issues of ANC data recording and reporting systems. In this study, 19 midwives' questionnaire responses were considered as preliminary data in the analysis, so as to enhance the future qualitative aspect of the study.

2.5. Statistical Analyses.
Descriptive statistics were deployed to assess the performance of routine ANC data collection, particularly in documenting the key recommended maternal and foetal characteristics (Table 1). This was done by calculating the amount of available records of the identified ANC characteristics in both manual (retrospective study)

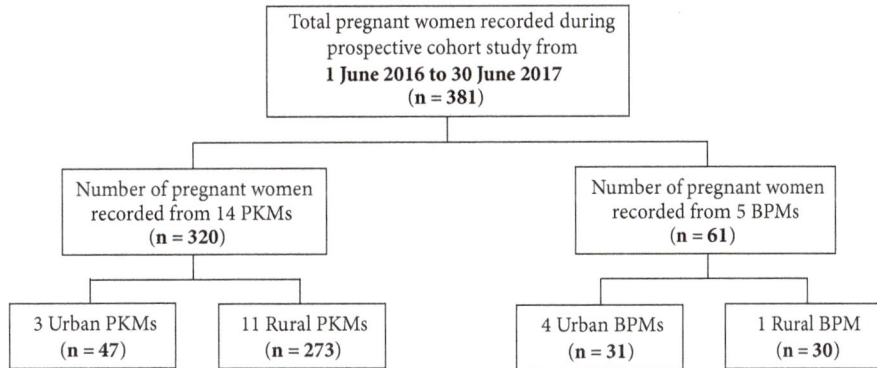

FIGURE 2: Description of prospective data.

and electronic (prospective study) pregnancy registers at each PHC centre. A two-sample t-test was used to compare the performance of data documentation process, before and after the training program, across PHC facilities. Data management and analyses were performed using Microsoft Excel 2010 and Minitab 17.

Analyses of the emerging codes, categories, and themes were conducted to investigate the causes of current ANC database gaps. The qualitative data were analysed using nonparametric statistics, frequencies, cross tabulations, and percentages. Cramer's V test was used to determine the degree of association between midwives' responses regarding factors affecting their ability to successfully complete the ANC data collection tasks. Data management and analyses were performed using Microsoft Excel 2010 and SPSS 23.

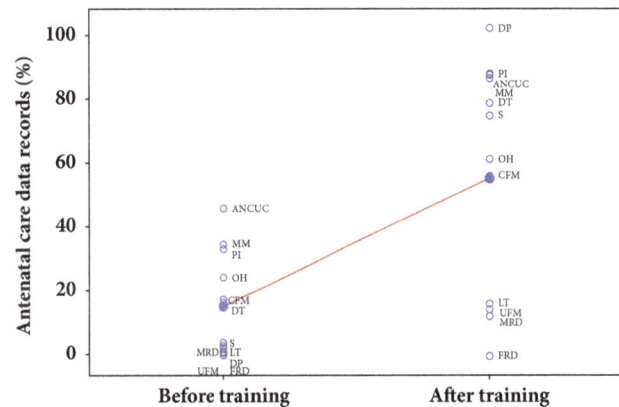

FIGURE 3: Individual plot of average ANC data records (%) before and after midwives' training across urban and rural PHC centres.

2.6. Ethics Approval and Consent to Participate. This study is a part of doctoral degree research and has obtained two ethics' clearances:

(1) The Ethical Committees of Medical Research, Medical Faculty, University of Lambung Mangkurat (ULM), Banjarmasin, South Kalimantan (Indonesia), on March 10, 2016, with registration number: 018/KEPK-FK UNLAM/EC/III/2016.

(2) The Science, Engineering, and Health College Human Ethics Advisory Network (CHEAN) of Royal Melbourne Institute of Technology (RMIT) University, Melbourne, Victoria (Australia), on March 16, 2016, with registration number: ASEHAPP 19-16/RM No: 19974.

Research permissions were also obtained from the Indonesian provincial and local governments. Information about the project and a consent form for recruitment to the study were given to the selected midwives and pregnant women (prospective study), who all agreed to participate.

3. Results

3.1. Midwives' Characteristics. Overall, the average age of the participating midwives was 41 years (29-56 years). The results revealed that 4 (21.1%) midwives were 46 years of age or older, 13 (68.4%) were 36-45 years old, and 2 (10.5%) were 25-35 years old. The average working experience of midwives in antenatal and midwifery services was 19 years. Their experience ranged from six to ten years ($n = 4$; 21.1%), eleven to twenty years ($n = 9$; 47.4%), twenty-one to thirty years ($n = 5$; 26.3%), and thirty-one or longer ($n = 1$; 5.3%).

3.2. The Impact of Scientific and Technical Training on Improving Routine Collection of ANC Data. Scientific and technical training has significantly improved the average amount of recorded ANC data suggested in Table 1 across PHC providers based on a two-sample t-test (from 17.5% to 62.1%, p-value <0.0005) (Table 2).

This significant improvement is presented in Figure 3 and listed in Table 3. The results show an overall improvement, particularly in documenting personal information, obstetric history, delivery plan, ANC utilisation criteria, maternal measurements, provision of supplements, clinical foetal measurements, and delivery time (from 0.8-47.9% to 57.4-99.2%). However, midwives' responsiveness on the importance of collecting and recording the results of laboratory tests, maternal risk detection, ultrasonic foetal measurements, and foetal risk detection suggest room for improvement (<12%).

TABLE 2: Two-sample t-test on the performance of ANC data collection before and after midwives' training across urban and rural PHC centres.

Treatment	Mean	Standard deviation	SE Mean	Estimate for difference	95% Confidence interval for difference		T value	P value	Pooled standard deviation
					Lower bound	Upper bound			
After training	62.1	40.4	1.7	44.6***	40.5	48.8	21.1	<0.0005	35.0
Before training	17.5	28.5	1.2						

***Significant at p-value < 0.0005.
**Significant at p-value < 0.05.
*Significant at p-value < 0.1.

TABLE 3: Average data records (%) of ANC category before and after midwives' training across urban and rural PHC centres.

12 recommended ANC categories	Before training (%)	After training (%)
Personal information (PI)	33.1	91.7
Obstetric history (OH)	25.9	64.4
Delivery plans (DP)	0.8	99.2
Antenatal care utilisation criteria (ANCUC)	47.9	91.0
Maternal measurements (MM)	32.3	82.1
Laboratory tests (LT)	1.5	11.3
Supplements (S)	5.0	69.9
Maternal risk detection (MRD)	2.4	6.5
Clinical foetal measurements (CFM)	18.0	57.4
Ultrasonic foetal measurements (UFM)	0.0	11.3
Foetal risk detection (FRD)	0.0	0.4
Delivery time (DT)	14.0	75.8

3.3. The Improvement of Database Adequacy for Maternal and Foetal Risk Assessment. This analysis is accompanied by Tables 4-14 (Appendix A in the Supplementary material) that compare the abilities of midwives in recording the results of the recommended ANC examinations (Table 1) before and after the training program. The results can be used to assess the impact of training on improving database adequacy for maternal and foetal risk detection during pregnancy.

The ANC categories are presented in the first column together with their characteristics. The second and third main columns provide the type of PHC centres: PKMs and BPMs. These columns have been divided into two subcolumns to represent urban and rural areas. Urban areas (subcolumns 1 and 3) consist of 3 midwives representing PKMs and 4 midwives representing BPMs, respectively. Rural areas (subcolumns 2 and 4) comprising of 11 midwives representing PKMs and 1 midwife representing BPM, respectively. In each subcolumn, the amount of recorded ANC data (%) of the identified characteristics has been calculated. The relevant summary of detailed data collection's performance is given below.

3.3.1. Maternal Risk Assessment. Maternal risks can be assessed from their personal information, obstetric history, delivery plans, maternal measurements, laboratory tests, and nutritional interventions/supplements.

Personal Information (PI). A significant improvement of midwives' abilities in documenting personal information is indicated in Table 4, particularly in data access to educational background, occupation, ownership of health insurance, ownership of MCH booklets, prepregnancy weight, prepregnancy height, prepregnancy BMI, and blood type (from 0.0-54.3% to 63.8-100.0%).

Obstetric History (OH). Midwives' competencies were improved in data collection tasks on obstetric history, particularly in recording the number of still births and premature births (Table 5). They were also more responsive in documenting gravidity, parity, number of deliveries, abortions, and live births, while a rural BPM's midwife collected substantially more data on prepregnancy contraception, pregnancy interval, the last birth attendance, the last TT immunisation, and the last mode of delivery (from 0.0% to 70-96.7%). However, midwives were less aware of the importance of documenting complication history (<17%) and chronic diseases and allergies (<7%).

Delivery Plans (DP). The performance of midwives in documenting information on birth preparedness was significantly improved across urban and rural centres (from 0.0-4.1% to 95.2-100.0%) (Table 6). This involved plans for birth attendance, birth place, birth companion, transportation, and blood donor.

Maternal Measurements (MM). The responsiveness of urban and rural midwives in collecting and recording the results of maternal measurements during pregnancy was significantly improved (Table 8). The examinations included anamnesis, patellar reflex, maternal MUAC, nutritional status, blood pressure, body temperature, pulse, and breath (from 0.0-88.0% to 66.1-100.0%). Improvement was also seen in the assessment of abdominal palpation and fundal height (from 0.0-69.8% to 42.5-100.0%).

Laboratory Tests (LT). The average amount of recorded laboratory data before (1.5%) and after (11.3%) the training program remained low (Table 3). However, urban and rural midwives have attempted to improve the data accessibility of laboratory test results. This is particularly true for the haemoglobin test (from 0.0-20.2% to 4.8-35.6%, Table 9) and the blood test (from 0.0-29.7% to 93.41-100.0%, Table 4), which are highly recommended to be routinely performed during pregnancy [5].

Supplements (S). Midwives' abilities in documenting the provision of supplements was substantially improved, particularly among rural midwives (from 0.0-42.5% to 81.0-100.0%) (Table 10), except TT immunisation records (< 45%). Less well documented was coverage and documentation of this characteristic across PHC facilities.

Maternal Risk Detection (MRD). Midwives have made efforts to improve information on maternal complications, yet the amount of records remained low (<26%) across PHC centres (Table 11). This resulted in a lack of documentation on appropriate interventions (<32%) and referral tasks (<15%).

3.3.2. Foetal Risk Assessment. Foetal risks can be assessed through available information on foetal measurements based on clinical and ultrasonic methods.

Foetal Measurements: Clinical (CFM) and Ultrasonic (UFM) Methods. Overall, midwives' competencies have improved in clinically documenting foetal growth (Table 12). Rural midwives tended to provide more information on the number of gestation, foetal weight estimation, foetal heart rate, foetal presentation, and foetal station/descent level than urban midwives (from 0.0-61.0% to 57.3-100.0%). A rural BPM's midwife was more responsive in collecting and recording the results of foetal measurements through ultrasound (from 0.0% to 0.9 -70.4%).

Foetal Risk Detection (FRD). Comparable to maternal risk detection, the competence of midwives in gathering information on foetal complications was persistently low (< 1%) (Table 13). As a result, data documentation on appropriate interventions and referral tasks was also low (< 2%).

3.3.3. ANC Service Utilisation and Pregnancy Outcomes.
ANC service utilisation and pregnancy outcomes can be assessed through available ANC utilisation criteria and maternal and neonatal information recorded at delivery time.

Antenatal Care Utilisation Criteria (ANCUC). The responsiveness of urban and rural midwives in collecting and recording the criteria of ANC utilisation during pregnancy was significantly improved (from 47.9% to 91.0%) (Table 3). The criteria included measurement of GA, method of ANC enrolment, date of consultation, date of the next consultation, and number of ANC visits.

Delivery time (DT). The performance of midwives in documenting maternal and neonatal information at delivery time was significantly improved across urban and rural centres (from 14.0% to 75.8%) (Table 3). The information included GA (from 8.8-34.9% to 100.0%), newborn gender (from 17.3-67.1% to 95.7-100.0%), birth weight (from 18.0-68.5% to 100.0%), and survival status of mother and newborn (from 7.7-47.7% to 100.0%) (Table 14). However, data documentation on neonatal anthropometric characteristics and delivery complications should be further improved.

3.4. Midwives' Perspectives on Challenges in Timely Collecting and Recording the Results of ANC Examinations.
Table 15 (Appendix B in the Supplementary material) is a cross tabulation analysis of midwives' opinions of the existing ANC data recording and reporting systems. The table includes their feedback on the scientific and technical training. The first column lists the main open questions with the respective categories of answers. The second column describes the percentage of responses across urban and rural PKMs and BPMs. The third column represents the percentage of responses for each category of identified answers. The last column shows the Cramer's V test value carried out to identify whether there is an association between midwives' responses with respect to factors affecting their ability to successfully complete the ANC data documentation tasks. A 5% significant level is used for the Cramer's V test.

Combination between pregnancy registers, mothers' medical cards, and MCH booklets are the most commonly used manual formats among midwives to collect and record ANC data (26.3-31.6%) (Table 15). Twenty-one per cent of the midwives believed that the design and infrastructure of these formats should be further improved. Supervision and monitoring on the completeness of ANC data have been routinely undertaken (78.9%). Almost half of the midwives have been trained for ANC data management. However, surprisingly, fewer than 20% of them were aware of and using the existing electronic database formats, either SIKDA Generic (5.3%) or PWS KIA Kartini (15.8%).

Poor recording and reporting systems (31.3%), unawareness of the pregnancy (25.0%), and time limitations (25.0%) were the main contributing factors for midwives not completing ANC data records (Table 15). Almost 60.0% of the midwives had to manually prepare multiple reports every month. Lack of awareness (46.2%), high workload (30.8%), and insufficient skills and facilities (15.4%) were the main reasons for the delay in collecting and reporting routine ANC data. Seventeen midwives (89.5%) responded to the effectiveness of the training and 52.6% of them responded to the importance of the developed electronic register, particularly if it could be computationally and automatically linked with the monthly ANC reporting formats.

4. Discussion

4.1. Age and Experience of the Midwives.
Most midwives' ages ranged between 29 and 56 years, implying that the participants were senior midwives. The midwives' working experience ranged between 6 and 36 years in antenatal and midwifery services across urban and rural PHC facilities.

4.2. The Impact of Scientific and Technical Training on Improving Routine Collection of ANC Examination Results.
Scientific and technical training has significantly equipped Indonesian urban and rural midwives, as pivotal health practitioners to ANC service [14, 42, 43], with the knowledge of the importance of ANC data documentation. It is documented that investments on continuous training among midwives are vital to ending preventable deaths [14]. The improvement of their basic midwifery care in documenting the results of ANC examinations was overall higher (62.1%) (Table 3) than the current national report (42.5%) [11]. This was particularly the case in collecting and recording the key quality characteristics of mother and foetus used to assess the risks during pregnancy.

Routine collection of ANC data is vital to improving maternal and foetal health. If good quality of care can be associated with its effective data collection during labour [14], then it is also crucial to having real-time data collection at different stages of pregnancy to optimize the quality of ANC. Such data collection is important to promoting evidence-based approaches to ANC for positive, transparent, and respectful pregnancy experiences and improvement of pregnancy outcomes [3].

Currently, local health registers rather than periodic household surveys are used to identify risk factors to reduce maternal and neonatal mortality [9, 10, 44]. With the adoption of a decentralisation policy in Indonesia [9, 10], access to routine and consistent local data collection of maternal and foetal measurements during ANC is urgently required. Given appropriate training, supervision, quality control, and technology to strengthen the records maintenance, local maternal, foetal, and neonatal health data can be used as reliable baseline information to improve the quality of care services [44].

4.3. The Improvement of Database Adequacy for Maternal and Foetal Risk Assessment. Access to individual (disaggregate) information on maternal and foetal health during pregnancy and at delivery is vital to strengthen accountability of routine health information systems. Our training has significantly improved midwives' responsiveness in consistently documenting the key characteristics of individual mother and foetus at different stages of pregnancy and delivery. The use of this information enables midwives to improve the quality of risk assessment tasks and pregnancy outcomes and to target informed planning, interventions, and referrals. It is for the purpose of preventing maternal, neonatal, and child mortality [8, 11, 14] and promoting equality [13], particularly in rural areas.

It is well documented that maternal lifestyle and chronic disease history are factors that contribute to spontaneous preterm births, stillbirths, and LBW [7, 14, 45] influencing maternal, foetal, and neonatal health [5]. Although tobacco and substance uses are recommended to be investigated during maternal assessment at every ANC visit [38], there are no specific columns, in the current manual pregnancy register, that allow midwives to document such information, except under the chronic diseases and allergies column. Therefore, we recommend additional columns be provided for recording smoking habits and alcohol consumption separately to improve maternal risk detection.

Midwives' unawareness in documenting information on a delivery plan potentially caused birth preparedness to be one of the remaining and emerging challenges in reducing maternal and neonatal mortality in Indonesia [11]. The training has significantly improved midwives' responsiveness in recording this information (from 0.8% to 99.2%) (Table 3). This would increase community demand for the use of care and consequently improve the quality continuum and effectiveness of obstetric care.

In the current national ANC standard, MUAC is measured once only, in the first trimester of pregnancy, to screen the risk of chronic energy deficiency or malnutrition among pregnant women [5]. We highly recommend that MUAC be measured routinely at different trimesters of pregnancy based on the following reasons. MUAC has a significant relationship with BMI which corresponds to maternal weight and height [46]; hence, it may be affected by the changes of maternal weight. MUAC is well documented to be a factor that contributes to spontaneous preterm births [7] and relates to LBW which is one of the main causes of neonatal deaths

[5, 11]. This becomes a focus to end preventable stillbirths [8]. This recommendation can potentially be considered a new baseline for evaluation in the future, particularly in the effort of reducing neonatal mortality and achieving the target of Sustainable Development Goals (SDGs) 2030 [11].

Data collection of laboratory test results during pregnancy is crucial. Keeping these records is highly recommended [5, 7, 44] since it can be used as an information base to improve detection of infections caused by microorganisms during pregnancy, particularly for those who are living in vulnerable and epidemic areas [37]. For instance, maternal infections and anaemia are well-documented to be one of the risk factors in the occurrence of spontaneous preterm births [7], stillbirths [14], and neonatal deaths [11]. Although the training program has improved laboratory data accessibility, the average amount of records across PHC services remained low. These findings may indicate that some of the laboratory tests are not necessarily performed. For example, malaria, syphilis, and HIV tests should be routinely undertaken only in high-prevalence settings [5, 37, 47] where in our study population this was not the case. In addition, urine protein, blood sugar level, and tuberculosis tests are only performed when symptoms occur [5].

Midwives' competencies in documenting the provision of nutritional interventions/supplements (iron, folic acid, calcium, and vitamin C) for pregnant women were significantly improved after the training program (from 0.0-42.5% to 34.0-100.0%) (Table 10). Daily intake of these supplements is highly recommended to prevent anaemia, sepsis, LBW, preterm births, stillbirths, and preeclampsia; consequently, it improves pregnancy outcomes [3, 5, 14, 38, 48]. Attention should be directed to the documentation of TT immunisation across PHC centres which remained below 45%. This is due to the fact that the vaccination is not necessary if a pregnant woman has previously been vaccinated or if her TT immunisation is known [5, 38].

Serial ultrasonic scanning has been recommended in the national and international ANC standards as a means to detect foetal growth abnormalities [4, 24, 25, 38, 41, 49]. However, the fields to record such measurements do not exist in the manual pregnancy register (Table 12). These findings indicate that the ultrasonic method is not accessible in the current practice of ANC services across Indonesian PHC centres because it requires intensive resources [38]. Even if it was accessible, there were no columns to facilitate the documentation of the measurements. In the developed electronic register, we have provided such columns to enable a rural midwife who was trained for ultrasound to record the results of the examination during pregnancy even though the percentage of recorded data in the current ANC needs further improvement.

Information on maternal and foetal complications, which can be derived from risk assessment analysis during pregnancy, is vital to improving the quality of ANC service and positive pregnancy outcomes [3]. Midwives, as the pivotal practitioners to ANC, are expected to record this information based on their integrated analyses of maternal and foetal characteristics [5, 14]. Nevertheless, the amount of recorded information across PHC centres was not sufficient (0.0%)

even after the training (6.5%) (Table 3). These results clearly indicate gaps in undertaking the risk analysis. The gaps are potentially due to the fact that midwives are required to record the signs of abnormalities only if they are present. The other significant reason is that screening tools, such as foetal growth charts, are currently not available to assist midwives in carrying out the systematic risk analysis during pregnancy.

4.4. Midwives' Perspectives on Challenges in Successfully Completing Routine ANC Data Documentation Tasks. Most midwives have reportedly complied with the standard ANC examination procedures in Indonesia [5]. However, some of them agreed that the design and infrastructure of the existing data recording and reporting formats need to be further improved to support accuracy and complete documentation, storage ability, and record maintenance. This result is similar to findings reported by other researchers [1].

The midwives stated that supervision and monitoring on ANC data collection have been initiated but were carried out irregularly. They were also trained for ANC data management yet many of them remained unfamiliar with the existing electronic applications, such as SIKDA Generic and PWS KIA Kartini. Lack of knowledge on these database systems was also described by other researchers [50].

The midwives informed several factors triggering incomplete and delayed ANC data recording and reporting tasks. These included high workload, lack of time for routine ANC examinations, limited skills and training, and lack of awareness about the importance of recording the examination results. This is consistent with those of Burke et al. [44] and Sibiya et al. [1] who found similar factors hindering complete and timely documentation of the recommended ANC examination results.

The midwives positively responded to the effectiveness of the training and the importance of keeping the results of ANC examinations electronically. They also recommended that the training should be routinely conducted among other midwives so that they have an equal chance to update their knowledge and improve their capabilities in timely recording and reporting ANC data from local to provincial and national levels. Ongoing education (raising awareness) and training might then be an integral part of investment programs in midwives to further reduce maternal and neonatal mortality [11, 20].

5. Conclusion

Risk assessment of maternal and foetal complications during pregnancy is vital to preventing potential adverse pregnancy outcomes. Adequate use of ANC information and its systematic analysis during different stages of pregnancy is crucial to assessing the prevalence of maternal and foetal risk factors. The statistical analysis shows that scientific and technical training has increased Indonesian midwives' awareness of the importance of monitoring and measuring the key characterists of mother and foetus during pregnancy and at delivery as well as collecting and maintaining the records electronically.

Strong commitment and consistent education/training coupled with routine supervision of data documentation and records maintenance can significantly improve midwives' competencies to report the results of ANC examinations in a timely manner. This will lead to improvement of the quality and quantity of routine collection of ANC data, promote a reliable and transparent local data recording and reporting system as baseline information, and allow the task of vital data transformation. Consequently, the national health information system needs to be strengthened and made more reliable to be used as an evidence-based guideline in targeting appropriate resource planning and allocations, interventions, and referrals. The ultimate aim is to end preventable maternal and neonatal mortality.

Abbreviations

ANC:	Antenatal care
PHC:	Primary healthcare
PKM:	Public primary healthcare centre
BPM:	Private primary healthcare centre (midwifery clinics)
LBW:	Low birth weight
PI:	Personal information
OH:	Obstetric history
DP:	Delivery plans
ANCUC:	Antenatal care utilisation criteria
MM:	Maternal measurements
LT:	Laboratory tests
S:	Supplements
MRD:	Maternal risk detection
CFM:	Clinical foetal measurement method
UFM:	Ultrasonic foetal measurement method
FRD:	Foetal risk detection
DT:	Delivery time
GA:	Gestational age
MCH:	Maternal and child health
TT:	Tetanus toxoid
MUAC:	Middle upper arm circumference
BMI:	Body mass index
HIV:	Human immunodeficiency virus
FH:	Fundal height
FS:	Foetal station/descent level
SIKDA:	Regional health information system
PWS KIA:	Local monitoring system of maternal and child health
SDGs:	Sustainable Development Goals.

Consent

The manuscript does not contain any individual person's data; hence, consent for publication is not applicable.

Disclosure

This research did not receive any specific grant from funding agencies in the public, commercial, or not-for-profit sectors. However, the Australian Agency for International Development (AusAID) has granted Dewi Anggraini a Ph.D. scholarship in Mathematical Sciences at the School of Science, RMIT University, Melbourne, Australia. This analysis is part of Dewi Anggraini's thesis.

Conflicts of Interest

The authors have no conflicts of interest to declare.

Authors' Contributions

Dewi Anggraini and Mali Abdollahian contributed in the conception and design of the study. Dewi Anggraini and Supri Nuryani provided the literature review and information summary on relevant research articles and policies in Indonesia. Dewi Anggraini, Supri Nuryani, Fadly Ramadhan, Rezky Putri Rahayu, Irfan Rizki Rachman, and Widya Wurianto performed data collection, preprocessing data, analysis, and interpretation. Dewi Anggraini prepared the manuscript. Mali Abdollahian and Kaye Marion provided data analysis, advice, proofreading, and critical revision of the manuscript. All of the authors read and approved the final manuscript.

Acknowledgments

The authors are grateful to the Australian Agency for International Development (AusAID) for funding Dewi Anggraini's Ph.D. scholarship in Mathematical Sciences at the School of Science, RMIT University, Melbourne, Australia. The authors are extremely thankful to the Head of the Provincial Health Department of South Kalimantan, Dr. Achmad Rudiansjah, M.S., who supported and permitted time release for the representative midwives to attend the training. They also thank Nani Lidya, SKM, for her participation in the training as the representative of the Provincial Health Department of South Kalimantan and Dr. Bambang Abimanyu, Sp.OG, KFM and Dr. Andy Yussianto, M.Epid, for their role in providing information about foetal biometric characteristics measured by ultrasound and current maternal and child health surveillance in Indonesia, respectively. They are immensely appreciative to the Head of the Provincial Midwifery Association (IBI) of South Kalimantan, Tut Barkinah, S.Si.T., M.Pd., and one of her members, Nurtjahaya, S.ST., who supported and selected the representative midwives to participate in the training. The authors are greatly indebted to the Higher Degree Research (HDR) Language and Learning Advisors of RMIT University (Dr. Judy Maxwell, Dr. Ken Manson, and Dr. Sarah McLaren) and a Linguistics Lecturer of Universitas Pendidikan Indonesia (R. Dian Dia-an Muniroh) for their roles in providing language help and proofreading the article. They are greatly appreciative to the midwives team (**midwives team:** Ariati, S.ST (Banjarmasin), Sari Milayanti, AMd.Keb and Masjudah, S.ST (Banjarbaru), Rini, AMd.Keb (Banjar), Rahmi Widiati, AM.Keb (Barito Kuala), Suwarni, AM.Keb (Tapin), Hiriana, AMd.Keb (Hulu Sungai Selatan), Yanti Pertiwi, AMd. Keb (Hulu Sungai Tengah), Siska Yunita, AM.Keb (Hulu Sungai Utara), Nurjanah, S.Si.T (Balangan), Suparti, S.Si.T (Tabalong), Rina, AM.Keb (Tanah Laut), Sri Wahyuningsih, AMd.Keb (Tanah Bumbu), Yani Kristanti, AMd. Keb (Kotabaru), Raihatul Jannah, AMd. Keb (BPM Banjarmasin), Rinawati, AMd. Keb (BPM Banjarmasin), Eka Septina, AMd. Keb (BPM Banjarmasin), Noorjannah, S.ST (BPM Banjarmasin), and Fauziah Olfah, S.ST (BPM Kotabaru)), for their roles in gathering the retrospective and prospective data from their assigned workplace. They also impressively thank the technical assistants (**technical assistants:** Widya Wurianto, Rowin Natalia Sihotang, Wuri Setyana Sari, S.Mat., Fauzan Helman, Jainal, S.Mat., and Nuer Vita Sari, S.Si.), for their roles in providing technical support for the participating midwives and the data entry group (**data entry group:** Akhmad Basuki, Muhammad Meidy Maulana, Nurul Istiqamah, Nurul Iftitah, Tri Wahyuni, Rizky Hidayatullah, S.Mat., Rezky Putri Rahayu, S.Mat., Widya Wurianto, Siti Hartinah, Filza Buana Putra, Rowin Natalia Sihotang, Muhammad Nizar Zulfi, Fadly Ramadhan, S.Mat., Linda Astuti, Muhammad Rifai, Yogi Apriyanto, and Irfan Rizki Rachman, S.Mat.), for their role in electronically recording the retrospective data.

Supplementary Materials

Appendix A: performance of data collection on 12 categories of recommended ANC examinations across urban and rural PHC centres before and after midwives' training. Table 4: personal information. Table 5: obstetric history. Table 6: delivery plans. Table 7: antenatal care utilisation criteria. Table 8: maternal measurements. Table 9: laboratory tests. Table 10: supplements. Table 11: maternal risk detection. Table 12: foetal measurements: clinical and ultrasonic. Table 13: foetal risk detection. Table 14: delivery time. Appendix B: perceptions on challenges of timely collecting and recording the results of ANC examinations. Table 15: midwives' perceptions on the current ANC data recording and reporting systems and the training program. *(Supplementary Materials)*

References

[1] M. N. Sibiya, R. J. Cele, and T. S. P. Ngxongo, "Assessment of the use of the new maternity case record in improving the quality of ante natal care in eThekwini District, KwaZulu-Natal," *International Journal of Africa Nursing Sciences*, vol. 2, pp. 53–58, 2015.

[2] A. Huang, K. Wu, W. Zhao, H. Hu, Q. Yang, and D. Chen, "Attendance at prenatal care and adverse birth outcomes in China: A follow-up study based on Maternal and Newborn's Health Monitoring System," *Midwifery*, vol. 57, pp. 26–31, 2018.

[3] O. Tuncalp, J. P. Pena-Rosas, T. Lawrie et al., "WHO recommendations on antenatal care for a positive pregnancy experience-going beyond survival," *BJOG: An International Journal of Obstetrics and Gynaecology*, vol. 124, no. 6, pp. 860–862, 2017.

[4] MoH, *Mother's Handbook of Health Services in Primary Health Facilities and Referral (Buku Saku Pelayanan Kesehatan Ibu di*

Fasilitas Kesehatan Dasar dan Rujukan), Ministry of Health, Republic of Indonesia, 2013.

[5] "Regulation of the Minister of Health of the Republic of Indonesia Number 97 Year 2014 About Health Service Before Pregnant, Pregnancy, Labor, And Easy After Birth, Contraceptive Implementation Services, and Sexual Health Care Services (Peraturan Menteri Kesehatan Republik Indonesia Nomor 97 Tahun 2014 Tentang Pelayanan Kesehatan Masa Sebelum Hamil, Masa Hamil, Persalinan, Dan Masa Sesudah Melahirkan, Penyelenggaraan Pelayanan Kontrasepsi, Serta Pelayanan Kesehatan Seksual)," 2014.

[6] W. H. Organization, *Strategic plan for strengthening health systems in the WHO Western Pacific Region*, WHO Regional Office for the Western Pacific, Manila, 2008.

[7] H. Blencowe, S. Cousens, D. Chou et al., "Born too Soon: the global epidemiology of 15 million preterm births," *Reproductive Health*, vol. 10, no. 1, article S2, 2013.

[8] J. E. Lawn, H. Blencowe, P. Waiswa et al., "Stillbirths: rates, risk factors, and acceleration towards 2030," *The Lancet*, vol. 387, no. 10018, pp. 587–603, 2016.

[9] N. R. Council, *Reducing Maternal and Neonatal Mortality in Indonesia: Saving Lives, Saving the Future*, National Academies Press, 2013.

[10] T. H. Hull, *Reducing maternal and neonatal mortality in Indonesia: saving lives, saving the future*, Taylor and Francis, Eds., 2015.

[11] E. Achadi and G. Jones, *Health Sector Review: Maternal, Neonatal and Child Health*, Ministry of National Development Planning/Bappenas, Republic of Indonesia, Jakarta, 2014.

[12] A. E. P. Heazell, D. Siassakos, H. Blencowe et al., "Stillbirths: Economic and psychosocial consequences," *The Lancet*, vol. 387, no. 10018, pp. 604–616, 2016.

[13] S. G. Moxon, H. Ruysen, K. J. Kerber et al., "Count every newborn; A measurement improvement roadmap for coverage data," *BMC Pregnancy and Childbirth*, vol. 15, article no. S8, 2015.

[14] L. De Bernis, M. V. Kinney, W. Stones et al., "Stillbirths: Ending preventable deaths by 2030," *The Lancet*, vol. 387, no. 10019, pp. 703–716, 2016.

[15] MoH, "Basic Health Research (Riset Kesehatan Dasar) 2013," Balitbangkes, Ministry of Health, Republic of Indonesia, Jakarta, 2013.

[16] A. Abdullah, E. Elizabeth, U. Wungouw, I. Kerong, Y. Butu, and I. Lobo, *Knowledge and skills of midwife supervisors and midwives in NTT and changes post training*, Australia Indonesia Partnership of Maternal and Neonatal Health (AIPMNH), Jakarta, 2015.

[17] K. J. Kerber, M. Mathai, G. Lewis et al., "Counting every stillbirth and neonatal death through mortality audit to improve quality of care for every pregnant woman and her baby," *BMC Pregnancy and Childbirth*, vol. 15, article no. S9, 2015.

[18] F. Bégin and V. M. Aguayo, "First foods: Why improving young children's diets matter.," *Maternal & Child Nutrition*, vol. 13, p. e12528, 2017.

[19] MoH, *Indonesia Health Profile (Profil Kesehatan Indonesia) 2012*, Ministry of Health, Republic of Indonesia, Jakarta, 2013.

[20] W. Van Lerberghe, Z. Matthews, E. Achadi et al., "Country experience with strengthening of health systems and deployment of midwives in countries with high maternal mortality," *The Lancet*, vol. 384, no. 9949, pp. 1215–1225, 2014.

[21] MoH, "Antenatal Integrated Guidelines (Pedoman Pelayanan Antenatal Terpadu," in *Jakarta:, Directorate General of Public Health Directorate of Maternal Health, Ministry of Health, Republic of Indonesia*, 2010.

[22] MoH, "Antenatal Integrated Guidelines (Pedoman Pelayanan Antenatal Terpadu," in *Jakarta:, Directorate General of Nutrition and Maternal and Child Health, Ministry of Health, Republic of Indonesia*, 2012.

[23] MoH, *Guidelines for Local Area Monitoring Maternal and Child Health (Pedoman Pemantauan Wilayah Setempat Kesehatan Ibu dan Anak (PWS-KIA))*, Jakarta, 2009.

[24] A. Papageorghiou, S. Kennedy, L. Salomon, E. Ohuma, L. Cheikh Ismail, and F. Barros, "International standards for early fetal size and pregnancy dating based on ultrasound measurement of crown–rump length in the first trimester of pregnancy," *Ultrasound in Obstetrics & Gynecology*, vol. 44, pp. 641–648, 2014.

[25] A. T. Papageorghiou, E. O. Ohuma, and D. G. Altman, "Erratum: International standards for fetal growth based on serial ultrasound measurements: the Fetal Growth Longitudinal Study of the INTERGROWTH-21 Project (Lancet (2014) 384 (869-879))," *The Lancet*, vol. 384, no. 9950, p. 1264, 2014.

[26] K. Beeckman, F. Louckx, G. Masuy-Stroobant, S. Downe, and K. Putman, "The development and application of a new tool to assess the adequacy of the content and timing of antenatal care," *BMC Health Services Research*, vol. 11, article no. 213, 2011.

[27] K. Beeckman, F. Louckx, S. Downe, and K. Putman, "The relationship between antenatal care and preterm birth: the importance of content of care," *European Journal of Public Health*, vol. 23, no. 3, pp. 366–371, 2013.

[28] K. Beeckman, F. Louckx, and K. Putman, "Content and timing of antenatal care: Predisposing, enabling and pregnancy-related determinants of antenatal care trajectories," *European Journal of Public Health*, vol. 23, no. 1, pp. 67–73, 2013.

[29] R. W. Johnson, "Calculations in estimating fetal weight," *American Journal of Obstetrics & Gynecology*, vol. 74, no. 4, p. 929, 1957.

[30] J. Gardosi, A. Chang, B. Kalyan, D. Sahota, and E. M. Symonds, "Customised antenatal growth charts," *The Lancet*, vol. 339, no. 8788, pp. 283–287, 1992.

[31] J. Gardosi, "Customized Charts Their Role in Identifying Pregnancies at Risk Because of Fetal Growth Restriction," *Journal of Obstetrics and Gynaecology Canada*, vol. 36, no. 5, pp. 408–415, 2014.

[32] J. Gardosi, S. Giddings, S. Buller, M. Southam, and M. Williams, "Preventing stillbirths through improved antenatal recognition of pregnancies at risk due to fetal growth restriction," *Public Health*, vol. 128, no. 8, pp. 698–702, 2014.

[33] J. Gardosi, M. Mongelli, M. Wilcox, and A. Chang, "An adjustable fetal weight standard," *Ultrasound in Obstetrics & Gynecology*, vol. 6, no. 3, pp. 168–174, 1995.

[34] J. E. Lawn, H. Blencowe, R. Pattinson et al., "Stillbirths: where? When? Why? How to make the data count?" *The Lancet*, vol. 377, no. 9775, pp. 1448–1463, 2011.

[35] A. C. C. Lee, J. Katz, H. Blencowe et al., "National and regional estimates of term and preterm babies born small for gestational age in 138 low-income and middle-income countries in 2010," *The Lancet Global Health*, vol. 1, no. 1, pp. e26–e36, 2013.

[36] H. Blencowe, S. Cousens, M. Z. Oestergaard et al., "National, regional, and worldwide estimates of preterm birth rates in the year 2010 with time trends since 1990 for selected countries: a systematic analysis and implications," *The Lancet*, vol. 379, no. 9832, pp. 2162–2172, 2012.

The Impact of Scientific and Technical Training on Improving Routine Collection of Antenatal Care...

205

[37] J. V. de Bernabé, T. Soriano, R. Albaladejo, M. Juarranz, M. a. E. Calle, and D. Marti, "Risk factors for low birth weight: A review," *European Journal of Obstetrics Gynecology and Reproductive Biology*, vol. 116, pp. 3–15, 2004.

[38] W. H. Organization, *WHO recommendations on antenatal care for a positive pregnancy experience*, World Health Organization, 2016.

[39] A. T. Papageorghiou, E. O. Ohuma, M. G. Gravett et al., "International standards for symphysis-fundal height based on serial measurements from the Fetal Growth Longitudinal Study of the INTERGROWTH-21(st) Project: Prospective cohort study in eight countries," *BMJ*, vol. 355, Article ID i5662, 2016.

[40] A. Yussianto, *Manual PWS KIA Electronic (Pemantauan Wilayah Setempat Kesehatan Ibu dan Anak) Kartini Version 3.0*, Jakarta, 2013.

[41] V. A. Postoev, A. M. Grjibovski, E. Nieboer, and J. Ø. Odland, "Changes in detection of birth defects and perinatal mortality after introduction of prenatal ultrasound screening in the Kola Peninsula (North-West Russia): Combination of two birth registries," *BMC Pregnancy and Childbirth*, vol. 15, no. 1, article no. 308, 2015.

[42] M. J. Renfrew, C. Homer, S. Downe, A. McFadden, N. Muir, T. Prentice et al., "Midwifery: an executive summary for the Lancets series," *Lancet*, vol. 384, p. 8, 2014.

[43] A. R. Rumbold, R. S. Bailie, D. Si et al., "Delivery of maternal health care in Indigenous primary care services: Baseline data for an ongoing quality improvement initiative," *BMC Pregnancy and Childbirth*, vol. 11, article no. 16, 2011.

[44] L. Burke, D. L. Suswardany, K. Michener et al., "Utility of local health registers in measuring perinatal mortality: A case study in rural Indonesia," *BMC Pregnancy and Childbirth*, vol. 11, article no. 20, 2011.

[45] S. Bar-Zeev, L. Barclay, S. Kruske, and S. Kildea, "Factors affecting the quality of antenatal care provided to remote dwelling Aboriginal women in northern Australia," *Midwifery*, vol. 30, no. 3, pp. 289–296, 2014.

[46] N. Benítez Brito, J. P. Suárez Llanos, M. Fuentes Ferrer et al., "Relationship between mid-upper arm circumference and body mass index in inpatients," *PLoS ONE*, vol. 11, no. 8, Article ID e0160480, 2016.

[47] W. H. Organization, *WHO child growth standards: methods and development: length/height-for-age, weight-for-age, weight-for-length, weight-for-height and body mass index-for-age*, World Health Organization, Geneva, 2006.

[48] V. Khanal, Y. Zhao, and K. Sauer, "Role of antenatal care and iron supplementation during pregnancy in preventing low birth weight in Nepal: Comparison of national surveys 2006 and 2011," *Archives of Public Health*, vol. 72, no. 1, 2014.

[49] A. T. Papageorghiou, B. Kemp, W. Stones, E. O. Ohuma, S. H. Kennedy, and M. Purwar, "Ultrasound based gestational age estimation in late pregnancy," *Ultrasound in Obstetrics Gynecology*, 2016.

[50] K. Isnawati, E. Nugroho, and L. Lazuardi, "Implemetation of the application of generic district health information system (SIKDA) in UPT. Puskesmas Gambut, Banjar District (Implementasi aplikasi sistem informasi kesehatan daerah (SIKDA) generik di UPT. Puskesmas Gambut Kabupaten Banjar," *Journal of Information Systems for Public Health*, vol. 1, pp. 64–71, 2016.

25

Estimating HIV Incidence during Pregnancy and Knowledge of Prevention of Mother-to-Child Transmission with an Ad Hoc Analysis of Potential Cofactors

Thomas Obinchemti Egbe,[1,2] **Rose-Mary Asong Tazinya,**[3] **Gregory Edie Halle-Ekane,**[1,2] **Eta-Nkongho Egbe,**[4] **and Eric Akum Achidi**[5]

[1]*Department of Obstetrics and Gynecology, Douala General Hospital, Douala, Cameroon*
[2]*Faculty of Health Sciences, University of Buea, Buea, Cameroon*
[3]*Mbingo Baptist Hospital Annexe, Douala, Cameroon*
[4]*District Hospital Poli, Poli, Cameroon*
[5]*Faculty of Science, University of Buea, Buea, Cameroon*

Correspondence should be addressed to Thomas Obinchemti Egbe; toegbe@gmail.com

Academic Editor: Vorapong Phupong

Background. We determined the incidence of HIV seroconversion during the second and third trimesters of pregnancy and ad hoc potential cofactors associated with HIV seroconversion after having an HIV-negative result antenatally. We also studied knowledge of PMTCT among pregnant women in seven health facilities in Fako Division, South West Region, Cameroon. *Method*. During the period between September 12 and December 4, 2011, we recruited a cohort of 477 HIV-negative pregnant women by cluster sampling. Data collection was with a pretested interviewer-administered questionnaire. Sociodemographic information, knowledge of PMTCT, and methods of HIV prevention were obtained from the study population and we did Voluntary Counselling and Testing (VCT) for HIV. *Results*. The incidence rate of HIV seroconversion during pregnancy was 6.8/100 woman-years. Ninety percent of the participants did not use condoms throughout pregnancy but had a good knowledge of PMTCT of HIV. Only 31.9% of participants knew their HIV status before the booking visit and 33% did not know the HIV status of their partners. *Conclusion*. The incidence rate of HIV seroconversion in the Fako Division, Cameroon, was 6.8/100 woman-years. No risk factors associated with HIV seroconversion were identified among the study participants because of lack of power to do so.

1. Background

Vertical transmission of Human Immunodeficiency Virus (HIV) is still a major challenge in the world, especially in the developing countries (USAID) [1]. It is estimated that 90% of HIV infections in children result from mother-to-child-transmission (WHO (Switzerland)) [2]. In the absence of any intervention to prevent MTCT (PMTCT), the MTCT rate varies between 13% and 48% [3, 4]. Maternal combination antiretroviral therapy (ART) together with postnatal interventions has demonstrated its efficacy in substantially reducing the risk of MTCT in African breastfed children to less than 5% (USAID 2013) [3, 5].

However, access to ART and the uptake of PMTCT programs remain limited and children continue to be HIV infected (Abidjan, Cote d'Ivoire) [2].

The World Health Organisation (WHO) guidelines recommend that all pregnant women should be tested for HIV in the first trimester and that a second test be considered in the third trimester by 34 weeks of gestational age [1, 6–8]. Guidelines in resource-limited settings are increasingly recommending HIV testing as early as possible during pregnancy and repeat testing towards the end of pregnancy or during labour, a strategy that has proven to be cost effective [8]. Despite these recommendations, recent studies show relatively high rates of seroconversion during pregnancy in

Africa. Brubaker et al. report HIV incidence rates of 10.8% in serodiscordant couples in Kenya whenever a pregnancy occurred [9]. Keating et al. further report a lower seroconversion rate of 1% amongst pregnant women in Malawi [10]. More recently, a meta-analysis published in 2014 reports an aggregate seroconversion rate of 3.8 per 100 person-years in African countries by Drake et al. in Washington USA [11].

HIV testing during labour has remained a challenge over the years in Cameroon. In 2009, of the 94,406 women with a previous negative result who presented in the labour rooms of the clinics carrying out PMTCT activities, only 2,643 were retested, giving a proportion of 2.8% [12].

In Cameroon, the prevalence of HIV was estimated to be 4.3% in the general population; a serosurveillance survey among pregnant women showed an HIV prevalence of 7.6% in 2010 [13]. As a result, the number of new pediatric infections continues to grow in Cameroon and there are still thousands of new infections each year [14]. In 2011, the UNAIDS launched the Global Plan towards eliminating new HIV infections among children and keeping their mothers alive, making Cameroon, where overall MTCT risk was reported to be around 24% [1], one of the 21 priority countries.

Since 2011, Cameroon has tripled its coverage of PMTCT prophylaxis, ranging from 6.9% to 36.5% in 2011, leading to 30% fewer new HIV infections among children [15]. In 2011, Cameroon opted for the WHO Option A regimen for PMTCT prophylaxis. Continuing access of pregnant women living with HIV to prenatal HIV services and increasing access to HIV treatment for eligible children and pregnant women will reduce maternal and child mortality [15]. Cameroon has focused on strengthening PMTCT services and caring of pediatric HIV cases for the 2011–2015 period; 99.4% of health districts were equipped to provide HIV treatment services for pregnant women and children living with HIV in 2011. However, even where the most effective PMTCT interventions are available, many women and infants are lost at different steps of the PMTCT cascade [16]; and the low cumulative uptake of PMTCT services does not allow controlling the extent of MTCT in Cameroon. The HIV seroprevalence in the SWR is 11.9%. This is one of the highest in Cameroon, closely followed by the East Region with 9.3% [17].

There is a high rate of MTCT of HIV with seroconversion in pregnancy [10, 18]. In Cameroon, particularly in the South West Region, there are no reports regarding the incidence of HIV seroconversion during pregnancy. There is a probability that many cases that seroconvert in pregnancy go without appropriate management, resulting in high MTCT as reported by Muffih in 2011 [12].

Data on the seroconversion rate after initial negative HIV test result in pregnancy would be useful in improving the management of HIV in pregnancy in Fako Division, SWR, Cameroon.

The aim of this study was to determine the incidence of HIV seroconversion during the second and third trimesters of pregnancy and ad hoc potential cofactors associated with HIV seroconversion after having an HIV-negative test result in the booking visit. We also studied knowledge of PMTCT

among pregnant women in seven health facilities in Fako Division, South West Region (SWR), Cameroon.

2. Materials and Methods

2.1. Study Design, Population, and Setting. This was a hospital based cohort study of women attending antenatal care (ANC) clinics and labour rooms of the maternity units of seven healthcare facilities in the Fako Division, South West Region, Cameroon, during the period between September 12 and December 4, 2011. Study participants were women who attended their booking or first antenatal care visit in any of the seven selected health facilities in the last six months and for whom an HIV test was done using the Determine test strips on this booking (first) ANC visit between 16 and 20 weeks of gestation. HIV seroconversion in pregnancy (HSP) was defined as maternal self-report of an HIV-negative test during the first antenatal care visit during this pregnancy, no documented use of antiretroviral drugs, and a positive HIV rapid test (Determine) done ≥3 months after the first antenatal care (booking) test.

The gestational age of the pregnancy was calculated from the last normal menstrual period (LNMP). All the women who were found to be HIV-negative at this first visit consented (written consent after study procedure and objectives had been explained to them) to participate in the study (Table 1). All study participants were counselled to repeat the HIV test within an interval of 3 to 6 months following the test of the booking ANC visit. All participants were those residing within a 10 Km radius from health facility for easy follow-up. The main outcome of interest was HIV seroconversion at second test during the ongoing pregnancy.

2.2. Sample Size and Sampling Procedure. Sample size was calculated by using the WHO-steps approach [19] with the assumptions of 95% confidence limits, 5% proportion of seroconverting women [18], and 2% margin of error. The minimum sample size was calculated to be 457 participants, but considering a nonresponse rate of 4%, we enrolled 477 participants for study.

A total of seven health facilities were selected by simple random sampling (balloting) for study. Participants who met the inclusion criteria were then selected by cluster sampling; and in each cluster, participants were included individually and consecutively to maximize confidentiality.

2.3. Data Collection Procedures. Data collection was done during a period of 12 weeks, from September 12 to December 4, 2011. During this period, the study participants were met at their various antenatal clinic sites on specific days of the week when these activities were carried out. A total of 4 weeks were spent per health facility with at least two facilities targeted at once depending on their ANC days (Table 2).

Information from each participant was collected through a pretested interviewer-administered survey questionnaire. Sociodemographic information (maternal age, gravidity, marital status and marital type, employment status, level of education, and residence), knowledge of PMTCT, and

TABLE 1: Prevalence of HIV among pregnant women at first (booking) antenatal care visit in the various health facilities used for the study.

Health facility	Number of women tested	Number positive	Number negative	Percentage of positive cases
Baptist Hospital Mutengene	559	83	476	14.8
CDC Tiko Cottage Hospital	97	13	84	13.4
CDC Camp 7 Clinic Tiko	83	13	70	15.6
Down Beach Health Centre Limbe	504	27	477	5.4
Buea Road Health Centre	269	26	243	9.7
Buea Medicalised Health Centre	165	10	155	6.1
Limbe Regional Hospital	277	29	248	10.5
Total	**1954**	**201**	**1753**	**10.3**

TABLE 2: Demographic characteristics of the study population ($n = 477$).

Variable	Category	Frequency	Percentage (%)
Age group (years)	<26	235	49.3
	26–35	215	45.1
	>35	27	5.7
	Total	**477**	**100**
Marital status	Married	364	76.3
	Single	113	23.7
	Total	**477**	**100**
Marriage type	Monogamy	350	96.2
	Polygamy	14	3.8
	Total	**364**	**100**
Parity	0–2	394	83.1
	3-4	62	13.1
	>4	18	3.8
	Total	**474**	**100.0**
Gestational age	Second trimester (13–28 weeks)	87	18.2%
	Third trimester (29–40 weeks)	390	81.8%
	Total	**477**	**100%**
Level of education	Primary or less	144	30.3
	Secondary or more	332	69.7
	Total	**476**	**100.0**
Employment status	Employed	265	55.6
	Unemployed	212	44.4
	Total	**477**	**100.0**

methods, if any, of HIV prevention were obtained from the study population.

Furthermore, Voluntary Counselling and Testing (VCT) for HIV was done on each study participant, whereby pretest counselling was done followed by the collections of 2-3 mL of venous blood by venipuncture into a dry vacutainer tube which was then allowed to settle for about 20 minutes to obtain serum from whole blood. The supernatant serum from the dry tube was then tested using Determine HIV-1/2 rapid test (Abbott Laboratories, Abbott Park, Illinois, USA) in the laboratory of the health facilities by trained laboratory personnel, experienced in HIV testing, according to manufacturer's test procedure. The same brand of test kits was used across all the health facilities that participated in the study. Following testing, a posttest counselling was done and results were delivered about one hour after testing. For

participants who were positive for Determine HIV 1/2 rapid test, a second-line test, SD Bioline HIV 1/2 3.0 (Standard Diagnostics, Inc.), was done according to manufacturer's instructions to differentiate between HIV-1 and HIV-2.

A participant was only considered positive if both tests were positive, negative if Determine was negative, and indeterminate if Determine was positive and then Bioline test was negative [20–22].

All the participants who were diagnosed HIV-positive were treated according to Cameroon's national guidelines for the PMTCT [23], which at the time recommended Option B involving either AZT + 3TC + NVP or D4T + 3TC + NVP.

2.4. Data Management and Analysis. The Epi info 3.4.5 and Microsoft Excel 2010 software were used for statistical analysis. Numerical variables like age, parity, and gestational age

TABLE 3: Incidence of HIV seroconversion in the seven healthcare facilities.

Number of participants	Time span between 1st and 2nd test (months)	Number of participants who seroconverted	Percentage of participants who seroconverted	Woman-years follow-up
262	3.0	8.0	3.1	65.5
123	4.0	1.0	0.81	41.0
63	5.0	1.0	1.59	26.25
29	6.0	0.0	0.00	14.5
Total = 477				147.25

Incidence of HIV seroconversion: 2.1% (147.25 woman-years).
Incidence rate of HIV seroconversion: 6.8/100 woman-years.

were classified into groups and their frequencies expressed in percentage were presented; meanwhile, categorical variables like marital status, educational level, and occupation were expressed as frequencies. Comparison of seroconversion incidence to other variables was done using Fisher's exact test reported with P values that were considered significant if P was less than 0.05. Univariable analysis was done using logistic regression to identify the potential factors associated with seroconversion in pregnancy, and then those with a P value less than 0.2 were included in the final model for multivariable logistic regression. Results were reported as adjusted odds ratios (OR) together with their 95% confidence intervals (CI).

2.5. Ethical Consideration. Ethical clearance was obtained firstly from the Faculty of Health Sciences Institutional Review Board (FHS/IRB) as well as the Cameroon Baptist Convention (CBC) Institutional Review Board before patient enrolment. Then, an authorisation was obtained from the Regional Delegation of Public Health for the South West Region. Permission was obtained from the health districts and the various health facilities for the study to be carried out in the desired health facilities. A signed informed consent was also obtained from all the study participants. The respondents were only identified by registration numbers instead of names. All information obtained from respondents remained strictly confidential.

3. Results

3.1. Study Participants

3.1.1. Characteristics of Study Population

Table 1. A total of 1954 antenatal women in seven healthcare facilities were tested for HIV to provide annual prevalence data in their first antenatal (booking) visit. Among this sample, 201 (10.3%) women were tested HIV-positive and were excluded from study. Amongst the remaining 1753 HIV-seronegative pregnant women, 477 (27.2%) were enrolled into the study in the second and third trimesters to study the incidence of seroconversion.

Table 2. The majority, 308 participants (64.65%), were in the age group 21–30 and 364 (76.32%) were married. About

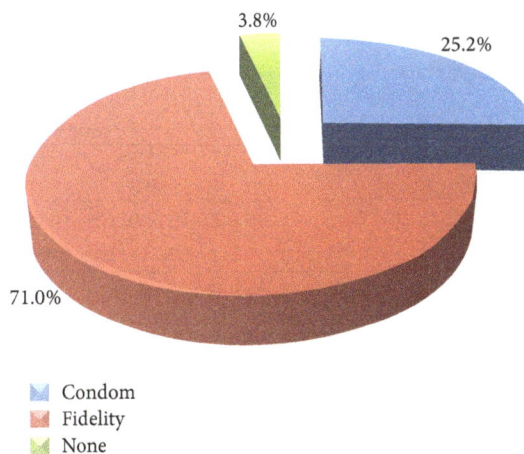

FIGURE 1: HIV prevention measures practiced by the participants.

350 (96.2%) of those who were married were monogamously married. Of the study population, 418 (87.6%) were urban dwellers, 394 (83.12%) had less than two children, three hundred and ninety (81.8%) were in the third trimester of pregnancy, and 388 (81.3%) had done secondary level of education and above.

Figure 1. Some women, 3.8%, had high risk behaviours. Most of the participants (99.6%) had one sexual partner.

3.2. Seroconversion Rates

Table 3. The incidence of participants who seroconverted was 2.1% (147.25 woman-years), giving an incidence rate of HIV seroconversion during pregnancy of 6.8 per 100 woman-years. The majority, 3% (8/262), of the patients who seroconverted did the second test 3 months after the first test.

Table 4. A minority, 31.9%, of participants did not know their HIV status prior to the first antenatal care (booking) visit while 33.0% of participants did not also know the HIV status of their partners/husbands.

Table 5. It shows that no statistically significant relationship was found between sociodemographic factors and HIV seroconversion in pregnancy.

TABLE 4: Participants' knowledge of their HIV statuses and those of their partners before first antenatal care (booking) visit.

Variable	Category	Frequency	%
Did you know your HIV status before this pregnancy?	No	152	31.9
	Yes	324	68.1
	Total	**476**	**100**
Do you know your husband's/partner's HIV status?	No	157	33.0
	Yes	319	67.0
	Total	**476**	**100**

TABLE 5: Association between sociodemographic factors and HIV seroconversion in pregnancy.

Variable	Category	Negative N (%)	Positive N (%)	P values
Age group (in years)	<26	227 (97.8%)	5 (2.2%)	
	26–35	208 (97.7%)	5 (2.4%)	1.00
	>35	27 (100%)	0 (0.0%)	
Marital status	Unmarried	109 (97.3%)	3 (2.7%)	
	Married	353 (98.1%)	7 (1.9%)	0.71
Gestational age	13–28 (2nd trimester)	87 (100%)	0 (0.0%)	
	29–40 (3rd trimester)	375 (97.4%)	10 (2.6%)	0.22
Parity	0–2	381 (97.4%)	10 (2.6%)	
	3-4	60 (100%)	0 (0.0%)	0.58
	>4	18 (100%)	0 (0.0%)	
Level of education	Primary and below	138 (97.2%)	4 (2.8%)	
	Secondary and above	323 (98.2%)	6 (1.8%)	0.50
Employment status	Unemployed	208 (99.1%)	2 (1.0%)	
	Employed	254 (97.0%)	8 (3.1%)	0.2
Interval between HIV tests	≤4 months	372 (97.6%)	9 (2.4%)	
	>4 months	90 (98.9%)	1 (1.1%)	0.70

P values are based on Fisher's exact test.

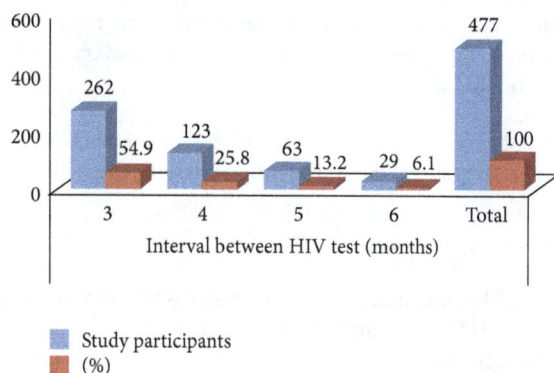

FIGURE 2: Time interval between repeat HIV test from booking test.

Study participants
(%)

Figure 2. The majority (54.9%) of participants had a repeat test 3 months after the first negative (booking) test result while 25.8%, 13.2%, and 6.1% had their repeat test done at 4, 5, and 6 months, respectively.

Eighty percent ($n = 8$) of those who seroconverted did so by the fourth month after the booking or first antenatal care visit HIV testing (Figure 2). Six (60%) of those who seroconverted were in a monogamous regime and 3 (30%) were single, while 1 (10%) was in a polygamous regime (one husband and two wives).

Table 6. Among the 10 participants who seroconverted in pregnancy, 8 knew about MTCT and PMTCT of HIV including when transmission could occur (either during pregnancy, labour/delivery, and breastfeeding or when the mother does not know she is HIV-positive). All the eight participants also knew it was possible to prevent MTCT ($P = 0.07$) and 7 out of 8 knew at least one correct method of PMTCT (avoiding breastfeeding, taking antiretroviral treatment, caesarean delivery, or mother being aware of her HIV serologic status before engaging in a pregnancy) ($P = 0.78$). This was not statistically significant.

Table 7. All the participants who seroconverted were having sexual intercourse during the current pregnancy ($P = 0.37$) and 9 (90%) were not users of the condom. All the participants who were HIV-positive had only one sexual partner throughout pregnancy ($P = 0.34$). This was not statistically significant, $P > 0.05$.

TABLE 6: Association between knowledge of PMTCT and seroconversion.

Variable	Category	Negative N (%)	Positive N (%)	P values
Do you know about mother-to-child transmission of HIV?	No	20 (90.9)	2 (9.1)	0.07
	Yes	442 (98.2)	8 (1.8)	
If yes, where did you hear about it?	Friend	8 (100)	0 (0.0)	0.7
	Hospital/health personnel	377 (98.2)	7 (1.8)	
	Media	32 (97.0)	1 (3.0)	
	Religious gathering	6 (100)	0 (0.0)	
	School	19 (100)	0 (0.0)	
When does mother-to-child transmission take place?	Correct response	396 (98.0)	8 (2.0)	1.0
	Wrong response	46 (100)	0 (0.0)	
Is it possible to prevent mother-to-child transmission of HIV?	No	40 (100)	0 (0.0)	1.0
	Yes	402 (98.1)	8 (1.9)	
If yes, by what means?	Wrong response	28 (96.6)	1 (3.4)	0.78
	Correct response	374 (98.2)	7 (1.8)	

P values are based on Fisher's exact test.
PMTCT: prevention of mother-to-child transmission.

TABLE 7: Association between HIV prevention practices and HIV seroconversion during pregnancy in a group of 477 pregnant women in Fako Division, Cameroon.

Variable	Category	Negative N (%)	Positive N (%)	P values
Which HIV prevention measure do you practice?	None	17 (94.4)	1 (6.2)	0.42
	Condom	117 (98.3)	2 (1.7)	
	One sex partner	327 (97.9)	7 (2.1)	
Did you know your HIV status before this pregnancy?	No	146 (97.3)	4 (2.7)	0.73
	Yes	315 (98.1)	6 (1.9)	
Do you know your partner/husband's HIV status?	No	152 (97.4)	4 (2.6)	0.74
	Yes	309 (98.1)	6 (1.9)	
Have you been having sex during this pregnancy?	No	70 (100)	0 (0.0)	0.37
	Yes	391 (97.5)	10 (2.5)	
If yes, have you had sex with another man other than your husband?	No	390 (97.5)	10 (2.5)	1.0
	Yes	1 (100)	0 (0.0)	
Did you use the condom?	No	376 (97.6)	9 (2.4)	0.34
	Yes	15 (93.8)	1 (6.2)	

P values are based on Fisher's exact test.
HIV: human immunodeficiency virus.

Table 8. In multivariate analysis, the odds of HIV seroconversion during pregnancy were 5 times higher among pregnant women who did not know about PMTCT (aOR 5.4; 95% CI 1.06–27.56). Also, pregnant women who were employed were at a higher risk of seroconversion than those who were unemployed (aOR 3.2; 95% CI 0.68–15.4), though this was not statistically significant.

Figure 3. The majority, 407 (85.3%), of the participants who knew about PMTCT got the information from the hospital/health personnel mainly during antenatal consultations, while 36 (7.5%) got informed through the media.

4. Discussion

HIV incidence during pregnancy and postpartum significantly increases risk of MTCT and is an important public health problem in Africa. Understanding maternal HIV incidence during this time period can be helpful to guide prevention and repeat testing strategies and policies, and little data on HIV incidence in pregnancy from West Africa exist. This study measures HIV incidence during pregnancy in seven healthcare facilities in Fako Division, South Region of Cameroon, by repeat testing later in pregnancy.

Women in the South West Region, like those in most other low-income countries, come to health facilities for

TABLE 8: Risk factors for HIV seroconversion in a multivariate model.

Variable	aOR	95% CI	P value
Employment status			
Employed	3.2	0.68–15.4	0.142
Unemployed	1.0	—	
Do you know about MTCT of HIV?			
Yes	1.0	—	
No	5.4	1.06–27.56	0.042

Prev.: prevalence within a group (row); aOR: adjusted odds ratios; CI: confidence interval; MTCT: mother-to-child transmission.

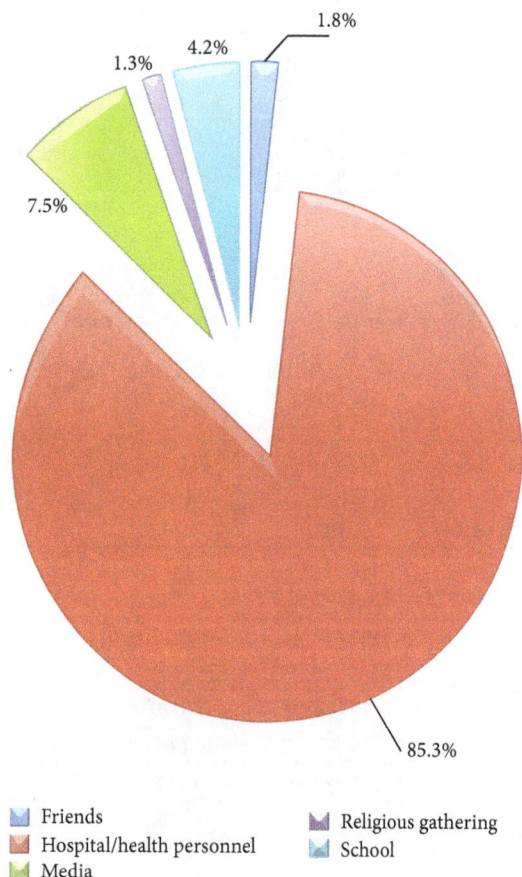

FIGURE 3: Source of information of participants regarding PMTCT.

antenatal care very late in pregnancy, usually in the second trimester [24]. At the same time, they prefer to give birth in a health facility because they perceive labour and delivery as a time of significant health risks that require biomedical attention [24]. For this reason we sometimes find it difficult to have women tested for HIV in the first trimester of pregnancy, especially in the rural areas.

4.1. Incidence of HIV Seroconversion in Pregnancy. The incidence of HIV seroconversion during pregnancy in this study was 2.1% (147.25 woman-years), yielding an incidence rate of 6.8/100 woman-years. These results are lower than that reported by Moodley et al. in 2009 in Uganda who

showed that, among 2377 HIV-negative women retested, 1099 (46.2%) and 1278 (53.4%) were tested at urban and rural health facilities, respectively. Seventy-two women (3%) were HIV-positive (679 woman-years of exposure), yielding an HIV incidence rate of 10.7/100 woman-years (95% confidence interval (CI) 8.2–13.1) [18]. HIV incidence in pregnancy was higher but not statistically significant at the urban facilities (12.4/100 woman-years versus 9.1/100 woman-years) and at least two-fold higher among the 25–29- and 30–34-year age groups (3.8 and 4.5%, resp.) as compared with the less than 20-year age group (1.9%). Single women were at 2.5 times higher risk of seroconverting during pregnancy (*P* = 0.017) [18]. In another study, Humphrey et al. reported that breastfeeding associated transmission for mothers who seroconverted postnatally (*n* = 334) averaged 34.56 infant infections per 100 child-years (95% CI 26.60 to 44.91) during the first nine months after maternal infection, declined to 9.50 (95% CI 3.07 to 29.47) during the next three months, and was zero thereafter. Among women who seroconverted postnatally and in whom the precise timing of infection was known (≤90 days between last negative and first positive test) (*n* = 51), 62% (8/13) of transmissions occurred in the first three months after maternal infection and breastfeeding associated transmission was 4.6 times higher than in mothers who tested HIV-positive at baseline and whose infant tested HIV-negative with PCR at six weeks [25]. A 5% seroconversion incidence was reported in Zimbabwe in 2002 (unpublished data).

Our results conform with the 2.2% seroconversion rate reported by Qolohle et al. in 1995 at the King Edward VIII hospital in Durban, South Africa (2.6%) [26] and the 2.9% reported by Lockman and Creek in Francistown, Botswana, at 62 weeks postpartum [27].

With the 2.1% incidence of HIV or 6.8/100 woman-years incidence rate of HIV seroconversion during pregnancy in Fako Division, there would be a correspondingly increasing rate of MTCT of HIV, thereby increasing the pediatric HIV burden [28]. It has been estimated that 19% of infants born to HIV-positive mothers are HIV infected when tested at 19 months [29]. The percentage is even higher in cases of seroconversions in pregnancy. This high rate of infant infection can be attributed to the fact that maternal HIV infection during pregnancy and breastfeeding occasion equally high rates of MTCT of HIV-1.

All participants who seroconverted did so in the third trimester of pregnancy, when most of the study participants (81.8%) were recruited.

All the participants who seroconverted in our study had HIV-1 which is the type of HIV mainly responsible for MTCT of the virus [30]. Therefore, all cases of HIV seroconversion during pregnancy should be considered as potential risks for more pediatric HIV. Seventy percent of the participants who seroconverted were married; therefore, marriage does not protect women from HIV infection in pregnancy. This finding is in conformity with results obtained in Harare, Zimbabwe [31].

Eighty percent of the participants who seroconverted had 3-4-month interval between the two tests, while there was no case of seroconversion among women who had 6-month interval. These results differ from those obtained in the Tygerberg Hospital of Cape Town where it was reported that women especially at risk of seroconversion are those who book much earlier, thereby increasing the interval between the initial test at first ANC visit and the repeat test [29]. To identify cases of seroconversion more early, it will be advisable for repeat HIV testing to be done to pregnant women every three months until delivery, no matter the time of first ANC visit.

4.2. Risk Factors of HIV Seroconversion in Fako Division. The risk factors that were studied (age, marital status, residence, parity and knowledge of MTCT of HIV, HIV prevention, and HIV seroconversion in pregnancy) did not show any significant statistical variations. These results are not in conformity with those reported in Harare, Zimbabwe, where women aged 17 and below were at higher risk of seroconverting than the general population of HIV-negative pregnant women studied [31].

4.3. Knowledge of PMTCT in the Fako Division. In this study, 442 (98.2%) of participants who remained seronegative and 8 (1.8%) of those who seroconverted had a good knowledge of PMTCT techniques. This is probably because it has been a routine practice at all antenatal clinics to give the women talks on HIV and PMTCT, especially during the first ANC visit. Familiarity level with PMTCT practices in this study is similar to that obtained in Yaounde, Cameroon, in 2011 [32].

The majority of study participants, though aware of MTCT of HIV during pregnancy, did not take the necessary preventive measures. This was exemplified by the fact that some participants did not know their HIV status before the first antenatal care (booking) visit. This may be the result of inadequate sensitization of the population of the SWR or negligence on the part of the participants. This fact alone could have a negative impact on the PMTCT strategies put in place in Fako Division and based on recommendations of the WHO and the Government of Cameroon [7].

The limitations to this study include the fact that we did not study the male partners' or husbands' risk factors and relied on results of HIV tests done at the booking or first antenatal care visit in the different health facilities. Such tests could have produced faulty results. Also, seroconversions were determined using rapid tests, not HIV RNA tests, thus potentially underestimating incidence rates. Furthermore, the study was underpowered to detect cofactors for risk and only measured cofactors based on demographics and PMTCT knowledge. We did not assess many other potential cofactors for acquisition of HIV, such as STIs. Finally, the collection of data using an interviewer-administered questionnaire could have resulted in social desirability bias.

5. Conclusion

The incidence of HIV seroconversion among pregnant women in the study is 2.1%, yielding an incidence rate of 6.8/100 woman-years in Fako Division. Most of the participants seroconverted 3 months after the first test and therefore make up a potential risk for pediatric HIV.

The study was underpowered to study associated risk factors for seroconversion. Furthermore, there was adequate knowledge of PMTCT among pregnant women. Testing partners of pregnant women could be a major PMTCT strategy in our setting. Lastly, pregnancy did not stop the women from sexual activities and most of them had one sex partner.

Competing Interests

The authors declare that they have no competing interests.

Authors' Contributions

Thomas Obinchemti Egbe, Gregory Edie Halle-Ekane, and Eric Akum Achidi conceptualized the study. Rose-Mary Asong Tazinya and Eta-Nkongho Egbe conducted the data collection. Rose-Mary Asong Tazinya conducted the data analysis. Thomas Obinchemti Egbe wrote the paper. All the co-authors gave advice on presentation of the results and editing of the text and approved the final paper.

Acknowledgments

The authors would like to thank Drs. Julius Atashili and Elvis Temfack for their assistance during statistical analysis. The authors also thank the authorities and staff of the seven health facilities (Mutengene Baptist Hospital; Limbe Regional Hospital; Buea Road Health Centre, Mutengene; Down Beach Integrated Health Centre, Limbe; CDC Cottage Hospital Tiko; Camp 7 Clinic Tiko; and the Muea Integrated Health Centre) for their availability and support during data collection.

References

[1] M. Sidibé, *Global Plan towards the Elimination of New HIV Infections among Children by 2015 and Keeping Their Mothers Alive*, 2014.

[2] K. M. De Cock, M. G. Fowler, E. Mercier et al., "Prevention of mother-to-child HIV transmission in resource-poor countries: translating research into policy and practice," *The Journal of the American Medical Association*, vol. 283, no. 9, pp. 1175–1182, 2000.

[3] V. Leroy, D. K. Ekouevi, R. Becquet et al., "18-Month effectiveness of short-course antiretroviral regimens combined with alternatives to breastfeeding to prevent HIV mother-to-child transmission," *PLoS ONE*, vol. 3, no. 2, Article ID e1645, 2008.

[4] Global Report 2013, http://www.unaids.org/sites/default/files/en/media/unaids/contentassets/documents/epidemiology/2013/gr2013/UNAIDS_Global_Report_2013_en.pdf.

[5] B. Tonwe-Gold, D. K. Ekouevi, I. Viho et al., "Antiretroviral treatment and prevention of peripartum and postnatal HIV transmission in West Africa: evaluation of a two-tiered approach," *PLoS Medicine*, vol. 4, no. 8, pp. 1362–1373, 2007.

[6] N. Rollins, S. Mzolo, T. Moodley, T. Esterhuizen, and H. van Rooyen, "Universal HIV testing of infants at immunization clinics: an acceptable and feasible approach for early infant diagnosis in high HIV prevalence settings," *AIDS*, vol. 23, no. 14, pp. 1851–1857, 2009.

[7] "WHO PMTCT Guidelines 2014," https://www.google.cm/?gws_rd=cr&ei=Y5Q4VvvuIaf9ywOBzoK4DQ#q=who+pmtct+guidelines+2014.

[8] L. Tsague and E. J. Abrams, "Commentary: antiretroviral treatment for pregnant and breastfeeding women—the shifting paradigm," *AIDS*, vol. 28, supplement 2, pp. S119–S121, 2014.

[9] S. G. Brubaker, E. A. Bukusi, J. Odoyo, J. Achando, A. Okumu, and C. R. Cohen, "Pregnancy and HIV transmission among HIV-discordant couples in a clinical trial in Kisumu, Kenya," *HIV Medicine*, vol. 12, no. 5, pp. 316–321, 2011.

[10] M. A. Keating, G. Hamela, W. C. Miller, A. Moses, I. F. Hoffman, and M. C. Hosseinipour, "High hiv incidence and sexual behavior change among pregnant women in lilongwe, malawi: implications for the risk of hiv acquisition," *PLoS ONE*, vol. 7, no. 6, Article ID e39109, 2012.

[11] A. L. Drake, A. Wagner, B. Richardson, and G. John-Stewart, "Incident HIV during pregnancy and postpartum and risk of mother-to-child HIV transmission: a systematic review and meta-analysis," *PLoS Medicine*, vol. 11, no. 2, Article ID e1001608, 2014.

[12] T. P. Muffih, *Aids Care and Prevention: Program Annual Report*, vol. 1, CBC Health Board, 2009.

[13] Microsoft Word—Document de plaidoyer_Affirmative_Action 00 (Enregistré automatiquement Modif), http://www.plate-forme-elsa.org/wp-content/uploads/2014/05/Document_plaidoyer_MARPS_Affirmative-action.pdf.

[14] M. Penazzato, V. Bendaud, L. Nelson, J. Stover, and M. Mahy, "Estimating future trends in paediatric HIV," *AIDS*, vol. 28, pp. S445–S451, 2014.

[15] "2013 Progress Report on the Global Plan," http://www.unaids.org/sites/default/files/en/media/unaids/contentassets/documents/unaidspublication/2013/20130625_progress_global_plan_en.pdf.

[16] L. Tudor Car, S. Brusamento, H. Elmoniry et al., "The uptake of integrated perinatal prevention of mother-to-child HIV transmission programs in low- and middle-income countries: a systematic review," *PLoS ONE*, vol. 8, no. 3, Article ID e56550, 2013.

[17] "Cameroon National EMTCT Plan 2012," https://www.google.cm/search?sclient=psy-ab&site=&source=hp&q=Cameroon+national+EMTCT+plan+2012&oq=Cameroon+national+EMTCT+plan+2012&gs_l=hp.12...5474.5474.3.8379.1.1.0.0.0.0.0.0..0.0....0...1c.1.64.psy-ab..33.0.0.0.iSHl3-g6ofA&pbx=1&bav=on.2,or.r_cp.&bvm=bv.113370389,d.bGg&biw=1280&bih=358&dpr=1&ech=1&psi=oESzVsjfIIj6swGj3Y-oDw.1454590292157.11&ei=oESzVsjfIIj6swGj3Y-oDw&emsg=NCSR&noj=1.

[18] D. Moodley, T. M. Esterhuizen, T. Pather, V. Chetty, and L. Ngaleka, "High HIV incidence during pregnancy: compelling reason for repeat HIV testing," *AIDS*, vol. 23, no. 10, pp. 1255–1259, 2009.

[19] J. Eng, "Sample size estimation: how many individuals should be studied?" *Radiology*, vol. 227, no. 2, pp. 309–313, 2003.

[20] 15221_Policy Brief_Testing Strategies, http://apps.who.int/iris/bitstream/10665/179521/1/WHO_HIV_2015.15_eng.pdf?ua=1.

[21] C. Evans and E. Ndirangu, "The nursing implications of routine provider-initiated HIV testing and counselling in sub-Saharan Africa: a critical review of new policy guidance from WHO/UNAIDS," *International Journal of Nursing Studies*, vol. 46, no. 5, pp. 723–731, 2009.

[22] WHO, "Statement on HIV testing and counseling: WHO, UNAIDS re-affirm opposition to mandatory HIV testing," http://www.who.int/hiv/events/2012/world_aids_day/hiv_testing_counselling/en/.

[23] "Guide de Poche," 2006, http://www.remed.org/GUIDE_DE_POCHE_PTME_recommandations_PNLS_Cameroun_09.pdf.

[24] L. Myer and A. Harrison, "Why do women seek antenatal care late? Perspectives from rural South Africa," *Journal of Midwifery & Women's Health*, vol. 48, no. 4, pp. 268–272, 2003.

[25] J. H. Humphrey, E. Marinda, K. Mutasa et al., "Mother to child transmission of HIV among Zimbabwean women who seroconverted postnatally: prospective cohort study," *BMJ*, vol. 341, Article ID c6580, 2010.

[26] D. C. Qolohle, A. A. Hoosen, J. Moodley, A. N. Smith, and K. P. Mlisana, "Serological screening for sexually transmitted infections in pregnancy: is there any value in re-screening for HIV and syphilis at the time of delivery?" *Genitourinary Medicine*, vol. 71, no. 2, pp. 65–67, 1995.

[27] S. Lockman and T. Creek, "Acute maternal HIV infection during pregnancy and breast-feeding: substantial risk to infants," *Journal of Infectious Diseases*, vol. 200, no. 5, pp. 667–669, 2009.

[28] L. F. Johnson, K. Stinson, M.-L. Newell et al., "The contribution of maternal HIV seroconversion during late pregnancy and breastfeeding to mother-to-child transmission of HIV," *Journal of Acquired Immune Deficiency Syndromes*, vol. 59, no. 4, pp. 417–425, 2012.

[29] G. B. Theron, J. Schoeman, and E. Carolus, "HIV seroconversion during pregnancy in the Tygerberg region of Cape Town," *South African Medical Journal*, vol. 96, article 204, 2006.

[30] C. N. Nkenfou, E. E. Lobé, O. Ouwe-Missi-Oukem-Boyer et al., "Implementation of HIV early infant diagnosis and HIV type 1 RNA viral load determination on dried blood spots in Cameroon: challenges and propositions," *AIDS Research and Human Retroviruses*, vol. 28, no. 2, pp. 176–181, 2012.

[31] M. T. Mbizvo, J. Kasule, K. Mahomed, and K. Nathoo, "HIV-1 seroconversion incidence following pregnancy and delivery among women seronegative at recruitment in Harare, Zimbabwe," *Central African Journal of Medicine*, vol. 47, no. 5, pp. 115–118, 2001.

[32] A.-C. Zoung-Kanyi Bissek, I. E. Yakana, F. Monebenimp et al., "Knowledge of pregnant women on mother-to-child transmission of HIV in Yaoundé," *Open AIDS Journal*, vol. 5, no. 1, pp. 25–28, 2011.

26

Risk Factors for Neonatal Sepsis in Pregnant Women with Premature Rupture of the Membrane

Dwiana Ocviyanti ⓘ **and William Timotius Wahono** ⓘ

Department of Obstetrics and Gynecology, Faculty of Medicine,
Universitas Indonesia/Cipto Mangunkusumo Hospital, Jakarta, Indonesia

Correspondence should be addressed to William Timotius Wahono; william.wahono@gmail.com

Academic Editor: Marco Scioscia

Background. Premature rupture of the membrane (PROM) is associated with high maternal as well as perinatal morbidity and mortality risks. It occurs in 5 to 10% of all pregnancy while incidence of amniotic membrane infection varies from 6 to 10%. This study aimed to determine the incidence of neonatal sepsis in Cipto Mangunkusumo Hospital and the risk factors. *Methods.* A cross-sectional study was done in Cipto Mangunkusumo Hospital, Jakarta, from December 2016 to June 2017. The study used total sampling method including all pregnant women with gestational age of 20 weeks or more experiencing PROM, who came to the hospital at that time. Samples with existing comorbidities such as diabetes mellitus or other serious systemic illnesses such as heart disease or autoimmune condition were excluded from the analysis. *Results.* A total of 405 pregnant women with PROM were included in this study. There were 21 cases (5.2%) of neonatal sepsis. The analysis showed that risk of neonatal sepsis was higher in pregnant women with prolonged rupture of membrane for ≥ 18 hours before hospital admission (OR 3.08), prolonged rupture of membrane for ≥ 15 hours during hospitalization (OR 7.32), and prolonged rupture of membrane for ≥ 48 hours until birth (OR 5.77). The risk of neonatal sepsis was higher in preterm pregnancy with gestational age of <37 weeks (OR 18.59). *Conclusion.* Risk of neonatal sepsis is higher in longer duration of prolonged rupture of membrane as well as preterm pregnancy.

1. Introduction

Premature rupture of membrane (PROM) is the rupture of the amniotic membrane before the onset of labor [1]. PROM is associated with high maternal as well as perinatal morbidity and mortality risks [2]. It occurs in 5 to 10% of all pregnancy and 8 to 10% of term pregnancy. Amniotic membrane infection is one of pregnancy complications that may occur in pregnancy with PROM, in both preterm and term pregnancies. In term pregnancy, the incidence of amniotic membrane infection varies from 6 to 10% and occurs in 40% of prolonged PROM that persists for more than 24 hours [3]. In preterm pregnancy, preterm premature rupture of the membrane occurs in 2.0% to 3.5% of pregnancies and is the most common cause of preterm birth, present in 30% to 40% of cases [4]. Sequelae of amniotic membrane infection are potentially fatal in pregnant women and their babies [3].

In 2005, the WHO reported that 37% of child mortality occurs below 5 years of age, and neonatal sepsis accounted for 29% of deaths within that age group [5]. Results of an epidemiological study done by the WHO and UNICEF in 2010 found that there were 7.6 million cases of under-five mortality, in which 64% (4.879 million) occurred due to infection and the remaining 40.3% (3.072 million) occurred in neonates [6]. The latest SDKI report in 2012 showed that Infant Mortality Rate (IMR) in Indonesia is at 32/1,000 live births [7]. Sepsis or meningitis is one of the leading causes of neonatal death, accounted for 5.2% (0.393 million) [6].

The incidence of neonatal infection after rupture of membrane that persists for more than 24 hours is 1%, and after clinical inspection, the incidence mounts up to 3-5%. In general, tenfold increase in neonatal infection occurred in premature rupture of membrane cases without complications [8]. A multicenter study on PROM in term pregnancy, conducted in the US, Canada, UK, and Israel, found that prolonged rupture of membrane for ≥48 hours and 24 to 48 hours increases the risk of neonatal infection by 2.25 times [3]. Some studies on preterm PROM showed no association between prolonged rupture of membrane with neonatal infection. However, a meta-analysis study found significant association between antibiotic administration in mothers with incidence of neonatal infection (OR 0.68 [0.53-0.87]) [9–12]. Based on the previous data, we decide to perform this study to find out the true incidence of neonatal sepsis and risk factors related to them.

2. Materials and Methods

This study is a hospital-based analytical descriptive study done in Cipto Mangunkusumo Hospital, Jakarta, for 7 months, since December 2016 until June 2017. The study used total sampling method, in which all pregnant women with PROM and gestational age of more than 20 weeks admitted since 1st January to 31st December of 2016, as well as their babies, are included. In terms of maternal data, we collect age, level of education, working status, parity, gestational age, mode of delivery, and mother hemoglobin. In terms of neonatal data, we collect birthweight, length of stay, APGAR score, treatment with antibiotics, and neonatal death. Subjects with existing comorbidities and complications such as diabetes mellitus, intrauterine infection, and other serious systemic illnesses, e.g., lung and heart diseases, autoimmune conditions, fetal congenital abnormality, and multiple pregnancy, were excluded. Subjects with incomplete medical record were also excluded. Data was analyzed using Stata 12.

3. Results

There were 488 cases of pregnant women with PROM in Cipto Mangunkusumo Hospital throughout the year of 2016. Of that number, a total of 405 women met the inclusion criteria. The remaining 83 were excluded.

Of 405 PROM cases, 21 (5.2%) suffered from neonatal sepsis. Of all PROM cases, 186 (45.9%) occurred in term pregnancy, of which 56 cases (30.1%) were suspected neonatal sepsis and 130 cases (68.9%) were without neonatal sepsis. Of 56 cases with suspected neonatal sepsis, positive blood culture was found in only one case and alive. The other 55 cases showed negative blood cultures. Of this number, one died (1.8%) and the remaining 54 cases (98.2%) were alive.

PROM cases in preterm pregnancy occurred in 219 subjects (54.1%), of which neonatal sepsis was suspected in 128 cases (58.4%), and there was no sepsis in 91 cases (41.6%). Of 128 cases with suspected neonatal sepsis, 20 cases (15.6%) showed positive blood cultures. Of these, 8 neonates died (40%) and 12 were alive (60%). Meanwhile, of 108 cases with negative blood cultures, 97 neonates were alive (89.8%) and 11 died (10.2%). In cases without neonatal sepsis, neonatal death was found in 2 cases (2.2%) and the remaining 89 were alive (97.8%). The characteristics of subjects were presented on Table 1.

Neonatal sepsis occurred in only one subject with gestational age of ≥ 37 weeks (0.5%), compared to 20 subjects (9.1%) with gestational age of < 37 weeks. In preterm pregnancy with gestational age of 34 to less than 37 weeks, neonatal sepsis was found in 2 subjects (2.4%), while, in gestational

TABLE 1: Subjects characteristics of patient with PROM.

Characteristic (n=405)	n (%)
Maternal age	
< 20 yo	34 (8.4)
20 – 35 yo	308 (76.0)
> 35 yo	63 (15.6)
Level of education	
≤ 6 year	13 (3.2)
> 6 - ≤ 12 year	100 (24.7)
> 12 year	35 (8.6)
No data available	257 (63.5)
Working status	
Working	119 (29.4)
Not working / Housewife	249 (61.5)
No data available	37 (9.1)
Parity	
Multiparity	239 (59.0)
Nulliparity	166 (41.0)
Gestational age (2 categories)	
Preterm < 37 weeks	219 (54.1)
Aterm ≥ 37 weeks	186 (45.9)
Gestational age (4 categories)	
< 28 weeks	17 (4.2)
28 - < 34 weeks	120 (29.6)
34 - < 37 weeks	82 (20.3)
≥ 37 weeks	186 (45.9)
Mode of delivery	
Cesarean section	305 (75.3)
Vaginal delivery	100 (24.7)
Mother hemoglobin	
< 7 g/dL	4 (1.0)
7 – 11 g/dL	135 (33.3)
> 11 g/dL	266 (65.7)

Data are expressed in n(%) and mean ± standard deviation or median (min-max).

age of 28 to less than 34 weeks, it was found in 13 subjects (10.8%). In gestational age of less than 28 weeks, neonatal sepsis was found in 5 subjects (29.4%). The distribution of risk factors based on neonatal sepsis incidence is presented in Table 2.

The average birth weight of babies with neonatal sepsis was 1,420 grams, compared to 2,560 grams in babies without neonatal sepsis. Babies with neonatal sepsis were hospitalized for 32 days on average, compared to 3 days in babies without the condition. Antibiotics were administered in all cases of neonatal sepsis (100%), whereas in those without the condition, 109 neonates (28.4%) were given. Administered antibiotics were ampicillin-sulbactam dan gentamycin, for duration of 10-14 days.

Neonatal death occurred in 8 cases (38.1%) with neonatal sepsis compared to 14 cases (3.7%) without the condition. The distribution of neonatal outcomes in pregnant women with PROM was presented in Table 3.

TABLE 2: Distribution of risk factors based on incidence of neonatal sepsis.

Variable	With neonatal sepsis n = 21 (5.2)	Without neonatal sepsis n = 384 (94.8)
Gestational age		
≥ 37 weeks	1 (0.5)	185 (99.5)
< 37 weeks	20 (9.1)	199 (90.9)
34 - < 37 weeks	2 (2.4)	80 (97.6)
28 - < 34 weeks	13 (10.8)	107 (89.2)
< 28 weeks	5 (29.4)	12 (70.6)
Duration from PROM to hospital admission (hour)	20 (1-72)	9 (0-600)
< 18 hour	9 (3.2)	268 (96.8)
≥ 18 hour	12 (9.4)	116 (90.6)
Duration from PROM to delivery (hour)	63 (6-247)	26 (2-647)
Duration from PROM during hospitalization (hour)	43 (3-223)	10 (1-164)

Data are expressed in n(%) and mean ± standard deviation or median (min-max).

TABLE 3: Distribution of neonatal outcome in pregnant women with PROM.

Variable	With neonatal sepsis n = 21 (5.2)	Without neonatal sepsis n = 384 (94.8)
Birthweight	1,420 (±410.3)	2,560 (±688.2)
Length of stay (day)	32 (3-79)	3 (0-85)
APGAR score		
First minute		
0 - 7	14 (13)	94 (87)
8 - 10	7 (2.4)	290 (97.6)
Fifth minute		
0 – 7	4 (17.4)	19 (82.6)
8 – 10	17 (4.5)	365 (95.5)
Treatment with antibiotics to neonates	21 (100)	109 (28.4)
Neonatal death	8 (38.1)	14 (3.7)

Data are expressed in n(%) and mean ± standard deviation or median (min-max).

To determine the effect of prolonged rupture of membrane upon neonatal sepsis incidence, Youden index was used to identify the cut-off point of Receiver Operating Characteristics (ROC) curve index. Cut-off point with the most optimum sensitivity and specificity value was then selected. Because of this, the cut-off point appeared on the graphs and tables were slightly different. In all PROM cases, cut-off point was 18 hours (Sn 60%, Sp 66.33%), 15 hours (Sn 80.95%, 63.28%), and 48 hours (Sn 66.67%, Sp 76.56%) for prolonged rupture of membrane before hospital admission, during hospitalization, and until birth, respectively. Cut-off point of duration from PROM to hospital admission was illustrated in Figure 1 and ROC curve of duration from PROM to hospital admission was illustrated in Figure 2.

ROC curve for the number of vaginal examination variable can not be identified. Thus, no analysis was performed. Based on neonatal sepsis incidence, the distribution of vaginal examination was as follows: 0 in 14 cases, 1 time in 5 cases, 2 times in 1 case, and 9 times in 1 case.

To identify the association between prolonged rupture of membrane as well as gestational age with the incidence of neonatal sepsis, bivariate analysis was performed. Statistically significant association (p<0.05) was found in prolonged rupture of membrane before hospital admission (OR 3.08),

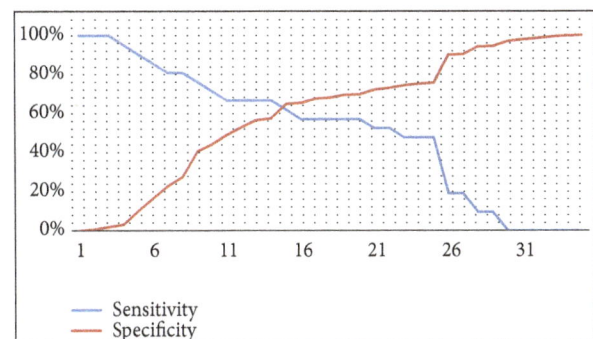

FIGURE 1: Cut-off point of duration from PROM to hospital admission in all PROM cases (18 hours).

during hospitalization (OR 7.32), and until birth (OR 5.77). Gestational age also showed statistically significant association (p<0.05) with OR 2.9. The association of these variables with neonatal sepsis incidence can be found in Table 4.

Subanalysis was performed on PROM cases occurring in preterm pregnancy. Youden index was again used to determine the cut-off point of ROC curve. In preterm pregnancy, the cut-off point on prolonged rupture of membrane was 18

TABLE 4: Bivariate analysis of duration of premature rupture of membrane with neonatal sepsis in all PROM cases in RSCM, 2016.

	Neonatal sepsis		P value	OR	95% CI	
	Positive (n=21)	Negative (n=384)			Min	Max
Duration from PROM to hospital admission						
≥ 18 hour	12 (9.4)	116 (90.6)	0.009	3.08	1.15	8.49
< 18 hour	9 (3.2)	268 (96.8)				
Duration from PROM during hospitalization						
≥ 15 hour	17 (10.8)	141 (89.2)	< 0.001	7.32	2.32	30.37
< 15 hour	4 (1.6)	243 (98.4)				
Duration from PROM to delivery						
≥ 48 hour	8 (17.8)	37 (82.2)	< 0.001	5.77	1.93	16.11
< 48 hour	13 (3.6)	347 (96.4)				
Gestational age (2 categories)						
Preterm < 37 weeks	20 (9.1)	199 (90.9)	<0.001	18.59	2.90	774.57
Aterm ≥ 37 weeks	1 (0.5)	185 (99.5)				
Gestational age (4 categories)						
< 28 weeks	5 (29.4)	12 (70.6)	<0.001	77.08	8.33	713.29
28 - <34 weeks	13 (10.8)	107 (89.2)	0.003	22.48	2.89	174.22
34 - <37 weeks	2 (2.4)	80 (97.6)	0.214	4.63	0.41	51.74
≥ 37 weeks	1 (0.5)	185 (99.5)				

TABLE 5: Bivariate analysis of duration of premature rupture of membrane with neonatal sepsis in preterm PROM <37 weeks in RSCM, 2016.

	Neonatal sepsis		p value	OR	95% CI	
	Positive (n=20)	Negative (n=199)			Min	Max
Duration from PROM to hospital admission						
≥ 18 hour	12 (15.2)	67 (84.8)	0.019	2.95	1.05	8.72
< 18 hour	8 (5.7)	132 (94.3)				
Duration from PROM during hospitalization						
≥ 38 hour	12 (18.2)	54 (81.8)	0.002	4.03	1.41	11.94
< 38 hour	8 (5.2)	145 (94.8)				
Duration from PROM to delivery						
≥ 59 hour	13 (21)	49 (79)	<0.001	5.69	1.96	17.67
< 59 hour	7 (4.5)	150 (95.5)				

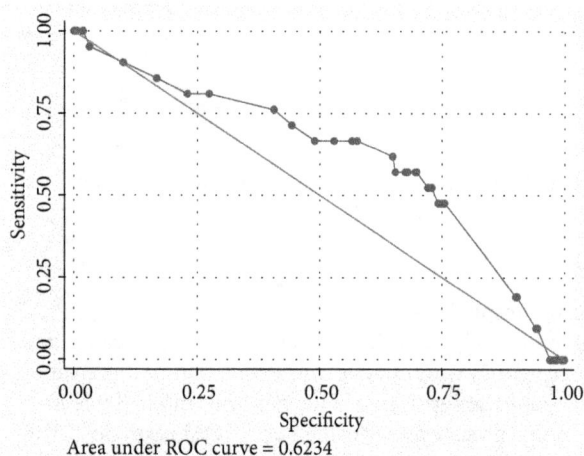

Area under ROC curve = 0.6234

FIGURE 2: ROC curve duration from PROM to hospital admission in all PROM cases.

hours, 38 hours, and 59 hours, respectively, before hospital admission, during hospitalization, and until birth.

Bivariate analysis of this subanalysis also showed significant association (p<0.05) between prolonged rupture of membrane before hospital admission (OR 2.95), during hospitalization (OR 4.03), and until birth (5.69) with neonatal sepsis incidence. The association of these variables with neonatal sepsis incidence in preterm pregnancy of less than 37 weeks can be found in Table 5.

4. Discussion

Our study shows that neonatal sepsis incidence proven by positive blood cultures was 5,2%. This number is slightly higher compared to study conducted by Van Der Ham et al. in 2014 where neonatal sepsis occurred in 3.4% of all PROM cases. Similar study by Popowski et al. showed neonatal sepsis incidence of 4.3% [13, 14]. Based on the 2015 report of Department of Child Health at Cipto Mangunkusumo Hospital, neonatal sepsis incidence in the hospital was 13.01% [15]. In contrast, studies from several local referral hospital showed that neonatal incidence in Indonesia varied between 1.5% and 3.7% [16].

This study showed that more than 50% of subjects with PROM had preterm pregnancy. This is quite reasonable since Cipto Mangunkusumo is a national referral hospital which provides NICU. In the hospital, delivery method was mostly done by caesarean section in most patients with PROM (75.3%). This number is higher than the study conducted by Pasquier et al. that was 58% [9]. Based on local guidelines at Cipto Mangunkusumo Hospital, for PROM cases in preterm pregnancy, after lung maturation patient without any immediate medical indication (such as pathological CTG) would be given informed choice to decide whether to have C-section or continue with induction of labor (with consequences of a longer duration of PROM due to induction). This might be the cause of high rate of caesarean section in PROM cases, because patient chose to have caesarean section to avoid further risk of neonatal infection.

However, caesarean section on maternal request is still a debatable topic. A study conducted by Indraccolo et al. in Italy found that OBGYNs and midwives agree that performing a planned caesarean section on maternal request (CSMR) without medical indication being considered an error. However, from lawyers point of view, following patient's own decision to have CSMR, independently from medical complication, is considered pivotal. The study also found that if patients ask for a caesarean but the OBGYN does not perform a planned CSMR, patients feel that the physician's decision in case of a vaginal delivery complication is juridically relevant, and it appears that patients would be more likely to lodge a claim in case of complications if the OBGYN does not perform a CSMR [17]. It is very important to develop a prediction model to predict neonatal sepsis in cases of PROM, which can help both the patient and clinician to decide which is best for maternal and neonatal outcome.

Regarding neonatal outcomes related to neonatal sepsis incidence, it was found that the average birth weight of babies suffering from neonatal sepsis was 1,420 grams, while for those without neonatal sepsis it was 2,560 grams. Since 95% of neonatal sepsis occurred in preterm pregnancy, low birth weight of babies was expected. Babies with neonatal sepsis also had longer length of stay in the hospital, with median of 32 days, compared to 3 days in those without the condition. This finding might as well be related to the preterm gestational age. It is also consistent with the study by Manuck et al., where duration of hospitalization is longer in preterm neonates [18].

Based on gestational age of mothers, neonatal sepsis in terms of pregnancy (≥ 37 weeks) was found in only 1 subject (0.5%) compared to 20 subjects (9.1%) in preterm pregnancy. It implies that prematurity is an important factor on the occurrence of neonatal sepsis. Manuck et al. also stated that preterm pregnancy of less than 37 weeks is the most frequent cause of neonatal morbidity [18]. Results from bivariate analysis showed that gestational age was significantly associated with neonatal sepsis incidence ($p < 0.05$). The OR for neonatal sepsis in preterm pregnancy was 18.59. When we tried to further divide preterm gestational age into 3 groups, i.e., <37 weeks, 34 to <37 weeks, and 28 to <34 weeks, an increasing trend of neonatal sepsis risk was observed in more preterm pregnancy. The odds are 4.63, 22.48, and 77.08, respectively. Similar trend was also found by Manuck et al., in which trends of neonatal morbidity and infection were higher at younger gestational age [18].

In all PROM cases, regardless of gestational age, bivariate analysis showed significant association ($p < 0.05$) between prolonged rupture of membrane before hospital admission, during hospitalization, and until birth with neonatal sepsis incidence. The odds ratio was 3.09, 7.32, and 5.77, respectively.

Subanalysis was then performed for PROM cases in preterm pregnancy of less than 37 weeks. It was again found that there was significant association ($p < 0.05$) between prolonged rupture of membrane before hospital admission, during hospitalization, and until birth with neonatal sepsis incidence. The odds ratio was 2.95, 4.03, and 5.69, respectively.

These findings showed that the longer the duration of membrane rupture, the higher the risk of neonatal sepsis. However, different results were shown by Drassinower et al., where prolonged rupture of membrane of ≥ 4 weeks was associated with lower incidence of neonatal sepsis. In this study, PROM with latent period of < 4 weeks occurred in younger gestational age (25.6 weeks). Meanwhile, PROM with latent period of ≥ 4 weeks occurred in older gestational age (28 weeks) where the birth weight was also greater [19].

5. Conclusion

Our study shows that risk of neonatal sepsis is higher in longer duration of prolonged rupture of membrane as well as preterm pregnancy.

Conflicts of Interest

The authors report no conflicts of interest.

References

[1] M. D. Hnat, B. M. Mercer, G. Thurnau et al., "Perinatal outcomes in women with preterm rupture of membranes between 24 and 32 weeks of gestation and a history of vaginal bleeding," *American Journal of Obstetrics & Gynecology*, vol. 193, no. 1, pp. 164–168, 2005.

[2] S. Surayapalem, V. Cooly, and B. Salicheemala, "A study on maternal and perinatal outcome in premature rupture of membranes at term," *International Journal of Reproduction, Contraception, Obstetrics and Gynecology*, vol. 6, no. 12, p. 5368, 2017.

[3] P. G. Seaward, M. E. Hannah, T. L. Myhr, D. Farine, A. Ohlsson, E. E. Wang et al., "International Multicentre Term Prelabor Rupture of Membranes Study: evaluation of predictors of clinical chorioamnionitis and postpartum fever in patients with prelabor rupture of membranes at termmembranes at term," *Am J Obstet Gynecol*, vol. 177, no. 5, pp. 1024–1029.

[4] M. H. Yudin, J. van Schalkwyk, and N. Van Eyk, "No. 233-Antibiotic Therapy in Preterm Premature Rupture of the Membranes," *Journal of Obstetrics and Gynaecology Canada*, vol. 39, no. 9, pp. e207–e212, 2017.

[5] J. Bryce, C. Boschi-Pinto, K. Shibuya, and R. E. Black, "WHO estimates of the causes of death in children," *The Lancet*, vol. 365, no. 9465, pp. 1147–1152, 2005.

[6] L. Liu, H. Johnson, and S. Cousens, "Global, regional and national causes of child mortality: an update systematic analysis for 2010 with time trends since 2000," *The Lancet*, vol. 379, no. 9832, pp. 2151–2161, 2012.

[7] BPS SI-. BPS-, BKKBN/Indonesia NP and FPB-, Health/Indonesia KK-. K-. M of, International ICF. Indonesia Demographic and Health Survey 2012. Jakarta, Indonesia: BPS, BKKBN, Kemenkes, and ICF International; 2013 . http://dhsprogram.com/pubs/pdf/FR275/FR275.pdf.

[8] P. H. Belady, L. J. Farkouh, and R. S. Gibbs, "Intra-Amniotic Infection and Premature Rupture of the Membranes," *Clinics in Perinatology*, vol. 24, no. 1, pp. 43–57, 1997.

[9] J. Pasquier, J. Picaud, M. Rabilloud et al., "Neonatal outcomes after elective delivery management of preterm premature rupture of the membranes before 34 weeks' gestation (DOMINOS study)," *European Journal of Obstetrics & Gynecology and Reproductive Biology*, vol. 143, no. 1, pp. 18–23, 2009.

[10] S. Kenyon, M. Boulvain, and J. Neilson, "Antibiotics for Preterm Rupture of the Membranes: A Systematic Review," *Obstet & Gynecol*, vol. 104, no. 5, pp. 1051–1057, 2004.

[11] R. W. Naef, J. R. Albert, E. L. Ross, B. Weber, R. W. Martin, and J. C. Morrison, "Premature rupture of membranes at 34 to 37 weeks' gestation: Aggressive versus conservative management," *American Journal of Obstetrics & Gynecology*, vol. 178, no. 1, pp. 126–130, 1998.

[12] H. Tanir, T. Sener, N. Tekin, A. Aksit, and N. Ardic, "Preterm premature rupture of membranes and neonatal outcome prior to 34 weeks of gestation," *International Journal of Gynecology & Obstetrics*, vol. 82, no. 2, pp. 167–172, 2003.

[13] T. Popowski, F. Goffinet, F. Maillard, T. Schmitz, S. Leroy, and G. Kayem, "Maternal markers for detecting early-onset neonatal infection and chorioamnionitis in cases of premature rupture of membranes at or after 34 weeks of gestation: a two-center prospective study," *BMC Pregnancy and Childbirth*, vol. 11, no. 1, 2011.

[14] D. P. van der Ham, S. van Kuijk, B. C. Opmeer et al., "Can neonatal sepsis be predicted in late preterm premature rupture of membranes? Development of a prediction model," *European Journal of Obstetrics & Gynecology and Reproductive Biology*, vol. 176, pp. 90–95, 2014.

[15] Clinical Practice Guidelines, Department of Pediatrics. Indonesia: Cipto Mangunkusumo Hospital; 2015.

[16] R. Rohsiswatmo, *Kontroversi diagnosis sepsis neonatorum. Update Neonatal Infect Jakarta*, Dep Ilmu Kesehat Anak FKUI-RSCM, 2005.

[17] U. Indraccolo, G. Scutiero, M. Matteo et al., "Cesarean section on maternal request: should it be formally prohibited in Italy?" *Ann dellIstituto Super di sanita*, vol. 51, no. 2, pp. 162–166, 2015.

[18] T. A. Manuck, M. M. Rice, J. L. Bailit, W. A. Grobman, U. M. Reddy, and R. J. Wapner, "Preterm neonatal morbidity and mortality by gestational age: a cohort," *Am J Obstet Gynecol*, vol. 215, no. 1, Article ID e1-103.e14, 2016.

[19] D. Drassinower, A. M. Friedman, S. G. Običan, H. Levin, and C. Gyamfi-Bannerman, "Prolonged latency of preterm premature rupture of membranes and risk of neonatal sepsis," *American Journal of Obstetrics & Gynecology*, vol. 214, no. 6, pp. 743–743.e6, 2016.

27

Breastfeeding after Gestational Diabetes: Does Perceived Benefits Mediate the Relationship?

Jordyn T. Wallenborn,[1] **Robert A. Perera,**[2] **and Saba W. Masho**[1]

[1]*Division of Epidemiology, Department of Family Medicine and Population Health, School of Medicine,*
 Virginia Commonwealth University, 830 East Main Street, Suite 821, P.O. Box 980212, Richmond, VA 23298-0212, USA
[2]*Department of Biostatistics, School of Medicine, Virginia Commonwealth University, 830 East Main Street,*
 P.O. Box 980032, Richmond, VA 23298-0032, USA

Correspondence should be addressed to Jordyn T. Wallenborn; wallenbornjt@vcu.edu

Academic Editor: Rosa Corcoy

Introduction. Breastfeeding is recognized as one of the best ways to decrease infant mortality and morbidity. However, women with gestational diabetes mellitus (GDM) may have breastfeeding barriers due to the increased risk of neonatal and pregnancy complications. While the prevalence of GDM is increasing worldwide, it is important to understand the full implications of GDM on breastfeeding outcomes. The current study aims to investigate the (1) direct effect of GDM on breastfeeding duration and (2) indirect effect of GDM on breastfeeding duration through perceived benefits of breastfeeding. *Methods.* Prospective cohort data from the Infant Feeding and Practices Study II was analyzed ($N = 4,902$). Structural equation modeling estimated direct and indirect effects. *Results.* Perceived benefits of breastfeeding directly influenced breastfeeding duration ($\beta = 0.392$, $p \leq 0.001$). GDM was not directly associated with breastfeeding duration or perceived benefits of breastfeeding. Similarly, GDM did not have an indirect effect on breastfeeding duration through perceived benefits of breastfeeding. *Conclusions.* Perceived benefits of breastfeeding are an important factor associated with breastfeeding duration. Maternal and child health care professionals should enhance breastfeeding education efforts.

1. Introduction

Breastfeeding helps infants reach their full health, development, and psychosocial potential [1]. Breastfeeding not only reduces the rate of morbidity and mortality in children [2, 3], but also reduces the likelihood of certain cancers and chronic diseases in mothers [4, 5]. Despite the widespread benefits, approximately half (51.8%) of mothers in the United States breastfeed for six months [6]—the recommended duration according to the American Academy of Pediatrics [7].

Research has demonstrated that a variety of factors including race/ethnicity [8], and Type 1 diabetes [9], impact breastfeeding practices. However, women with gestational diabetes mellitus (GDM) may have an increased risk of breastfeeding for a shorter duration since higher rates of neonatal and pregnancy complications are reported among women with GDM [10]. Moreover, women with GDM may have delayed lactogenesis that could lead to lower rates of breastfeeding [11].

While the prevalence of GDM increases worldwide, it is estimated that up to 14% of pregnancies in the United States (US) are impacted by GDM [12]. Despite recent trends of GDM, research investigating the relationship between GDM and breastfeeding is limited. To the authors' knowledge, two studies have been conducted on GDM and breastfeeding [13, 14], both of which utilized international samples. Results from a retrospective cohort analysis conducted in Ontario reported that women with GDM were less likely to breastfeed (odds ratio (OR) = 0.77; 95% confidence interval (CI) = 0.68–0.87) compared to women without GDM after controlling for potential confounders [13]. Because of the differences in breastfeeding practices between countries and the demonstrated relationship between breastfeeding and infant outcomes for mothers with GDM [15, 16], further

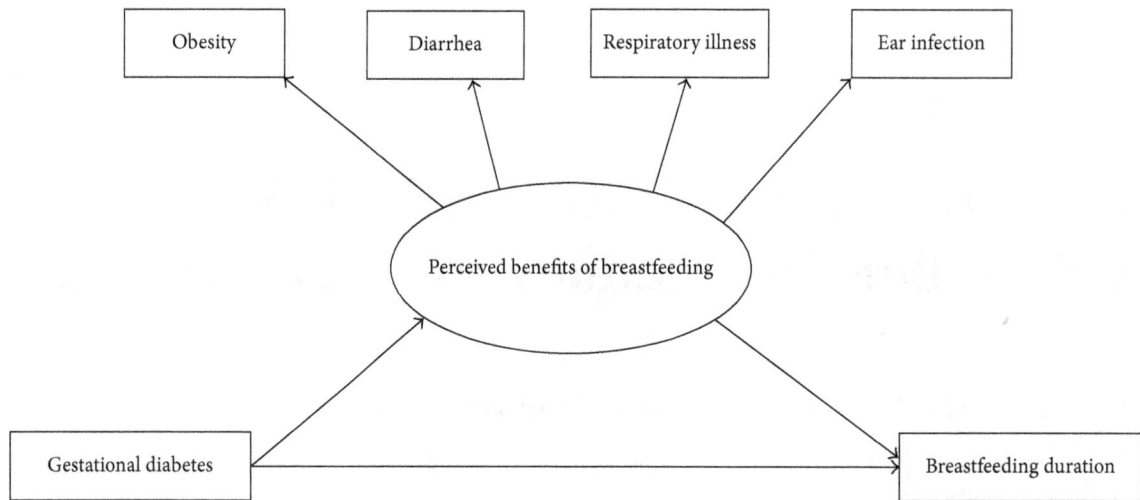

FIGURE 1: Gestational diabetes, perceived benefits of breastfeeding, and breastfeeding duration conceptual model.

research is needed to understand the relationship between GDM and breastfeeding duration in the US.

The current research is supported by the framework of the health belief model (HBM), which asserts that health behavior is dependent upon (1) a desire to avoid illness and (2) a belief that the threat of illness will be prevented through a health action [17]. In addition to these variables, the HBM also incorporates perceived factors such as susceptibility, severity, benefits, and barriers [17]. In the context of breastfeeding, the HBM suggests that women who believe that breastfeeding prevents illness will be more likely to initiate breastfeeding and breastfeed for a longer duration. Consistent with the HBM, a prospective study showed a strong correlation ($r = 0.455$, $p = 0.0001$) between perceived benefits of breastfeeding and breastfeeding practices [18].

Since women with GDM have to monitor their blood glucose levels [19], they may attend more prenatal care visits compared to women without GDM. This could result in an increased knowledge of breastfeeding benefits due to the increase in available educational interventions and contact with health care providers. Therefore, we hypothesize that perceived benefits are a mediator in the association between GDM and breastfeeding. Despite showing associations between GDM and breastfeeding [13, 14], only two studies of international populations have investigated this relationship. In order to provide insight into the relationship between GDM and breastfeeding outcomes in the US, this study aims to investigate (1) the direct effect of GDM on breastfeeding duration and (2) the indirect effect of GDM on breastfeeding duration through perceived benefits of breastfeeding (Figure 1).

2. Materials and Methods

The current study utilized longitudinal data from the Center for Disease Control and Prevention's Infant Feeding and Practices Study II (IFPS II). Data for IFPS II was collected from May 2005 to June 2007 in the US. Participants were

identified using a nationally representative consumer opinion panel of households that resulted in a sample of 4,902 women. To be included in the study, mothers and their children must have been in good health, defined as "neither the mother nor the infant could have a medical condition at birth that would affect feeding and that the infant had to have been born after at least 35 weeks' gestation, weigh at least 5 lb, be a singleton, and not have stayed in the intensive care for >3 days [20]." The survey also excluded mothers who were less than 18 years old at the time of the first questionnaire or whose infants later developed a condition or illness that impacted feeding in the first year of life. Information was collected on maternal and child health, infant feeding behaviors, and a mother's diet. Further description on the IFPS II methodology and questionnaires [20] can be found elsewhere.

The exposure and mediator variables were ascertained from the prenatal questionnaire. Gestational diabetes (yes; no), the exposure variable, was based on the survey item: "Have you had gestational diabetes with this pregnancy?" Perceived benefits of breastfeeding, the latent mediator variable, was measured using the survey items: "How strongly do you agree or disagree with the following statements: If a baby is breastfed, he or she will be less likely to (get an ear infection; get a respiratory illness; get diarrhea; become obese)." Participants responded using a five-item Likert scale of strongly agree to strongly disagree. The outcome, breastfeeding duration (continuous), was based upon three postnatal survey questions pertaining to breastfeeding: "Did you ever breastfeed this baby (or feed this baby your pumped milk)?," "Have you completely stopped breastfeeding and pumping milk for your baby?," and "How old was your baby when you completely stopped breastfeeding and pumping milk?" If mothers were still breastfeeding at last questionnaire (12 months postpartum) ($N = 917$), the following survey question was asked at the six-year follow-up and was used to determine breastfeeding duration: "How old was your 6-year-old when the following happened? He or she stopped being fed breast milk, including pumped breast milk."

Various factors were considered as historical confounders for both endogenous and exogenous variables as determined in the literature. These included marital status (married; not married), maternal race (White; Black; Hispanic; other, including Asian/pacific islander), maternal age (continuous), maternal education (less than high school; high school graduate; 1–3 years of college; college graduate), income (less than \$20,000; \$20,000–49,999; at least \$50,000), prepregnancy body mass index (underweight ($<18.5\,\text{kg/m}^2$); normal weight (18.5–$24.9\,\text{kg/m}^2$); overweight (25.0–$29.9\,\text{kg/m}^2$); obese ($30.0+\,\text{kg/m}^2$)), and health insurance or health care plan (yes; no).

Descriptive statistics were used to examine the distribution of data. Structural equation modeling (SEM) was conducted. A single factor model using the indicators for perceived benefits of breastfeeding will be fit using the two-step approach [21]. SEM was the most appropriate approach for examining the association between GDM and breastfeeding because of the ability to simultaneously estimate the direct and indirect mediation effect that GDM has on breastfeeding duration. The two-step approach starts with a confirmatory factor analysis (CFA) followed by a structural model if there is evidence of good fit. The factor loading of ear infection, an indicator variable for the latent factor (perceived benefits of breastfeeding), was fixed to 1 for model identification. Once the CFA was determined to have good fit, then the structural model was developed. Considered fit indices and their prespecified goodness of fit cutoffs included root mean square error of approximation (RMSEA; <0.05), comparative fit index (CFI; >0.90), chi-square test ($p <$ 0.05), and weighted root mean residual (WRMR; <1.00). Parameters were estimated using robust diagonally weighted least squares (DWLS) which is the preferred approach for analyzing categorical variables [22]. The mediation effect of GDM on breastfeeding duration through perceived benefits was tested using the indirect effect with a percentile bootstrap confidence interval (CI). Descriptive statistics were calculated using SAS version 9.4 statistical software (SAS, Cary, NC), and SEM analyses were performed in R [23] using the Lavaan package [24].

3. Results

The majority of the respondents were white (82.8%), were married (75.5%), had at least a high school diploma (75.3%), and reported initiation of breastfeeding (85.7%). Approximately a quarter (24.8%) reported being overweight, and a third (32.4%) were aged 25–29 years. Over half of participants disagreed or neither agreed nor disagreed that breastfed babies would be less likely to have diarrhea (50.7%) or become obese (63.8%). Maternal characteristics were similar between GDM groups. However, a higher proportion of women who reported having GDM were older and obese (Table 1).

The measurement model showed evidence of good fit (χ^2 (DF = 8) = 86.331; $p <$ 0.001; CFI = 0.999; RMSEA (90% CI) = 0.06 (0.049, 0.072); WRMR = 1.617), allowing us to fit the structural model that is saturated. Fit statistics for the structural model are identical to the measurement model as the structural model is saturated. The final model

included 2,739 observations. The crude model showed no direct effect of GDM on either breastfeeding duration or perceived benefits of breastfeeding. Similarly, there was no indirect effect of GDM on breastfeeding duration through perceived benefits of breastfeeding (Table 2). However, there was a direct effect of perceived benefits of breastfeeding on breastfeeding duration (β = 0.392, $p \leq$ 0.001). After adjusting for marital status, race, education, income, insurance, age, and prepregnancy body mass index, the relationship between knowledge of breastfeeding benefits and breastfeeding duration remained significant while all GDM paths were not significant (Table 3).

4. Discussion

The current findings suggest that GDM does not impact breastfeeding duration directly or indirectly through perceived benefits of breastfeeding; however, perceived benefits of breastfeeding are associated with breastfeeding duration. Our finding that perceived benefits are associated with increased breastfeeding is consistent with the HBM and can be supported through the existing, although limited, literature examining the relationship between perceived benefits of breastfeeding and breastfeeding outcomes. A study conducted by Chezem et al. (2003) found a strong correlation between breastfeeding knowledge and breastfeeding duration [18]. Furthermore, Kornides and Kitsantas (2013) found that mothers with greater knowledge of breastfeeding benefits were 11.2 times more likely to initiate breastfeeding and 5.6 times more likely to breastfeed for a longer duration [25]. These findings can be explained using the HBM, which predicts that a health behavior such as breastfeeding is dependent upon the belief that a health action can prevent illness [17].

Even though the current study did not find an association between GDM and breastfeeding duration, these findings are important to disseminate especially in light of current studies that suggest GDM can impact breastfeeding practices. Specifically, a review study investigating Type 2 diabetes and GDM stated that women with GDM have higher rates of pregnancy and neonatal complications that can create barriers to breastfeeding. Further, GDM is more common in obese women which may be an additional barrier to breastfeeding [26]. Various factors such as hormonal response [27], latching challenges [28], body image, and embarrassment have been reported to influence breastfeeding practices among overweight or obese women [29].

To the authors' knowledge, this is one of the first studies to closely examine the pathway between GDM and breastfeeding duration. This study utilized a prospective cohort design that allowed clear temporal sequence. Findings from the current study make a valuable contribution to the literature by demonstrating the direct effect of perceived benefits on breastfeeding duration and by disputing the limited research examining GDM and breastfeeding. Lastly, research on GDM is especially timely and salient due to current GDM trends and a national push to increase breastfeeding rates.

Despite its strengths, this study is not without limitations. Data from IFPS II may not be generalizable due to

TABLE 1: Distribution of maternal characteristics by study population and gestational diabetes mellitus[a].

Characteristic	Overall Percent	GDM Percent ($N = 310$)	No GDM Percent ($N = 4134$)	χ^2 (p value)
Age				*<0.0001*
18–24 years	28.3	17.2	28.2	
25–29 years	32.4	27.9	33.0	
30–34 years	25.0	27.0	25.3	
35–52 years	14.4	27.9	13.5	
Marital status				0.43
Married	75.5	77.9	75.8	
Not married	24.5	22.1	24.2	
Maternal race				0.12
White, non-Hispanic	82.8	79.5	81.6	
Black, non-Hispanic	5.3	4.4	6.4	
Hispanic	6.7	9.1	6.8	
Other	5.1	7.1	5.2	
Maternal education				0.80
Less than high school	4.8	4.4	4.5	
High school	19.9	21.9	19.4	
1–3 years of college	41.1	39.3	41.3	
College graduate	34.2	34.4	34.8	
Income				0.55
<$20,000	15.6	15.8	16.1	
$20,000–$49,999	41.4	40.7	43.4	
≥$50,000	43.0	43.6	40.5	
Health insurance				0.63
Yes	94.7	95.4	94.8	
No	5.3	4.6	5.2	
Prepregnancy BMI				*<0.0001*
Underweight (<18.5 kg/m2)	5.3	1.7	5.5	
Normal weight (18.5–24.9 kg/m2)	46.3	26.7	47.9	
Overweight (25.0–29.9 kg/m2)	24.8	26.1	24.8	
Obese (30.0+)	23.6	45.5	21.8	
Breastfeeding duration				*0.06*
Never breastfed	14.3	20.4	14.2	
Breastfed less than 6 months	42.7	39.8	45.0	
Breastfed 6 or more months	43.0	39.8	38.0	
Breastfeeding prevents diarrhea[b]				0.79
Strongly disagree	5.7	6.1	5.7	
Somewhat disagree	8.9	9.0	9.0	
Neither agree or disagree	36.1	38.4	35.4	
Somewhat agree	26.6	26.1	27.0	
Strongly agree	22.8	20.3	22.8	
Breastfeeding prevents obesity[b]				0.48
Strongly disagree	10.9	13.6	10.7	
Somewhat disagree	10.1	8.4	10.3	
Neither agree or disagree	42.8	43.2	42.5	
Somewhat agree	19.7	19.0	19.7	
Strongly agree	16.5	15.8	16.9	

TABLE 1: Continued.

Characteristic	Overall Percent	GDM Percent ($N = 310$)	No GDM Percent ($N = 4134$)	χ^2 (p value)
Breastfeeding prevents ear infections[b]				0.16
Strongly disagree	5.3	6.8	5.2	
Somewhat disagree	6.5	9.4	6.3	
Neither agree nor disagree	25.4	23.4	25.0	
Somewhat agree	31.2	29.2	31.5	
Strongly agree	31.6	31.2	32.0	
Breastfeeding prevents respiratory illness[b]				0.45
Strongly disagree	5.1	6.5	5.0	
Somewhat disagree	6.0	7.8	6.0	
Neither agree nor disagree	25.6	25.3	25.1	
Somewhat agree	32.5	29.9	33.1	
Strongly agree	30.7	30.5	30.7	

GDM = gestational diabetes mellitus, BMI = body mass index.
[a]Not all percentages sum to 100% due to rounding.
[b]The following category is from an IFPS II survey question asking, "How strongly do you agree or disagree with the following statements: If a baby is breastfed, he or she will be less likely to (get an ear infection; get a respiratory illness; get diarrhea; become obese)".

TABLE 2: Parameter estimates of the indirect effect of GDM on breastfeeding duration through perceived benefits of breastfeeding.

Parameter	Estimate	Bootstrap CI
Crude model		
Indirect effect of GDM on breastfeeding duration through breastfeeding benefits	0.52 (0.59)	−0.62–1.69
Fully adjusted model[a]		
Indirect effect of GDM on breastfeeding duration through breastfeeding benefits	0.01 (0.64)	−1.16–1.19

GDM = gestational diabetes mellitus; CI = confidence interval.
[a]Adjusted for marital status, race, education, income, insurance, age, and prepregnancy body mass index.

TABLE 3: Parameter estimates of direct effects.

Parameter	Estimate (standard error)	Z-value	p
Crude model			
Direct effect of GDM on breastfeeding duration	1.18 (1.44)	0.82	0.411
Direct effect of breastfeeding benefits on breastfeeding duration	1.98 (0.09)	21.18	<0.0001
Direct effect of GDM on breastfeeding benefits	0.26 (0.29)	0.89	0.373
Fully adjusted model[a]			
Direct effect of GDM on breastfeeding duration	1.27 (1.51)	0.85	0.398
Direct effect of breastfeeding benefits on breastfeeding duration	1.91 (0.10)	19.78	<0.0001
Direct effect of GDM on breastfeeding benefits	0.01 (0.32)	0.02	0.988

GDM = gestational diabetes mellitus; CI = confidence interval.
[a]Adjusted for marital status, race, education, income, insurance, age, and prepregnancy body mass index.

participants having a higher mean education level, being of older age, being white, being more likely to have middle income, being employed, being less likely to smoke, and having fewer children compared to a representative sample from the National Survey of Family Growth [20]. However, the homogenous population reduces potential bias from residual confounding. Social desirability bias may influence mothers to overestimate their breastfeeding duration leading to nondifferential misclassification bias, which could bias the estimate towards from the null—however, previous research has demonstrated that self-reported breastfeeding duration is a reliable measure. Lastly, potential confounding factors such as substance abuse, breastfeeding self-efficacy, and perceived milk supply were not available in the dataset and could not be assessed.

benefits of breastfeeding have a direct effect on breastfeeding duration. Healthcare and public health professionals can utilize this information to strengthen current and future interventions by educating women about the benefits of breastfeeding which may increase breastfeeding rates. Due to inconsistent findings in the few studies investigating GDM and breastfeeding, further research is warranted.

5. Conclusions

Our results suggest that GDM does not have a direct or indirect effect on breastfeeding duration; however, perceived

Conflicts of Interest

The authors declare that there are no conflicts of interest regarding the publication of this paper.

References

[1] L. M. Gartner, J. Morton, R. A. Lawrence et al., "Breastfeeding and the use of human milk," *Pediatrics*, vol. 115, no. 2, pp. 496–506, 2005.

[2] M. M. McDowell, C. Wang, and J. Kennedy-Stephenson, *Breastfeeding in the United States: Findings from the National Health and Nutrition Examination Surveys, 1999-2006*, US Department of Health and Human Services, Centers for Disease Control and Prevention, National Center for Health Statistics, 2008.

[3] J.-A. Blaymore Bier, T. Oliver, A. Ferguson, and B. R. Vohr, "Human milk reduces outpatient upper respiratory symptoms in premature infants during their first year of life," *Journal of Perinatology*, vol. 22, no. 5, pp. 354–359, 2002.

[4] P. A. Newcomb, B. E. Storer, M. P. Longnecker et al., "Lactation and a reduced risk of premenopausal breast cancer," *The New England Journal of Medicine*, vol. 330, no. 2, pp. 81–87, 1994.

[5] K. A. Rosenblatt and D. B. Thomas, "Lactation and the risk of epithelial ovarian cancer. The WHO collaborative study of neoplasia and steroid contraceptives," *International Journal of Epidemiology*, vol. 22, no. 2, pp. 192–197, 1993.

[6] Centers for Disease Control and Prevention, Breastfeeding report card, https://www.cdc.gov/breastfeeding/data/reportcard.htm.

[7] Section on Breastfeeding, "Breastfeeding and the use of human milk," *Pediatrics*, vol. 129, no. 3, pp. e827–e841, 2012.

[8] A. C. Celi, J. W. Rich-Edwards, M. K. Richardson, K. P. Kleinman, and M. W. Gillman, "Immigration, race/ethnicity, and social and economic factors as predictors of breastfeeding initiation," *Archives of Pediatrics and Adolescent Medicine*, vol. 159, no. 3, pp. 255–260, 2005.

[9] S. Hummel, C. Winkler, S. Schoen et al., "Breastfeeding habits in families with type 1 diabetes," *Diabetic Medicine*, vol. 24, no. 6, pp. 671–676, 2007.

[10] J. S. Taylor, J. E. Kacmar, M. Nothnagle, and R. A. Lawrence, "A systematic review of the literature associating breastfeeding with type 2 diabetes and gestational diabetes," *Journal of the American College of Nutrition*, vol. 24, no. 5, pp. 320–326, 2005.

[11] E. P. Gunderson, "Breastfeeding after gestational diabetes pregnancy: subsequent obesity and type 2 diabetes in women and their offspring," *Diabetes Care*, vol. 30, supplement 2, pp. S161–S168, 2007.

[12] G. K. Poomalar, "Changing trends in management of gestational diabetes mellitus," *World Journal of Diabetes*, vol. 6, no. 2, p. 284, 2015.

[13] S. A. Finkelstein, E. Keely, D. S. Feig, X. Tu, A. S. Yasseen, and M. Walker, "Breastfeeding in women with diabetes: Lower rates despite greater rewards. A population-based study," *Diabetic Medicine*, vol. 30, no. 9, pp. 1094–1101, 2013.

[14] S. Hummel, M. Hummel, A. Knopff, E. Bonifacio, and A. Ziegler, "Stillverhalten bei frauen mit gestationsdiabetes," *Deutsche Medizinische Wochenschrift*, vol. 133, no. 5, pp. 180–184, 2008.

[15] I. R. A. Chertok, I. Raz, I. Shoham, H. Haddad, and A. Wiznitzer, "Effects of early breastfeeding on neonatal glucose levels of term infants born to women with gestational diabetes," *Journal of Human Nutrition and Dietetics*, vol. 22, no. 2, pp. 166–169, 2009.

[16] B. E. Metzger, T. A. Buchanan, D. R. Coustan et al., "Summary and recommendations of the Fifth International Workshop-Conference on Gestational Diabetes Mellitus," *Diabetes Care*, vol. 30, supplement 2, pp. S251–S260, 2007.

[17] N. K. Janz and M. H. Becker, "The health belief model: a decade later," *Health Education & Behavior*, vol. 11, no. 1, pp. 1–47, 1984.

[18] J. Chezem, C. Friesen, and J. Boettcher, "Breastfeeding knowledge, breastfeeding confidence, and infant feeding plans: effects on actual feeding practices," *Journal of Obstetric, Gynecologic, & Neonatal Nursing*, vol. 32, no. 1, pp. 40–47, 2003.

[19] B. E. Metzger, D. R. Coustan, and Organizing Committee, "Summary and recommendations of the fourth international workshop-conference on gestational diabetes mellitus," *Diabetes Care*, vol. 21, no. 2, pp. B161–B167, 1998.

[20] Center for Disease Control and Prevention, Infant feeding practices study II and its year six follow-up, http://www.cdc.gov/breastfeeding/data/ifps/index.htm.

[21] J. C. Anderson and D. W. Gerbing, "Structural equation modeling in practice: a review and recommended two-step approach," *Psychological Bulletin*, vol. 103, no. 3, pp. 411–423, 1988.

[22] J. Newsom, "Practical approaches to dealing with nonnormal and categorical variables," 2005.

[23] R Core Team, *R: A Language and Environment for Statistical Computing*, R Foundation for Statistical Computing, 2013.

[24] Y. Rosseel, "Lavaan: an R package for structural equation modeling," *Journal of Statistical Software*, vol. 48, no. 2, pp. 1–36, 2012.

[25] M. Kornides and P. Kitsantas, "Evaluation of breastfeeding promotion, support, and knowledge of benefits on breastfeeding outcomes," *Journal of Child Health Care*, vol. 17, no. 3, pp. 264–273, 2013.

[26] S. W. Masho, M. R. Morris, and J. T. Wallenborn, "Role of marital status in the association between prepregnancy body mass index and breastfeeding duration," *Women's Health Issues*, vol. 26, no. 4, pp. 468–475, 2016.

[27] K. M. Rasmussen and C. L. Kjolhede, "Prepregnant overweight and obesity diminish the prolactin response to suckling in the first week postpartum," *Pediatrics*, vol. 113, no. 5, pp. e465–e471, 2004.

[28] D. J. Chapman and R. Pérez-Escamilla, "Identification of risk factors for delayed onset of lactation," *Journal of the American Dietetic Association*, vol. 99, no. 4, pp. 450–454, 1999.

[29] L. E. Hauff and E. W. Demerath, "Body image concerns and reduced breastfeeding duration in primiparous overweight and obese women," *American Journal of Human Biology*, vol. 24, no. 3, pp. 339–349, 2012.

28

Maternal-Cord Blood Vitamin D Correlations Vary by Maternal Levels

Ganesa Wegienka,[1] Hareena Kaur,[1] Roopina Sangha,[2] and Andrea E. Cassidy-Bushrow[1]

[1]Department of Public Health Sciences, Henry Ford Hospital, Detroit, MI 48202, USA
[2]Department of Women's Health, Henry Ford Hospital, Detroit, MI 48202, USA

Correspondence should be addressed to Ganesa Wegienka; gwegien1@hfhs.org

Academic Editor: Albert Fortuny

Vitamin D levels of pregnant women and their neonates tend to be related; however, it is unknown whether there are any subgroups in which they are not related. 25-Hydroxyvitamin D [25(OH)D] was measured in prenatal maternal and child cord blood samples of participants ($n = 241$ pairs) in a birth cohort. Spearman correlations were examined within subgroups defined by prenatal and delivery factors. Cord blood as a percentage of prenatal 25(OH)D level was calculated and characteristics compared between those who did and did not have ≥25% and ≥50% of the maternal level and those who did and did not have a detectable 25(OH)D level. The correlation among Black children was lower than in White children. When the maternal 25(OH)D level was <15 ng/mL, the overall correlation was $r = 0.16$. Most children had a 25(OH)D cord blood level less than half of their mother's; 15.4% had a level that was <25% of their mother's. Winter birth and maternal level were associated with the level being less than 25%. Children with undetectable levels were more likely to be Black and less likely to be firstborn. These data suggest mothers may reduce their contribution to the fetus's 25(OH)D supply once their own level becomes low.

1. Introduction

Vitamin D is important for its many health benefits for adults and children. The best evidence for the role of vitamin D in health is related to its importance to bone health [1, 2]. Vitamin D may also be related to other health conditions. For example, early life supplementation in children has been associated with decreased risks of type 1 diabetes and influenza [3, 4]. Despite its positive role in health, vitamin D deficiency is a pandemic [5].

Given the important role of vitamin D in health, there has been much discussion about the best ways to prevent and treat vitamin D deficiency [3, 6]. Prevention in children is a priority as it may relate to skeletal and immune development. Previous research has demonstrated that the vitamin D levels of women and their neonates are highly related [7–11]. The goal of this work was to examine whether there are any particular subgroups in which the mother's prenatal 25-hydroxyvitamin D [25(OH)D] level and her child's cord blood level of 25(OH)D are not strongly related. These

analyses could identify pregnant women who need a prenatal vitamin D intervention tailored to them based on the various characteristics, as well as identifying children who may have a lower level of 25(OH)D at birth and may be prioritized for vitamin D screening.

2. Methods

2.1. Study Population. The birth cohort studied here is part of an NIH and institutionally funded cohort study that enrolled pregnant women receiving care at obstetrics clinics in a health system in the Detroit, Michigan, USA, area for longitudinal study of their children through early childhood with the goal of examining early life exposures related to childhood allergies and asthma. These children and their mothers served as the source population for the analyses. Details of cohort creation have been published [12–14]. Briefly, women were enrolled in their 3rd trimester at which time they provided a blood sample and completed an interview about their health. The child's cord blood was collected at delivery. Only maternal-child pairs in which the child was Black/African American or White/Non-Hispanic/Non-Middle Eastern had their 25(OH)D levels determined as there were insufficient maternal-child pairs for analyses in other race and ethnicity groups. This work was approved by the health system's IRB.

2.2. Vitamin D. 25(OH)D, representing the sum of $25(OH)D_2$ (ergocalciferol which is diet related) and $25(OH)D_3$ (cholecalciferol which is sun related), was measured in frozen plasma samples ($-80°C$) in the laboratory of Dr. Neil Binkley at the University of Wisconsin. An HPLC method was used and has been used in previously published research [15–22]. 25(OH)D is expressed in ng/mL. 25(OH)D was measured in the stored samples from pregnancy (3rd trimester) and delivery (cord blood). For those with 25(OH)D levels below the lowest detectable limit of 5 ng/mL, a value of 2.5 ng/mL was assigned. This assignment is a common practice with lab values in research as it allows results to be retained in analyses of continuous measures rather than being removed from analyses due to lack of an actual value.

For the analyses, we examined whether maternal-child correlations in subgroups would vary between those in which maternal 25(OH)D was and was not low. We chose the *a priori* cutpoints of 20 ng/mL and 15 ng/mL. While 20 ng/mL defines deficiency [3], we knew that many of the mothers in the analyses had even lower levels of 25(OH)D. Thus, we also chose to examine the cutpoint of 15 ng/mL. Although limited by sample size, we also examined the associations when maternal levels were less than 40 ng/mL versus levels at least 40 ng/mL ($n = 218$ and $n = 23$, resp.) as it has previously been shown that 40 ng/mL is the level at which 25(OH)D conversion to 1,25-dihydroxyvitamin D_3 [$1,25(OH)_2D_3$] is maximized [23].

2.3. Prenatal Medical Chart Review. The maternal prenatal chart was reviewed for key information used in the analyses including maternal height, parity, delivery type, gestational age at delivery, and the child's birthweight. The maternal weight taken at the first prenatal appointment was recorded and this measurement occurred an average of 7.5 (SD = 5.6) months prior to the child's birth; maternal weight was defined as obese if body mass index (BMI) $\geq30 kg/m^2$ or as classes II-III obese if BMI $\geq35 kg/m^2$. Child race was based on maternal report in a study-specific interview.

2.4. Maternal Atopic Status. Allergen-specific IgE (sIgE) levels in mothers' prenatal blood samples were assessed for a set of allergens (*Dermatophagoides farinae*, dog, cat, timothy grass, ragweed, *Alternaria alternata*, egg, and German cockroach). Maternal atopy was defined as having at least one sIgE $\geq0.35 IU/mL$.

2.5. Statistical Analyses. Descriptive statistics were calculated to provide an overview of the factors and the 25(OH)D levels. We then took a multistep approach to examine the association between the maternal prenatal and cord blood 25(OH)D levels. First, we examined the Spearman

correlations for all children and within subgroups. Subgroups were defined by child race (Black or White), delivery type (c-section or vaginal), winter birth (December, January, or February), firstborn status (yes/no), maternal BMI (kg/m^2 at first prenatal appointment, $<30 kg/m^2/\geq30 kg/m^2$, and $<35 kg/m^2/\geq35 kg/m^2$), preterm birth (<37 weeks/≥37 weeks), birth weight ($\leq2500 g/>2500 g$), maternal prenatal 25(OH)D, and maternal atopic status (yes/no). These variables were chosen as they are among the most commonly studied characteristics of pregnancy and delivery. Maternal atopic status was included because the primary goal of the cohort was to study allergic outcomes in the children and prenatal and early life vitamin D levels have been investigated for their role in allergic disease development [22, 24–27]. We then calculated cord blood as a percentage of the prenatal level and compared characteristics between those who did and did not have a percentage at least 25% and 50% of the maternal level. Finally, we compared characteristics of those who were and were not above the lowest limit of detection. Factors compared between the groups include child race, winter birth, delivery type, firstborn status, maternal atopic status, birthweight, gestational age, and maternal prenatal level of 25(OH)D.

3. Results

There were 241 maternal-child pairs who contributed samples to the analyses. Maternal average age was 30.3 (SD = 5.4) years and most of the children were Black ($n = 175$, 72.6%) and were not born in the winter (81.7%). Almost half the women were obese (46.4%, BMI $> 30 kg/m^2$), about a third of the pregnancies were by c-section (36.5%) and most of the children were not firstborn (81.3%).

Descriptive information about the overall prenatal and cord blood levels of 25(OH)D is provided in Table 1. The mean cord blood 25(OH)D level (10.9 ng/mL) is nearly half of the mean maternal prenatal level (23.6 ng/mL). White children and their mothers tended to have higher 25(OH)D levels compared to Black children and their mothers (Tables 1 and 2). Lower prenatal and cord blood levels were found in those who were not firstborn, those mothers with low 25(OH)D levels ($<40 ng/mL$, $<20 ng/mL$, and $<15 ng/mL$), and those who were obese ($\geq30 kg/m^2$ and $\geq35 kg/m^2$). Lower prenatal levels were found among mothers who had a low birthweight infant. No statistically significant differences were found between those who were and were not born in the winter and were of preterm or low birthweight, or by delivery mode or by maternal atopic status.

Spearman correlations between the prenatal-cord blood levels are presented in Table 3. The prenatal and cord blood levels were highly correlated, overall ($r = 0.75$) and for most subgroups including those defined by winter birth, firstborn status, maternal BMI, preterm birth, low birth weight status, delivery type, and maternal atopic status. The correlation among Black children was less than that of the White children, although both correlations were quite strong ($r = 0.65$ and 0.87, resp.). However, there was a notable exception. When maternal levels of 25(OH)D were low,

TABLE 1: Descriptive information for 25(OH)D levels in the 241 maternal-child pairs. Values are given in ng/mL*.

	Mean	SD	Median	Minimum	Maximum	Number below lowest detectable limit
Prenatal	23.6	11.9	22.7	2.5*	64.9	4.98%
Cord blood	10.9	7.4	10.5	2.5*	47.5	24.9%
Child is Black ($n = 175$)						
Prenatal	20.1	10.3	19.8	2.5*	49.9	6.9%
Cord blood	9.1	6.6	8.5	2.5*	47.5	30.2%
Child is White ($n = 66$)						
Prenatal	32.9	10.8	34.1	13.1	64.9	0
Cord blood	15.6	7.2	15.6	2.5*	28.7	10.6%

*2.5 ng/mL is assigned when the 25(OH)D value is less than the lowest detectable value of 5 ng/mL.

TABLE 2: 25(OH)D levels for prenatal 25(OH)D and cord blood 25(OH)D. Values are in ng/mL.

	N	Prenatal		Cord	
		Mean (SD)	Range	Mean (SD)	Range
Baby is Black	175	20.1 (10.3)	2.5–49.9	9.1 (6.6)	2.5–47.5
Baby is White	66	32.9 (10.8)	13.1–64.9	15.6 (7.2)	2.5–28.7
Baby is firstborn	45	27.7 (11.6)	2.5–51.3	13.2 (6.8)	2.5–28.2
Baby is not firstborn	196	22.7 (11.8)	2.5–64.9	10.4 (7.4)	2.5–47.5
Winter birth	44	24.1 (12.2)*	2.5–51.3	10.5 (7.4)*	2.5–28.2
Nonwinter birth	197	23.5* (11.8)	2.5–64.9	11.0* (7.4)	2.5–47.5
Maternal prenatal 25(OH)D <40 ng/mL	218	21.3 (9.6)	2.5–39.5	9.8 (6.5)	2.5–47.5
Maternal prenatal 25(OH)D ≥40 ng/mL	23	46.1 (6.0)	40.3–64.9	21.9 (6.2)	2.5–28.7
Maternal prenatal 25(OH)D <20 ng/mL	95	12.2 (5.2)	2.5–19.8	6.0 (6.2)	2.5–47.5
Maternal prenatal 25(OH)D ≥20 ng/mL	146	31.0 (8.7)	20.1–64.9	14.1 (6.2)	2.5–28.7
Maternal prenatal 25(OH)D <15 ng/mL	60	9.2 (4.1)	2.5–14.8	5.7 (7.5)	2.5–47.5
Maternal prenatal 25(OH)D ≥15 ng/mL	181	28.4 (9.5)	15.2–64.9	12.6 (6.5)	2.5–28.7
Maternal BMI at 1st prenatal visit <30 kg/m²	126	26.8 (12.7)	2.5–64.9	12.1 (7.5)	2.5–35.9
Maternal BMI at 1st prenatal visit ≥30 kg/m²	109	20.0 (9.8)	2.5–50.2	9.9 (7.0)	2.5–47.5
Maternal BMI at 1st prenatal visit <35 kg/m²	170	25.8 (12.2)	2.5–64.9	11.8 (7.3)	2.5–35.9
Maternal BMI at 1st prenatal visit ≥35 kg/m²	65	18.1 (9.1)	2.5–42.2	9.1 (7.3)	2.5–47.5
Preterm birth (<37 weeks)	20	23.1 (14.6)*	2.5–51.3	13.8 (9.5)*	2.5–35.9
Full term birth (≥37 weeks)	218	23.5 (11.6)*	2.5–64.9	10.6 (7.1)*	2.5–47.5
Low birth weight (≤2500 g)	17	17.2 (10.5)	2.5–38.9	10.2 (8.1)*	2.5–35.9
Not low birth weight (>2500 g)	207	24.0 (12.0)	2.5–64.9	10.9 (7.4)*	2.5–47.5
Baby born vaginally	153	24.4 (12.8)*	2.5–64.9	11.3 (7.4)*	2.5–35.9
Baby born via c-section	88	22.3 (10.0)*	2.5–51.3	10.3 (7.3)*	2.5–47.5
Mother is atopic	144	22.9 (10.8)*	2.5–58.1	11.1 (7.3)*	2.5–47.5
Mother is not atopic	90	24.6 (13.6)*	2.5–64.9	10.5 (7.6)*	2.5–28.7

*Indicates no statistically significant difference in 25(OH)D levels between those with and without that characteristic at that time point ($p \geq 0.05$, Wilcoxon Rank Sum test).

the correlation with the cord blood was weak. For example, when the maternal level was less than 15 ng/mL, the correlation was only 0.16. The correlation was stronger, albeit not as strong as the overall, when the maternal prenatal level was less than 20 ng/mL ($r = 0.29$).

Most of the children had a 25(OH)D cord blood level that was 50% or less of their mother's prenatal level ($n = 149$, 61.8%) and 37 children (15.4%) had a level that was less than 25% of their mother's level. No factors were associated with the level being less than 50% (data not shown); however, there were two factors associated with the level being less than 25%: winter birth and maternal prenatal level. Those children with the percentage less than 25% were more likely to be born in the winter months (29.7% versus 16.2%, $p = 0.05$) and have a lower prenatal maternal level (mean maternal prenatal level = 18.9 ng/mL versus 24.5 ng/mL, $p = 0.003$).

We also examined the characteristics of those children whose 25(OH)D levels were above and below the lowest detectable limit (Table 4). Children who had levels below the detectable limit were more likely to be Black and less likely to

TABLE 3: Spearman correlations between prenatal 25(OH)D and cord blood 25(OH)D.

	r	p
All children	0.75	<0.001
Baby is Black	0.65	<0.001
Baby is White	0.87	<0.001
Baby is firstborn	0.78	<0.001
Baby is not firstborn	0.75	<0.001
Winter birth	0.81	<0.001
Nonwinter birth	0.74	<0.001
Maternal prenatal 25(OH)D <40 ng/mL	0.71	<0.001
Maternal prenatal 25(OH)D ≥40 ng/mL	0.65	<0.001
Maternal prenatal 25(OH)D <20 ng/mL	0.29	0.004
Maternal prenatal 25(OH)D ≥20 ng/mL	0.73	<0.001
Maternal prenatal 25(OH)D <15 ng/mL	0.16	0.22
Maternal prenatal 25(OH)D ≥15 ng/mL	0.77	<0.001
Maternal BMI at 1st prenatal visit <30 kg/m^2	0.78	<0.001
Maternal BMI at 1st prenatal visit ≥30 kg/m^2	0.78	<0.001
Maternal BMI at 1st prenatal visit <35 kg/m^2	0.79	<0.001
Maternal BMI at 1st prenatal visit ≥35 kg/m^2	0.70	<0.001
Preterm birth (<37 weeks)	0.54	0.015
Full term birth (≥37 weeks)	0.77	<0.001
Low birth weight (≤2500 g)	0.43	0.08
Not low birth weight (>2500 g)	0.77	<0.001
Baby born vaginally	0.78	<0.001
Baby born via c-section	0.71	<0.001
Mother is atopic	0.73	<0.001
Mother is not atopic	0.78	<0.001

be firstborn or have an atopic mother. The mean prenatal level tended to be higher for those who had a detectable 25(OH)D level.

4. Discussion

In these analyses of this birth cohort, the correlation between maternal prenatal and cord blood 25(OH)D is quite strong overall. However, the maternal-child correlation is much weaker when the maternal level is low. White maternal-child pairs had higher correlations than the Black maternal-child pairs and Black children had lower percentages of their maternal prenatal 25(OH)D levels. These results are likely due to the generally lower level of 25(OH)D among Black women and suggest that mothers may insufficiently contribute to the child's 25(OH)D supply once their own level falls too low (lower threshold). The data also demonstrate that it is inappropriate to use a prenatal 25(OH)D level to represent the 25(OH)D in a child's early life.

Furthermore, these data suggest that children who are not firstborn will have a lower percentage of their maternal level. This could be attributed to the fact that maternal prenatal 25(OH)D levels were higher in women carrying their firstborn child. This could also reflect that (1) maternal stores may be depleted from prior births and have not recovered and (2) prenatal supplementation in parous women may not be sufficient to eliminate low 25(OH)D levels. In a study of 92 pregnant women in Saudi Arabia, women with two or more previous births were significantly more likely to have lower 25(OH)D$_3$ levels compared with those with one previous birth ($p < 0.05$) [28]. The authors also reported a significant correlation between maternal serum and neonatal 25(OH)D$_3$ ($r = 0.89$, $p = 0.01$).

Our results complement and, by adding extensive subgroup analyses, add an additional important dimension to previously published analyses of examinations of prenatal-cord correlations and factors predicting cord blood 25(OH)D levels [7, 29]. Nicolaidou et al. reported that neonatal vitamin D had a positive correlation with maternal vitamin D levels ($r = 0.69$, $p < 0.001$) in those mothers with normal vitamin D levels but not in those with hypovitaminosis ($n = 123$ maternal-child pairs) [29]. Godang found a strong positive association between maternal 25(OH)D and cord 25(OH)D ($\beta = 0.42$, $p < 0.001$) in a subset of 202 Scandinavian women but did not examine the association in subgroups [30]. Bodnar et al. examined whether prepregnancy obesity predicted poor vitamin D status in neonates in their study of 400 women in Pittsburgh, Pennsylvania [7]. Prenatal (4–22 weeks) levels of 25(OH)D were lower for women who were obese before pregnancy compared to women who were lean even after adjusting for season and other factors. This difference likely led to the result in which women who were obese before pregnancy were more likely to have delivered a child with vitamin D deficiency compared to women who had a normal BMI (odds ratio = OR = 2.1, 95% confidence interval = CI 1.2, 3.6). While we did not see differences by antenatal BMI, the work of Bodnar et al. also highlights the importance of examining subgroups.

A limitation of our study is that maternal prenatal 25(OH)D, while measured in the 3rd trimester, was not measured at the same time in the 3rd trimester for all women. We did not have maternal prepregnancy weights and relied on the weight measured at the time of the first prenatal care visit; however, Holland et al. suggest similar BMI categorization based on first measured pregnancy weight and self-reported prepregnancy weight [31]. Furthermore, there may be maternal characteristics that were not collected for these analyses that may identify other subgroups with variable prenatal-cord correlations.

Our goal was to examine whether the maternal-child 25(OH)D correlation varied within subgroups rather than to examine predictors of a child's cord blood 25(OH)D level as previous studies have already highlighted the importance of the maternal level [8, 9, 11, 30]. The results from this birth cohort suggest that a child's 25(OH)D level is only a fraction of their mother's prenatal level. Furthermore, the degree to which the newborn's level is associated with their mother's prenatal level varies by several interrelated factors

TABLE 4: Characteristics of children with 25(OH)D levels above and below the lowest detectable limit.

	Child's level below lowest detectable limit $N = 60$	Child's level *not* below lowest detectable limit $N = 181$	p
Baby is Black	88.3%	67.4%	<0.05
Winter birth	23.3%	16.6	0.24
C-section delivery	40%	35.4%	0.52
Child is firstborn	6.7%	22.7%	<0.05
Mother is atopic	50.9%	65.1%	0.05
Birthweight (in grams)	3397 (711)	3370 (608)	0.85
Gestational age (weeks)	38.9 (1.5)	38.7 (2.0)	0.87
Prenatal level (ng/mL)	14.0 (8.7)	26.8 (11.0)	<0.05

Winter is defined as December, January, or February.
p for Chi-square (categorical) or Wilcoxon Rank Sum test (continuous).

including maternal race, birth order, and the actual maternal level. Not only do these studies indicate that use of the prenatal level of 25(OH)D to represent the child's early life vitamin D level is not specific, but also the data suggest that a maternal threshold exists below which the mother limits her contribution of 25(OH)D to the fetus. The designs and analytical plans of future studies of prenatal dietary interventions should consider the possibility of a threshold effect when considering the maternal contribution to the fetus. Furthermore, children who are Black and not firstborn and those born to women with very low 25(OH)D may identify a priority group for vitamin D deficiency screening.

5. Conclusions

The degree to which a newborn's vitamin D [25(OH)D] level is associated with their mother's prenatal level varies by several interrelated factors including maternal race, birth order, and the actual maternal level. A maternal threshold may exist below which the mother limits her contribution of 25(OH)D to the fetus; low thresholds should be assessed for other prenatal nutrients. The designs and analytical plans of future studies of prenatal dietary interventions should consider the possibility of a threshold effect when considering the maternal contribution to the fetus. Children who are not firstborn, those who are Black, and those born to women with very low 25(OH)D may identify a priority group for vitamin D deficiency screening.

Conflict of Interests

The authors report no conflict of interests.

Acknowledgment

This work was funded by NIH.

References

[1] A. Hossein-Nezhad and M. F. Holick, "Optimize dietary intake of vitamin D: an epigenetic perspective," *Current Opinion in Clinical Nutrition and Metabolic Care*, vol. 15, no. 6, pp. 567–579, 2012.

[2] M. F. Holick, "The D-lightful vitamin D for child health," *Journal of Parenteral and Enteral Nutrition*, vol. 36, no. 1, supplement, pp. 9S–19S, 2012.

[3] M. F. Holick, N. C. Binkley, H. A. Bischoff-Ferrari et al., "Evaluation, treatment, and prevention of vitamin D deficiency: an endocrine society clinical practice guideline," *The Journal of Clinical Endocrinology & Metabolism*, vol. 96, no. 7, pp. 1911–1930, 2011.

[4] M. Urashima, T. Segawa, M. Okazaki, M. Kurihara, Y. Wada, and H. Ida, "Randomized trial of vitamin D supplementation to prevent seasonal influenza A in schoolchildren," *The American Journal of Clinical Nutrition*, vol. 91, no. 5, pp. 1255–1260, 2010.

[5] M. F. Holick, "Vitamin D: extraskeletal health," *Rheumatic Disease Clinics of North America*, vol. 38, no. 1, pp. 141–160, 2012.

[6] C. J. Rosen, S. A. Abrams, J. F. Aloia et al., "IOM committee members respond to endocrine society vitamin D guideline," *Journal of Clinical Endocrinology and Metabolism*, vol. 97, no. 4, pp. 1146–1152, 2012.

[7] L. M. Bodnar, J. M. Catov, J. M. Roberts, and H. N. Simhan, "Prepregnancy obesity predicts poor vitamin D status in mothers and their neonates," *Journal of Nutrition*, vol. 137, no. 11, pp. 2437–2442, 2007.

[8] L. M. Bodnar, H. N. Simhan, R. W. Powers, M. P. Frank, E. Cooperstein, and J. M. Roberts, "High prevalence of vitamin D insufficiency in black and white pregnant women residing in the northern United States and their neonates," *Journal of Nutrition*, vol. 137, no. 2, pp. 447–452, 2007.

[9] J. L. Josefson, J. Feinglass, A. W. Rademaker et al., "Maternal obesity and vitamin D sufficiency are associated with cord blood vitamin D insufficiency," *Journal of Clinical Endocrinology and Metabolism*, vol. 98, no. 1, pp. 114–119, 2013.

[10] B. W. Hollis and W. B. Pittard III, "Evaluation of the total fetomaternal vitamin D relationships at term: evidence for racial differences," *Journal of Clinical Endocrinology and Metabolism*, vol. 59, no. 4, pp. 652–657, 1984.

[11] A. Dawodu, H. F. Saadi, G. Bekdache, Y. Javed, M. Altaye, and B. W. Hollis, "Randomized controlled trial (RCT) of vitamin D supplementation in pregnancy in a population with endemic vitamin D deficiency," *The Journal of Clinical Endocrinology & Metabolism*, vol. 98, no. 6, pp. 2337–2346, 2013.

[12] G. Wegienka, S. Havstad, C. L. M. Joseph et al., "Racial disparities in allergic outcomes in African Americans emerge as early as age 2 years," *Clinical and Experimental Allergy*, vol. 42, no. 6, pp. 909–917, 2012.

[13] G. Wegienka, C. L. M. Joseph, S. Havstad, E. Zoratti, D. Ownby, and C. C. Johnson, "Sensitization and allergic histories differ between black and white pregnant women," *Journal of Allergy and Clinical Immunology*, vol. 130, no. 3, pp. 657–662.e2, 2012.

[14] N. Aichbhaumik, E. M. Zoratti, R. Strickler et al., "Prenatal exposure to household pets influences fetal immunoglobulin e production," *Clinical and Experimental Allergy*, vol. 38, no. 11, pp. 1787–1794, 2008.

[15] R. P. Heaney, L. A. G. Armas, J. R. Shary, N. H. Bell, N. Binkley, and B. W. Hollis, "25-Hydroxylation of vitamin D3: relation to circulating vitamin D3 under various input conditions," *The American Journal of Clinical Nutrition*, vol. 87, no. 6, pp. 1738–1742, 2008.

[16] B. W. Hollis, C. L. Wagner, M. K. Drezner, and N. C. Binkley, "Circulating vitamin D3 and 25-hydroxyvitamin D in humans: an important tool to define adequate nutritional vitamin D status," *Journal of Steroid Biochemistry and Molecular Biology*, vol. 103, no. 3–5, pp. 631–634, 2007.

[17] G. L. Lensmeyer, D. A. Wiebe, N. Binkley, and M. K. Drezner, "HPLC method for 25-hydroxyvitamin D measurement: comparison with contemporary assays," *Clinical Chemistry*, vol. 52, no. 6, pp. 1120–1126, 2006.

[18] N. Binkley and D. Krueger, "Evaluation and correction of low vitamin D status," *Current Osteoporosis Reports*, vol. 6, no. 3, pp. 95–99, 2008.

[19] N. Binkley, D. Krueger, D. Gemar, and M. K. Drezner, "Correlation among 25-hydroxy-vitamin D assays," *Journal of Clinical Endocrinology and Metabolism*, vol. 93, no. 5, pp. 1804–1808, 2008.

[20] N. Binkley, D. Krueger, and G. Lensmeyer, "25-Hydroxyvitamin D measurement, 2009: a review for clinicians," *Journal of Clinical Densitometry*, vol. 12, no. 4, pp. 417–427, 2009.

[21] N. Binkley, D. C. Krueger, S. Morgan, and D. Wiebe, "Current status of clinical 25-hydroxyvitamin D measurement: an assessment of between-laboratory agreement," *Clinica Chimica Acta*, vol. 411, no. 23-24, pp. 1976–1982, 2010.

[22] G. Wegienka, S. Havstad, E. M. Zoratti, H. Kim, D. R. Ownby, and C. C. Johnson, "Association between vitamin D levels and allergy-related outcomes vary by race and other factors," *Journal of Allergy and Clinical Immunology*, vol. 136, no. 5, pp. 1309–1314, 2015.

[23] B. W. Hollis, D. Johnson, T. C. Hulsey, M. Ebeling, and C. L. Wagner, "Vitamin D supplementation during pregnancy: double-blind, randomized clinical trial of safety and effectiveness," *Journal of Bone and Mineral Research*, vol. 26, no. 10, pp. 2341–2357, 2011.

[24] A. P. Jones, D. Palmer, G. Zhang, and S. L. Prescott, "Cord blood 25-hydroxyvitamin D3 and allergic disease during infancy," *Pediatrics*, vol. 130, no. 5, pp. e1128–e1135, 2012.

[25] A. P. Jones, M. K. Tulic, K. Rueter, and S. L. Prescott, "Vitamin D and allergic disease: sunlight at the end of the tunnel?" *Nutrients*, vol. 4, no. 1, pp. 13–28, 2012.

[26] A. L. Kozyrskyj, S. Bahreinian, and M. B. Azad, "Early life exposures: impact on asthma and allergic disease," *Current Opinion in Allergy and Clinical Immunology*, vol. 11, no. 5, pp. 400–406, 2011.

[27] A. A. Litonjua, "Childhood asthma may be a consequence of vitamin D deficiency," *Current Opinion in Allergy and Clinical Immunology*, vol. 9, no. 3, pp. 202–207, 2009.

[28] Y. F. Aly, M. A. El Koumi, and R. N. Abd El Rahman, "Impact of maternal vitamin D status during pregnancy on the prevalence of neonatal vitamin D deficiency," *Pediatric Reports*, vol. 5, no. 1, pp. 24–27, 2013.

[29] P. Nicolaidou, Z. Hatzistamatiou, A. Papadopoulou et al., "Low vitamin D status in mother-newborn pairs in Greece," *Calcified Tissue International*, vol. 78, no. 6, pp. 337–342, 2006.

[30] K. Godang, K. F. Frøslie, T. Henriksen, E. Qvigstad, and J. Bollerslev, "Seasonal variation in maternal and umbilical cord 25(OH) vitamin D and their associations with neonatal adiposity," *European Journal of Endocrinology*, vol. 170, no. 4, pp. 609–617, 2014.

[31] E. Holland, T. A. M. Simas, D. K. D. Curiale, X. Liao, and M. E. Waring, "Self-reported pre-pregnancy weight versus weight measured at first prenatal visit: effects on categorization of pre-pregnancy body mass index," *Maternal and Child Health Journal*, vol. 17, no. 10, pp. 1872–1878, 2013.

Permissions

List of Contributors

Mustafa Adelaja Lamina
Maternal and Fetal Health Research Unit, Department of Obstetrics and Gynaecology, Olabisi Onabanjo University Teaching Hospital, PMB 2001, Sagamu, Nigeria

Timothy O. Ihongbe
Division of Epidemiology, Department of Family Medicine and Population Health, School of Medicine, Virginia Commonwealth University, Richmond, VA, USA

Saba W. Masho
Division of Epidemiology, Department of Family Medicine and Population Health, School of Medicine, Virginia Commonwealth University, Richmond, VA, USA
Department of Obstetrics and Gynecology, School of Medicine, Virginia Commonwealth University, Richmond, VA, USA
Institute forWomen's Health, Virginia Commonwealth University, Richmond, VA, USA

David E. Harris, Nancy Baugh and Cheryl Sarton
School of Nursing, University of Southern Maine, Portland, ME 04104, USA

AbouEl-Makarim Aboueissa
Department of Mathematics and Statistics, University of Southern Maine, Portland, ME 04104, USA

Erika Lichter
Department of Applied Medical Sciences, University of Southern Maine, Portland, ME 04104, USA

Tesfaye Birhane
Meket District Health Office, Meket, Ethiopia

Gizachew Assefa Tessema
Department of Reproductive Health, Institute of Public Health, University of Gondar, Gondar, Ethiopia

Kefyalew Addis Alene and Abel Fekadu Dadi
Department of Epidemiology and Biostatistics, Institute of Public Health, University of Gondar, Gondar, Ethiopia

Katja Erjavec
Department of Obstetrics and Gynecology, University Hospital Merkur, Zajčeva 19, 10000 Zagreb, Croatia

Ratko Matijević
Department of Obstetrics and Gynecology, University Hospital Merkur, Zajčeva 19, 10 000 Zagreb, Croatia
Department of Obstetrics and Gynecology, School of Medicine, University of Zagreb, Šalata 3, 10000 Zagreb, Croatia

Tamara Poljičanin
Department of Medical Informatics and Biostatistics, Croatian Institute of Public Health, Rockefellerova 7, 10000 Zagreb, Croatia

Namrata Kashyap, Mandakini Pradhan, Neeta Singh and Sangeeta Yadav
Department of Maternal and Reproductive Health, Sanjay Gandhi Post Graduate Institute of Medical Sciences (SGPGIMS), Lucknow 226 014, India

J. Hazart, D. Le Guennec, N. Farigon, C. Lahaye and M. Miolanne-Debouit
CHU Clermont-Ferrand, Service de Nutrition Clinique, CRNH Auvergne, Universit´e Clermont Auvergne, 63000 Clermont-Ferrand, France

Y. Boirie
CHU Clermont-Ferrand, Service de Nutrition Clinique, CRNH Auvergne, Universit´e Clermont Auvergne, 63000 Clermont-Ferrand, France
INRA, Unit´e de Nutrition Humaine (UNH), CRNH Auvergne, Universit´e Clermont Auvergne, 63000 Clermont-Ferrand, France

M. Accoceberry and D. Lemery
CHU Clermont-Ferrand, Service de Gyn´ecologie-Obst´etrique, Universit´e Clermont Auvergne, 63000 Clermont-Ferrand, France

A. Mulliez
CHU Clermont-Ferrand, D´el´egation Recherche Clinique and Innovation, 63000 Clermont-Ferrand, France

Anne Møller
Department of Public Health, Aarhus University, Aarhus, Denmark
Center for Fetal Diagnostics, Aarhus University Hospital, Aarhus, Denmark

Ida Vogel
Center for Fetal Diagnostics, Aarhus University Hospital, Aarhus, Denmark

Department of Clinical Genetics, Aarhus University Hospital, Aarhus, Denmark

Olav Bjørn Petersen
Center for Fetal Diagnostics, Aarhus University Hospital, Aarhus, Denmark
Fetal Medicine Unit, Department of Obstetrics and Gynaecology, Aarhus University Hospital, Aarhus, Denmark

Stina Lou
Center for Fetal Diagnostics, Aarhus University Hospital, Aarhus, Denmark
DEFACTUM, Public Health and Health Services Research, Central Denmark Region, Aarhus, Denmark

Abduelmula R. Abduelkarem
College of Pharmacy, University of Sharjah, Sharjah, UAE

Hafsa Mustafa
AME Global FZE, Sharjah, UAE

Annick Denzler, Tilo Burkhardt and Roland Zimmermann
Department of Obstetrics, Zurich University Hospital, Frauenklinikstraße 10, 8091 Zurich, Switzerland

Giancarlo Natalucci
Department of Neonatology, Zurich University Hospital, Frauenklinikstraße 10, 8091 Zurich, Switzerland

Ben Willem Mol
Department of Obstetrics, Gynaecology and Fertility, Faculty of Medicine, University of Amsterdam (AMC-UvA), Meibergdreef 9, 1105 AZ Amsterdam, The Netherlands

Anneloes E. Ruifrok
Department of Obstetrics, Gynaecology and Fertility, Faculty of Medicine, University of Amsterdam (AMC-UvA), Meibergdreef 9, 1105 AZ Amsterdam, The Netherlands
Department of Obstetrics and Gynaecology, Faculty of Medicine, VU University Medical Center, 1007 MB Amsterdam, The Netherlands

Christianne J. M. de Groot
Department of Obstetrics and Gynaecology, Faculty of Medicine, VU University Medical Center, 1007 MB Amsterdam, The Netherlands

Ellen Althuizen, Nicolette Oostdam, Willem van Mechelen and Mireille N. M. van Poppel
Department of Public and Occupational Health, EMGO+ Institute for Health and Care Research, VU University Medical Center, Van der Boechorststraat 7, 1081 BT Amsterdam, The Netherlands

Nompumelelo Yende, Nora S. West and Jean Bassett
Witkoppen Health andWelfare Centre, Johannesburg, South Africa

Annelies Van Rie
Department of Epidemiology, University of North Carolina Gillings School of Global Health, Chapel Hill, NC, USA

Sheree R. Schwartz
Department of Epidemiology, Johns Hopkins Bloomberg School of Public Health, Baltimore, MD, USA

Valerie E. Whiteman and Mary Ashley Cain
Division of Maternal-Fetal Medicine, Department of Obstetrics and Gynecology, College of Medicine, University of South Florida, 2 Tampa General Circle, 6th Floor, Tampa, FL 33606, USA

Hamisu M. Salihu
Division of Maternal-Fetal Medicine, Department of Obstetrics and Gynecology, College of Medicine, University of South Florida, 2 Tampa General Circle, 6th Floor, Tampa, FL 33606, USA
Maternal and Child Health Comparative Effectiveness Research Group, Department of Epidemiology and Biostatistics, College of Public Health, University of South Florida, 13201 Bruce B. Downs BoulevardMDC 56, Tampa, FL 33612, USA

Jason L. Salemi
Maternal and Child Health Comparative Effectiveness Research Group, Department of Epidemiology and Biostatistics, College of Public Health, University of South Florida, 13201 Bruce B. Downs BoulevardMDC 56, Tampa, FL 33612, USA

Mulubrhan F. Mogos
Department of Community and Health Systems, School of Nursing, University of Indiana, 1111 Middle Drive, Indianapolis, IN 46202, USA

Muktar H. Aliyu
Department of Health Policy and Medicine, Vanderbilt University, 2525 West End Avenue, Suite 750, Nashville, TN 32703, USA

Reva Tripathi, Shakun Tyagi, Nilanchali Singh, Yedla Manikya Mala and Chanchal Singh
Department of Obstetrics and Gynaecology, Maulana Azad Medical College, New Delhi 110002, India

Preena Bhalla
Department of Microbiology, Maulana Azad Medical College, New Delhi, India

Siddhartha Ramji
Department of Paediatrics, Maulana Azad Medical College, New Delhi, India

Alemu Zenebe
Department of Pediatric OperationTheatre, Black Lion teaching Hospital, Addis Ababa, Ethiopia

Abebaw Gebeyehu
Department of Reproductive Health, Institute of Public Health, College of Medicine and Health Science, University of Gondar, Gondar, Ethiopia

Lemma Derseh
Department of Epidemiology and Biostatistics, Institute of Public Health, College of Medicine and Health Science, University of Gondar, Gondar, Ethiopia

Kedir Y. Ahmed
Department of Public Health, College of Medicine and Health Science, Debre Markos University, Debre Markos, Ethiopia

Viltė Daugirdaitė
Department of General Psychology, Philosophy Faculty, Vilnius University, Universiteto 9/1, Vilnius, LT-01513, Lithuania

Olga van den Akker
Department of Psychology, Middlesex University, The Burroughs, Hendon, London NW4 4BT, UK

Satvinder Purewal
Institute of Psychology, University ofWolverhampton, Wulfruna Street, WolverhamptonWV1 1LY, UK

Simona Johansson
Department of Clinical Sciences, Obstetrics and Gynecology, Sundsvalls Research Unit, Umeå University, Umeå 90185, Sweden

Marju Dahmoun
Department of Obstetrics and Gynecology, Sundsvall County Hospital, Sundsvall 85186, Sweden

Sahruh Turkmen
Department of Clinical Sciences, Obstetrics and Gynecology, Sundsvalls Research Unit, Umeå University, Umeå 90185, Sweden
Department of Obstetrics and Gynecology, Sundsvall County Hospital, Sundsvall 85186, Sweden

Mohammed Akibu and Sodere Nurgi
Department of Midwifery, Institute of Medicine and Health Sciences, Debre Berhan University, Debre Berhan, Ethiopia

Wintana Tsegaye
Concordia University, Montreal, Quebec, Canada

Tewodros Megersa
Obstetrics Unit, Gandhi Maternal Specialized Hospital, Addis Ababa, Ethiopia

Jordyn T. Wallenborn and Saba W. Masho
School of Medicine, Division of Epidemiology, Department of Family Medicine and Population Health, Virginia Commonwealth University, 830 East Main Street, Suite 821, Richmond, VA, USA

Diego F. Wyszynski
Pregistry, Los Angeles, CA 90045, USA

Wendy J. Carman
Epidemiology, OptumInsight, Waltham, MA 02451, USA

John Seeger
Epidemiology, OptumInsight, Waltham, MA 02451, USA
Department of Medicine, Division of Pharmacoeconomics and Pharmacoepidemiology, Brigham &Women's Hospital, Harvard Medical School, Boston, MA 02120, USA

Alan B. Cantor
Children's Hospital Boston, Boston, MA 02115, USA

John M. Graham Jr.
Medical Genetics Institute, Cedars Sinai Medical Center, Los Angeles, CA 90048, USA

Liza H. Kunz
Palo Alto Medical Foundation, Mountain View, CA 94040, USA

Anne M. Slavotinek
Department of Pediatrics, Division of Genetics, University of California, San Francisco, San Francisco, CA 94115, USA

Russell S. Kirby
College of Public Health, University of South Florida, Tampa, FL 33612, USA

J. A. Swift, J. Pearce, P. H. Jethwa, M. A. Taylor, A. Avery, S. Ellis and S. C. Langley-Evans
School of Biosciences, University of Nottingham, Sutton Bonington, Loughborough LE12 5RD, UK

S. McMullen
National Childbirth Trust, 30 Euston Square, London NW1 2FB, UK

Thorkild F. Nielsen
Department of Obstetrics and Gynecology, Sahlgrenska Academy, University of Gothenburg, Gothenburg, Sweden

Maria Bullarbo
Department of Obstetrics and Gynecology, Sahlgrenska Academy, University of Gothenburg, Gothenburg, Sweden
Department of Gynecology, Närhälsan, Mölndal, Sweden

Helena Mattson and Natalia Ödman
Women's Clinic, Södra Älvsborgs Hospital, Borås, Sweden

Anna-Karin Broman
Women's Clinic, Norra Älvsborgs Hospital, Trollhättan, Sweden

Milagros C. Rosal, Tiffany A. Moore Simas, Sybil L. Crawford and Katherine Leung
Department of Medicine, Division of Preventive and Behavioral Medicine, University of Massachusetts Medical School, 55 Lake Avenue North, Worcester, MA 01655, USA

Monica L. Wang
Boston University School of Public Health, 801 Massachusetts Avenue, Boston, MA 02215, USA
Harvard School of Public Health, 677 Huntington Avenue, Boston, MA 02215, USA

Jamie S. Bodenlos
Department of Psychology, Hobart andWilliam Smith Colleges, 217 Gulick Hall, Geneva, NY 14456, USA

Heather Z. Sankey
Department of Obstetrics and Gynecology, Baystate Medical Center, 759 Chestnut Street, Springfield, MA 01199, USA

Anteneh Amsalu, Getachew Ferede and Setegn Eshetie
Department of Medical Microbiology, University of Gondar, Gondar, Ethiopia

Agete Tadewos and Demissie Assegu
Department of Medical Laboratory Sciences, Hawassa University, Hawassa, Ethiopia

Mali Abdollahian and Kaye Marion
School of Science (Mathematical and Geospatial Sciences), College of Science, Engineering, and Health, RMIT University, Melbourne, VIC 3001, Australia

Dewi Anggraini
School of Science (Mathematical and Geospatial Sciences), College of Science, Engineering, and Health, RMIT University, Melbourne, VIC 3001, Australia
Study Program of Mathematics, Faculty of Mathematics and Natural Sciences, University of Lambung Mangkurat (ULM), Ahmad Yani Street, Km. 36, Banjarbaru, South Kalimantan 70714, Indonesia
Study Program of Statistics, Faculty of Mathematics and Natural Sciences, University of Lambung Mangkurat (ULM), Ahmad Yani Street, Km. 36, Banjarbaru, South Kalimantan 70714, Indonesia

Fadly Ramadhan, Rezky Putri Rahayu, Irfan Rizki Rachman and Widya Wurianto
Study Program of Mathematics, Faculty of Mathematics and Natural Sciences, University of Lambung Mangkurat (ULM), Ahmad Yani Street, Km. 36, Banjarbaru, South Kalimantan 70714, Indonesia

Supri Nuryani
Ulin Public Hospital, 43 Ahmad Yani Street, Km 2.5, Banjarmasin, South Kalimantan 70233, Indonesia
Abdi Persada Midwifery Academy, 365 Sutoyo S. Street, Banjarmasin, South Kalimantan 70115, Indonesia

Thomas Obinchemti Egbe and Gregory Edie Halle-Ekane
Department of Obstetrics and Gynecology, Douala General Hospital, Douala, Cameroon
Faculty of Health Sciences, University of Buea, Buea, Cameroon

Rose-Mary Asong Tazinya
Mbingo Baptist Hospital Annexe, Douala, Cameroon

Eta-Nkongho Egbe
District Hospital Poli, Poli, Cameroon

Eric Akum Achidi
Faculty of Science, University of Buea, Buea, Cameroon

Dwiana Ocviyanti and William Timotius Wahono
Department of Obstetrics and Gynecology, Faculty of Medicine, Universitas Indonesia/Cipto Mangunkusumo Hospital, Jakarta, Indonesia

Jordyn T. Wallenborn and Saba W. Masho
Division of Epidemiology, Department of Family Medicine and Population Health, School of Medicine, Virginia Commonwealth University, 830 East Main Street, Suite 821, Richmond, VA 23298-0212, USA

Robert A. Perera
Department of Biostatistics, School of Medicine, Virginia Commonwealth University, 830 East Main Street, Richmond, VA 23298-0032, USA

Ganesa Wegienka, Hareena Kaur and Andrea E. Cassidy-Bushrow
Department of Public Health Sciences, Henry Ford Hospital, Detroit, MI 48202, USA

Roopina Sangha
Department of Women's Health, Henry Ford Hospital, Detroit, MI 48202, USA

Index